OXFORD ASSESS AND PROGRESS
MEDICAL SCIENCES

Edited by

Jade Chow
Associate Dean of Undergraduate Education
St George's, University of London

John Patterson
Honorary Senior Lecturer
Barts and the London School of Medicine and Dentistry,
Queen Mary University of London

D0714424

OXFORD
UNIVERSITY PRESS

OXFORD
UNIVERSITY PRESS

Great Clarendon Street, Oxford OX2 6DP,
United Kingdom

Oxford University Press is a department of the University of Oxford.
It furthers the University's objective of excellence in research, scholarship,
and education by publishing worldwide. Oxford is a registered trade mark of
Oxford University Press in the UK and in certain other countries

© Oxford University Press 2012

The moral rights of the authors have been asserted
First Edition published in 2012

Impression: 1

British Library Cataloguing in Publication Data

Data available

Library of Congress Cataloging in Publication Data

Library of Congress Control Number: 2012933280

ISBN 978–0–19–960507–1

Printed in Great Britain
by Ashford Colour Press Ltd, Gosport, Hampshire

Oxford University Press makes no representation, express or implied, that the
drug dosages in this book are correct. Readers must therefore always check
the product information and clinical procedures with the most up-to-date
published product information and data sheets provided by the manufacturers
and the most recent codes of conduct and safety regulations. The authors and
the publishers do not accept responsibility or legal liability for any errors in the
text or for the misuse or misapplication of material in this work. Except where
otherwise stated, drug dosages and recommendations are for the non-pregnant
adult who is not breastfeeding.

Links to third party websites are provided by Oxford in good faith and
for information only. Oxford disclaims any responsibility for the materials
contained in any third party website referenced in this work.

SERIES EDITOR PREFACE

The Oxford *Assess and Progress* Series is a groundbreaking development in the extensive area of self-assessment texts available for medical students. The questions were specifically commissioned for the series, written by practising clinicians and medical students, extensively peer-reviewed by students and their teachers, and quality-assured to ensure that the material is up-to-date, accurate, and in line with modern testing formats.

The series has a number of unique features and is designed as much as a formative learning resource as a self-assessment one. The questions are constructed to test the same clinical problem-solving skills that we use as practising clinicians, rather than just testing theoretical knowledge, namely:

- Gathering and using data required for clinical judgement
- Choosing examination and investigations, and interpreting the findings
- Applying knowledge
- Demonstrating diagnostic skills
- Having the ability to evaluate undifferentiated material
- Having the ability to prioritize
- Making decisions and demonstrating a structured approach to decision making.

Each question is bedded in reality and is typically presented as a clinical scenario, the contents of which have been chosen to reflect the common and important conditions that most doctors are likely to encounter both during their training and in exams! The aim of the series is to build the reader's confidence around recognizing important symptoms and signs and suggesting the most appropriate investigations and management, and in so doing aid development of a clear approach to patient management which can be transferred to the wards.

The content of the series has deliberately been pinned to the relevant *Oxford Handbook* but in addition has been guided by a blueprint which reflects the themes identified in *Tomorrow's Doctors* and *Good Medical Practice* to include novel areas such as history-taking, recognition of signs including red flags, and professionalism.

Particular attention has been paid to giving learning points and constructive feedback on each question, using clear fact-based or evidence-based explanations as to why the correct response is right and why the incorrect responses are less appropriate. The question editorials are clearly referenced to the relevant sections of the accompanying *Oxford Handbook* and/or more widely to medical literature or guidelines. They are designed to guide and motivate the reader, being multi-purpose in nature, covering, for example, exam technique, approaches to difficult subjects, and links between subjects.

Another unique aspect of the series is the element of competency progression from being a relatively inexperienced student to a more experienced junior doctor. We have suggested the following four degrees of difficulty to reflect the level of training so the reader can monitor his or her own progress over time, namely:

★   Graduate should know

★ ★   Graduate nice to know

★ ★ ★   Foundation should know

★ ★ ★ ★   Foundation nice to know.

We advise the reader to attempt the questions in blocks as a way of testing knowledge in a clinical context. The series can be treated as a dress rehearsal for life on the ward by using the material to hone clinical acumen and build confidence by encouraging a clear, consistent, and rational approach, aiding proficiency in recognizing and evaluating symptoms and signs, making a rational differential diagnosis, and suggesting appropriate investigations and management.

Adopting such an approach can aid not only being successful in examinations, which really are designed to confirm learning, but, more importantly, being a good doctor. In this way we can deliver high-quality and safe patient care by recognizing, understanding, and treating common problems, but at the same time remaining alert to the possibility of less likely but potentially catastrophic conditions.

David Sales and Kathy Boursicot, Series Editors
November 2010

A NOTE ON SINGLE BEST ANSWER AND EXTENDED MATCHING QUESTIONS

Single best answer questions are currently the format of choice, being widely used by most undergraduate and postgraduate knowledge tests, and hence most of the assessment questions in this book follow this format.

Briefly, the single best answer question presents a problem, usually a clinical scenario, before presenting the question itself and a list of five options. Of these five, there is one correct answer and four incorrect options or 'distracters' from which the reader chooses a response.

Extended matching questions are also known as extended matching items and were introduced as a more reliable way of testing knowledge. They are still currently widely used in many undergraduate and postgraduate knowledge tests, and hence are included in this book.

An extended matching question is organized as one list of possible options followed by a set of items, usually clinical scenarios. The correct response to each item must be chosen from the list of options.

All of the questions in this book, which typically are based on an evaluation of symptoms, signs, or results of investigations either as single entities or in combination, are designed to test *reasoning* skills rather than straightforward recall of facts, and use cognitive processes similar to those used in clinical practice.

The questions all peer-reviewed and are written and edited in accordance with contemporary best assessment practice and their content has been guided by a blueprint pinned to all areas of *Good Medical Practice*, which ensures comprehensive coverage.

The answers and their rationales are evidence-based and have been reviewed to ensure that they are absolutely correct.

Incorrect options are selected as being plausible and indeed may look correct to the less knowledgeable reader. When answering questions, readers may wish to use the 'cover' method in which they read the scenario and the question but cover the options.

Kathy Boursicot and David Sales, Series Editors

VOLUME EDITOR PREFACE

This new volume in the *Assess and Progress* series of publications is linked to the *Oxford Handbook of Medical Sciences*, 2nd edition, and is designed to be used as a revision tool from the earliest days of an undergraduate's course right up to and even beyond final degree examinations.

The medical sciences are the foundation on which rests the ability of a doctor to apply clinical reasoning to work out in a systematic, scientific pathway from symptoms and signs, through diagnostic investigation, to an understanding of a patient's problems. This reasoning process confirms or refutes hypotheses about the patient's condition to arrive at a diagnosis on which treatment can be based.

Ever since the reforms following Abraham Flexner's highly critical review of North American medical education in 1910, medical schools across the globe have traditionally begun a medical education with studies of biomedical sciences—often taught on a subject-by-subject (anatomy, physiology, biochemistry) basis and sometimes divorced more or less completely from a clinical context. Nowadays, more enlightened curricula try to ensure that clinically relevant context is provided for undergraduates during the early phase of the course, so that as scientific knowledge is acquired it becomes linked to its clinical applications. This is the strategy which underpins the way this book is constructed.

Unlike some of the more specialist titles in the *Assess and Progress* series, this book is intended for use from the outset of medical studies through to qualifying as a doctor. In the postgraduate phase it can be used to revise medical sciences for membership and licensing examinations. This usefulness comes, in part, from the division of the book into three sections.

The six chapters in the first section cover much of the basic cell biology and other science needed to study medicine. Such material is common to many courses in the life and health sciences, and most undergraduate programmes in medicine include these topics to ensure that students entering from differing educational routes achieve a common knowledge base.

The second section has eight chapters which deal mainly with the various body systems, covering the ways in which medical sciences and clinical knowledge are intertwined. These chapters will fit well with modern medical curricula, where the early and middle years are delivered as systems-based modules rather than by traditional subject disciplines.

The third section of the book is a single chapter. Here, the questions diverge to some extent from the layout of the *Oxford Handbook of Medical Sciences*. In this, the final chapter, questions are deliberately made similar to those students may expect to encounter in examinations in the final stages of their course, and beyond. The questions cover themes of diagnosis, investigation, mechanisms of disease, and patient treatment and management, and, while highly clinical, they continue to test the ways in which medical sciences apply to clinical situations.

Another useful feature of the book is the way it has been written, namely by a group of contributors. No contributor has taken responsibility for an individual chapter; instead, we have worked together as a team, in much the same way that a team of examiners would construct an examination paper. For each chapter, several contributors have written a series of questions to cover one or more topics. All the contributors have then met to review and amend the questions before including them in the book. This approach provides questions in a variety of examiner styles, and uses a mixture of examiner subject expertise, much as might be seen in a real assessment. So close has this model been to that used in real examinations that in Section 3 we are able to demonstrate how a team of examiners works out the content of an assessment to achieve a balanced coverage, using a technique known as 'blueprinting'.

As in other books in the *Assess and Progress* series, this volume uses a combination of single best answer and extended matching question formats. Students are likely to encounter both forms in their assessments since while single best answers are considered a more accurate (or reliable) assessment format, extended matching questions, while also reliable, are rather better at differentiating (discriminating) different levels of candidate ability. For both types of question we not only provide the reasons why the best answer is correct, but also some explanation as to why other options are not the best choice. In this way the book reinforces knowledge to a much greater extent than would happen by simply by asking the reader to select a correct answer.

Finally, by helping to revise knowledge and develop reasoning skills, this text should help to build a student's confidence for the demanding examinations which pave the way to a professional qualification. Of necessity in a book of this size, questions will not cover all areas of the curriculum, and this book will be of greatest use to students and junior doctors who have already acquired a substantial knowledge of medicine and the medical sciences by directed and private study.

John Patterson and Jade Chow
June 2011

ACKNOWLEDGEMENTS

We thank Kathy Boursicot who, as one of the editors of the series *Assess and Progress* together with David Sales, suggested that we undertake this book. Our thanks also go to the staff at Oxford University Press, particularly Holly Edmondson and Geraldine Jeffers, who have provided constant guidance and support throughout the project; thanks also to John Vlachos and Alan Grundy of St George's Healthcare NHS Trust for some of the radiographic images.

Of course, our greatest thanks go to our team of contributors; the clinicians recruited by Jade from St George's University of London medical school and the medical scientists recruited by John from Barts and the London School of Medicine and Dentistry. In the midst of busy professional lives, these contributors gave freely of their time over the course of more than a year to writing the 400 or so questions in this book, to providing most of the illustrations and to spending several weekends discussing and improving the questions. While this was hard work, it was mostly very enjoyable and, it has to be said, we had some good parties and grew closer as colleagues and friends.

Finally we would like to thank our partners for their patience, forbearance, and support during the past 18 months, when much time has been taken away from our domestic lives.

Jade Chow and John Patterson
June 2011

FIGURE
ACKNOWLEDGEMENTS

1.2 Reproduced from *Oxford Handbook of Medical Sciences,* 2nd edn with permission.

1.3 Reproduced from *Oxford Handbook of Medical Sciences* with permission.

1.5 Reproduced from *Oxford Handbook of Medical Sciences* with permission.

4.4 Reproduced from *Oxford Handbook of Medical Sciences* with permission.

4.5 Reproduced from *Oxford Handbook of Medical Sciences* with permission.

5.3 Reproduced with permission from National Eye Institute, National Health Institutes.

8.3 Reproduced with permission from Pocock, G and Richards, CD (2004), *Human Physiology: The Basis of Medicine*, 2nd edn, Oxford University Press.

10.1 Reproduced from *Oxford Handbook of Medical Sciences* with permission.

10.3 Reproduced from Mackinnon and Morris, *Oxford Textbook of Functional Anatomy*, vol 2, p147 (Oxford, 2005) with permission from Oxford University Press.

12.1 Reproduced with permission from Pocock, G and Richards, CD (2004), *Human Physiology: The Basis of Medicine, 2nd edn*, Oxford University Press.

12.2 Reproduced from *Oxford Handbook of Medical Sciences,* 2nd edn with permission.

12.3 Reproduced from *Oxford Handbook of Medical Sciences,* 2nd edn with permission.

12.4 Reproduced from Mackinnon, Pamela and Morris, John, *Oxford Textbook of Functional Anatomy*, vol 2, p170 (Oxford, 2005) with permission.

12.5 Reproduced from *Oxford Handbook of Medical Sciences,* 2nd edn with permission.

CONTENTS

Section 3: Medical sciences in clinical reasoning

ABOUT THE EDITORS

Volume Editors

Jade Chow is Associate Dean of Undergraduate Education at St George's, University of London, and Reader and Honorary Consultant Histopathologist at St George's, University of London. She is also Chair of the Undergraduate Medical and Bioscience Committee. She is responsible for the three MBBS courses at SGUL: Biomedical Science, Intercalated BSc and Biomedical Informatics courses. Jade has extensive experience and expertise in assessment, having been chief examiner in the written final examinations at St George's for over 10 years and having played a pivotal role in the design of the overall assessment strategy. Dr Chow is a practising histopathologist and is currently a Regional Specialist Advisor for Histopathology for the Royal College of Pathologists and examiner for Fellowship of the Royal College of Pathologists.

John Patterson is an Honorary Senior Lecturer in the Centre for Medical Education, Barts and the London School of Medicine and Dentistry, Queen Mary University of London. At the time he retired in 2009 he was Associate Dean for Undergraduate Medical Studies and Head of MBBS Assessment, having been closely involved with curriculum development, assessment design and analysis, and degree regulations for more than half of his 30-year career as a physiologist at Barts and the London. He was three times elected 'best preclinical teacher' by the students and in 2001 was awarded a Queen Mary, University of London Drapers' Prize for Excellence in Teaching and Learning for curriculum and assessment development work. In retirement he continues to teach, to run workshops, and to provide advice on assessment theory and practice to Universities and Royal Colleges.

Series Editors

Katharine Boursicot is a Reader in Medical Education and Deputy Head of the Centre for Medical and Healthcare Education at St George's, University of London. Previously she was Head of Assessment at Barts and the London School of Medicine and Dentistry, and Associate Dean for Assessment at Cambridge University School of Clinical Medicine. She is consultant on assessment to several UK medical schools, royal medical colleges and international institutions as well as the General Medical Council PLAB Part 2 Panel and Fitness to Practise clinical skills testing.

David Sales is a general practitioner by training who has been involved in medical assessment for over 20 years, having previously been convenor of the MRCGP knowledge test. He has run item-writing workshops for a number of undergraduate medical schools and medical Royal Colleges, as well as internationally. For the General Medical Council he currently chairs the Professional and Linguistic Assessments Board Part 1 panel and is their consultant on fitness to practise knowledge testing.

CONTRIBUTORS

Mark Carroll is honorary Senior Lecturer in Biochemistry in the Centre for Medical Education, Barts and the London School of Medicine and Dentistry, Queen Mary University of London. Mark is an MBBS Year Leader, with responsibilities for course and assessment delivery. Mark was formerly Associate Dean for Education Quality

Olimpia Curran is Specialist Registrar in Histopathology, St George's Healthcare NHS Trust.

Catherine Molyneux is Senior Lecturer in Anatomy in the Centre for Medical Education, Barts and the London School of Medicine and Dentistry, Queen Mary University of London, and Director of Anatomical Studies.

Lesley Robson is Senior Lecturer in Anatomy in the Blizard Institute of Cellular and Molecular Biology, Barts and the London School of Medicine and Dentistry, Queen Mary University of London. Lesley is also an MBBS Year Leader with curriculum and assessment responsibilities and a special interest in the locomotor system.

Peter Shortland is Senior Lecturer in Neuroscience in the Blizard Institute of Cellular and Molecular Biology, Barts and the London School of Medicine and Dentistry, Queen Mary University of London. He is particularly concerned with teaching and assessment of modules dealing with brain and behaviour on both MBBS and intercalated BSc courses.

Brendan E. Tinwell is Consultant Histopathologist at St George's Healthcare NHS Trust. In addition to having a well-rounded basis in pathology, he has special expertise in urological and pulmonary pathology.

Claire E. Wells is Clinical Research Fellow, St George's, University of London and Co-Director of the MPharm course at St George's, University of London/Kingston University.

NORMAL AND AVERAGE VALUES

	Normal value
Haematology	
White cell count (WCC)	$4-11 \times 10^9$/L
Haemoglobin (Hb)	M: 13.5–18g/dL F: 11.5–16g/dL
Packed cell volume (PCV)	M: 0.4–0.54% F: 0.37–0.47%
Mean corpuscular volume (MCV)	76–96fL
Neutrophils	$2-7.5 \times 10^9$/L
Lymphocytes	$1.3-3.5 \times 10^9$/L
Eosinophils	$0.04-0.44 \times 10^9$/L
Basophils	$0-0.1 \times 10^9$/L
Monocytes	$0.2-0.8 \times 10^9$/L
Platelets	$150-400 \times 10^9$/L
Reticulocytes	$25-100 \times 10^9$/L
Erythrocyte sedimentation rate (ESR)	<20mm/h (but age-dependent; see OHCM p356)
Prothrombin time (PT)	10–14s
Activated partial thromboplastin time (aPTT)	35–45s
International normalized ratio (INR)	0.9–1.2
Biochemistry	
Alanine aminotransferase (ALT)	5–35IU/L
Albumin	35–50g/L
Alkaline phosphatase (ALP)	30–15IU/L
Amylase	0–180U/dL
Aspartate transaminase (AST)	5–35IU/L
Bilirubin	3–17μmol/L
Calcium (total)	2.12–2.65mmol/L

Chloride	95–105mmol/L
Cortisol	450–750nmol/L (am) 80–280nmol/L (midnight)
C-reactive protein (CRP)	<10mg/L
Creatine kinase	M: 25–195IU/L F: 25–170IU/L
Creatinine	70–<150µmol/L
Ferritin	12–200µg/L
Folate	2.1µg/L
γ-Glutamyl transpeptidase (GGT)	M: 11–51IU/L F: 7–33IU/L
Lactate dehydrogenase (LDH)	70–250IU/L
Magnesium	0.75–1.05mmol/L
Osmolality	278–305mOsmol/kg
Potassium	3.5–5mmol/L
Protein (total)	60–80g/L
Sodium	135–145mmol/L
Thyroid-stimulating hormone (TSH)	0.5–5.7mU/L
Thyroxine (T_4)	70–140nmol/L
Thyroxine (free)	9–22pmol/L
Urate	M: 210–480mmol/24h F: 150–39mmol/24h
Urea	2.5–6.7ng/l
Vitamin B_{12}	0.13–0.68ng/l
Arterial blood gases	
pH	7.35–7.45
P_aO_2	>10.6kPa
P_aCO_2	4.7–6.0kPa
Base excess	±2mmol/L
Urine	
Cortisol (free)	<280nmol/24h
Osmolality	350–1000mOsmol/kg
Potassium	14–120mmol/24h
Protein	<150mg/24h
Sodium	100–250mmol/24h

ABBREVIATIONS

A&E	Accident & Emergency
ACC	Anterior cingulated cortex
ACE	Angiotension converting enzyme
ACH	Acetylcholine
ACTH	Adrenocorticotrophic hormone
ADA	Adenosine deaminase deficiency
ADH	Antidiuretic hormone
ADP	Adenosine diphosphate
AER	Apical ectodermal ridge
AF	Atrial fibrillation
AIDS	Acquired immune deficiency syndrome
ALT	Alanine aminotransferase
AM	Amplitude-modulated
AMP	Adenosine monophosphate
AMPA	α-amino-3-hydroxy-5-methyl-4-isoazolepropionic acid
ANS	Autonomic nervous system
AO	Anti-sense oligonucleotides
APB	Abductor pollicis brevis
ARF	Acute renal failure
ARR	Aldosterone : renin ratio
ASD	Atrial septal defect
ASIS	Anterior superior iliac spine
AST	Aspartate transaminase
ATN	Acute tubular necrosis
ATP	Adenosine triphosphate
BCG	Bacille Calmette–Guérin
BMR	Basal metabolic rate
BNF	British National Formulary
Botox®	*Botulinum* toxin
cAMP	Cyclic adenosine monophosphate
CCK	Cholecystokinin
CD20	Cluster differentiation 20
CFTR	Cystic fibrosis transmembrane regulator

MB	Myoglobin
MCP	Metocarpophalangeal
MI	Myocardial infarction
MMC	Migrating motor complexes
MND	Motor neurone disease
MRI	Magnetic resonance imaging
mRNA	Messenger RNA
MRSA	Meticillin-resistant *Staphylococcus aureus*
MS	Multiple sclerosis
NAD	Nicotinamide adenine dinucleotide
NADPH	Reduced form of NAPD$^+$ (Nicotinamide adenine dinucleotide phosphate)
ncRNA	Non-coding RNA
NMDA	N-methyl-D-aspartic acid
NREM	Non- rapid eye movement
NS	Nephrotic syndrome
NSAID	Non-steroidal anti-inflammatory drug
OD	Once daily
OGTT	Oral glucose tolerance test
OHCM	*Oxford Handbook of Clinical Medicine*
OHMS	*Oxford Handbook of Medical Sciences*
PAF	Platelet activating factor
pANCA	Perinuclear antineutrophil cytoplasmic antibodies
PCR	Polymerase chain reaction
PDH	Pyruvate dehydrogenase
PEFR	Peak expiratory flow rate
PET	Positron emission tomography
PFC	Prefrontal cortex
PFK-1	Phosphofructokinase-1
PIPJ	Proximal interphalangeal joints
PKU	Phenylketonuria
PL	Prolactin
PML	Progressive multifocal leukoencephalopathy
PNS	Peripheral nervous system
PP	Precocious puberty
PTSD	Post traumatic stress disorder
rAAV	Recombinant adeno-associated viral vector
RBC	Red blood cells
REM	Rapid eye movement

RMP	Resting membrane potential
RNA	Ribonucleic acid
rRNA	Ribosomal RNA
RSV	Respiratory syncytial virus
RTA	Road traffic accident
RV	Residual volume
SAH	Subarachnoid haemorrhage
SCID	Severe combined immunodeficiency disease
SGLUT	Sodium glucose linked transporter proteins
SIRS	Systemic inflammatory response syndrome
SNARE	Soluble NSF attachment protein receptor
snoRNA	Small nucleolar RNA
SNP	Single nucleotide polymorphism
SPN	Solitary pulmonary nodule
SSR	Simple sequence repeats
SSRI	Selective serotonin re-uptake inhibitor
TB	Tuberculosis
TBM	TB meningitis
TCA	Tricarboxylic acid
TCA	Tricyclic anti-depressants
TfR	Transferrin receptor
TKI	Tyrosine kinase inhibitor
TLC	Total lung capacity
TNF	Tumour necrosis factor
TPR	Total peripheral resistance
TRH	Thyrotrophin releasing hormone
tRNA	Transfer RNA
TSH	Thyroid stimulating hormone
TVF	Tactile vocal fremitus
vCJB	variant Creutzfeldt–Jakob disease
VEGF	Vascular endothelial growth factor
VIP	Vasoactive intestinal peptide
VNTR	Variable number of tandem repeats
VR	Vocal resonance
VZV	Varicella-zoster virus
WBC	White blood cells
WHO	World Health Organization
ZPA	Zone of polarizing activity

HOW TO USE THIS BOOK

Oxford Assess and Progress, Medical Sciences has been carefully designed to ensure you get the most out of your revision. Here is a brief guide to some of the features and learning tools.

Organization of content

Chapter editorials will help you unpick tricky subjects, and when it's late at night and you need something to remind you why you're doing this, you'll find words of encouragement!

Following the editorial you will find Single Best Answer (SBA) questions and then Extended Matching Questions (EMQs), both indicated by this symbol [?]. The answers can be found at the end of each chapter and you will find these in the same order, i.e. Single Best Answer questions followed by Extended Matching Questions [?].

How to read an answer

Unlike other revision guides on the market, this one is full of feedback, so you should understand exactly why each answer is correct.

With every answer there is an explanation of why that particular choice is the most appropriate. For some questions there is additional explanation of why the distracters are less suitable. Where relevant you will also be directed to sources of further information, such as the *Oxford Handbook of Medical Sciences, second edition* (OHMS 2nd edn), or relevant textbooks.

Progression points

The questions in every chapter are ordered by level of difficulty and competence, indicated by the following symbols:

★ - Early years student should know

★★ - Middle to later years student should know

★★★ - Graduating student should know

★★★★ - Junior doctor level of knowledge.

Oxford Handbook of Medical Sciences, second edition (OHMS 2nd edn)

The OHMS 2nd edn page references are given with the answers to some questions. OHMS 2nd edn → p402 Please note that this reference is to the second edition of the OHMS, and that subsequent editions are unlikely to have the same material in exactly the same place.

Colour Illustrations

Please note that colour illustrations are placed in a colour plate section in the middle of the book. They are referred to in the text as both a figure and a plate number, for example, Fig. 1.2 (see Plate 1).

CELLS, TISSUES, AND MOLECULES

CHAPTER 1

CELL STRUCTURE AND FUNCTION

Almost every medical student in the United Kingdom, and in many other countries, begins his or her studies with a course on basic cellular structure and function. Such courses are often designed to help students from a variety of educational backgrounds to appreciate the concepts and vocabulary central to all of the life sciences. Over time this core knowledge will be supplemented by other, more specific, areas of medical science until the point is reached at which learners can apply their scientific understanding to those processes of clinical reasoning that lead to diagnosis and treatment. Medical science assists the process of diagnosis by explaining how underlying disease states produce characteristic symptoms and signs. It also facilitates safer treatment by explaining many of the properties, both beneficial and deleterious, of the increasing range of often potent therapeutic agents used in clinical management.

This chapter poses questions about the basic chemicals of life: proteins, lipids, and carbohydrates. It also covers significant features of the cell membrane and cellular organelles as well as cell division, cellular differentiation, and cell death. Understanding the basic principles of intracellular and intercellular communication and regulation provides the foundation for appreciating the role that these processes play in normal and abnormal neural and hormonal control, which will be considered in more detail in later chapters. All of these topics will eventually contribute to a medical student's grasp of normal structure and function and how it becomes disturbed in disease.

The current chapter also includes questions on basic pharmacokinetics. Knowing how each drug works—that is to say its kinetics and mode of action—is a first step in learning to prescribe safely. Other important principles will be added later in the medical student learning process: for example, the indications and contraindications for the use of a drug; any unwanted side-effects; the route of administration and dosages to produce optimal effects. All of this information must be mastered to help prevent the prescribing errors that are all too common in clinical practice. ■

1. The amino acid sequence of a polypeptide chain (its primary structure) dictates how it will fold to form secondary and tertiary structures. Typical secondary structures are α-helices and β-pleated sheets. Which single molecular interaction stabilizes protein secondary structures via forces linking the atoms of the peptide bonds? ★

A Disulphide bond

B Hydrogen bond

C Hydrophobic interaction

D Ionic bond

E Van der Waals force

2. Both haemoglobin and myoglobin bind and release oxygen in human cells. As with all proteins, their structure is optimized for their function. Which single property of the haemoglobin molecule distinguishes it from myoglobin? ★

A It contains an Fe^{2+} ion in a haem group

B It consists of more than one polypeptide chain

C It has a high proportion of α-helix

D It has a largely polar surface and a largely non-polar interior

E It is a water-soluble globular protein

3. Collagen is the most abundant protein found in the body. Its presence in the extracellular matrix of connective tissues provides tensile strength and it is particularly abundant in tendons and ligaments. The biological properties of collagen stem from its unique protein structure. Which single chemical feature of mature collagen accounts best for its tensile strength? ★

A It has a double helical structure

B It has a high proportion of α-helix

C It has a low proportion of the amino acid glycine

D It is stabilized by covalent cross-links

E It undergoes vitamin B-dependent hydroxylation of some proline residues

4. Under defined conditions, an enzyme has a characteristic Michaelis constant, K_m, and a maximal rate of reaction, V_{max}, as shown in Fig. 1.1. Which is the single defining property of the V_{max} value of an enzyme-catalysed reaction? ★

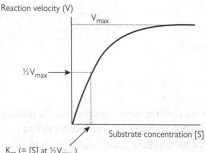

Fig. 1.1

A It increases with increasing enzyme concentration

B It decreases in the presence of a competitive inhibitor

C It is the rate at which the substrate concentration is twice the K_m value

D It is unchanged in the presence of a non-competitive inhibitor

E It may have units of millimoles per litre

5. Some medicinal drugs, for example the antibiotic penicillin, exert their effect by specifically inhibiting a target enzyme. The nature of this inhibition can be either competitive or non-competitive. Which single property of a non-competitive inhibitor of an enzyme-catalysed reaction best distinguishes it from a competitive inhibitor? ★ ★

A It bears a structural resemblance to the substrate

B It binds reversibly to the active site of the enzyme

C It changes the K_m value of the enzyme

D It forms a covalent complex with the enzyme

E It lowers the rate of the reaction except at high substrate concentration

6. Cholera toxin causes severe diarrhoea by binding to complex oligosaccharides of certain lipids in the plasma membrane of cells lining the lumen of the intestine. To which single type of membrane lipid does cholera toxin bind? ★ ★

A Cerebroside

B Cholesterol

C Ganglioside

D Phosphatidylinositol

E Sphingomyelin

7. Carbohydrates perform various functions in the human body: as metabolic fuels; in cell–cell recognition; as components of the extra-cellular matrix. Glycogen is an important store of metabolic energy, especially in liver and skeletal muscle. Which single property of glycogen is most important for its storage function? ★

A It contains β-1,4 and β-1,6 glycosidic bonds

B It contains one non-reducing end and many reducing ends

C It is a linear polysaccharide

D It is present in the mitochondria of hepatocytes (liver cells)

E It is sparingly soluble in aqueous solution

8. The structure and function of cell membranes is best described by the fluid mosaic model. In this model, lipids are associated with proteins in a characteristic way. Which single feature defines best the fluid mosaic model of membrane structure? ★

A Amphipathic lipids form a hydrophobic (non polar) bilayer

B Carbohydrate is present on both the extracellular and intracellular surfaces

C Fluidity is increased by incorporating more cholesterol

D Peripheral proteins bind covalently to integral proteins

E Protein is arranged on each surface in an extended conformation

9. Polypeptide hormones act on membrane-bound receptors located on target cells. This interaction generates a second messenger in the cytoplasm that brings about the physiological effects of the hormone. One important second messenger is cyclic adenosine monophosphate (cAMP). Which single option best describes the signalling properties of cyclic AMP? ★

A It activates a membrane-bound G-protein

B It is degraded by hydrolysis catalysed by the enzyme adenylate cyclase

C It is reduced in concentration in the presence of caffeine

D It is synthesized from adenosine triphosphate (ATP) by the enzyme phosphodiesterase

E It is the second messenger when glucagon acts on hepatocytes (liver cells)

10. The plasma membrane represents a barrier to the transmission of an external signal to the cell's interior. Many structures and mechanisms have evolved to facilitate chemical and electrical communication and coordination between cells. Which single effect is the immediate consequence of acetylcholine binding to a nicotinic receptor at a neuromuscular junction? ★

A Activation of a protein kinase

B Activation of gene transcription

C Opening of ion channels

D Release of Ca^{2+} ions

E Synthesis of a second messenger

11. Polar signalling molecules arriving at the target cell must transmit their 'message' across the plasma membrane to the cytoplasm. G-proteins are a key intermediate in this process. Which single property best characterizes G-proteins? ★

A They are a type of ligand-gated ion channel

B They are able to hydrolyse guanosine diphosphate (GDP)

C They are found in both stimulatory and inhibitory forms

D They are peripheral membrane proteins

E They are receptors for hormones and neurotransmitters

12. A 19-year-old male develops a high fever and a purpuric rash. During the evening before he complained to his friends of flu-like symptoms and a severe headache. Lumbar puncture reveals turbid cerebrospinal fluid (CSF) with low glucose, high protein, and high neutrophils. Which single type of structure, responsible for the special permeability properties of the blood–brain barrier, is most likely to have been disrupted in this case? ★

A Adherens junction (zonula adherens)

B Basal lamina

C Gap junction

D Podocyte

E Tight junction

Cell structure and function

13. Methotrexate is an antimetabolite which inhibits an enzyme essential for DNA replication. With which single phase(s) of the cell cycle does methotrexate interfere? ★

A G_0 phase

B G_1 phase

C G_2 phase

D M phase

E S phase

14. A 2-year-old girl has cutaneous syndactyly between the second and third toes of her left foot. Which single tissue process provides the mechanism that normally dissolves the interosseal web? ★

A Apoptosis

B Atrophy

C Oncosis

D Pyroptosis

E Necrosis

15. A 56-year-old Egyptian man is operated on for a large bladder tumour. The histopathologist reviews his previous bladder biopsies (retrieved from the archive of the large Cairo Hospital). Low and higher magnification photomicrographs of separate bladder biopsies taken some ten years previously are shown in Fig. 1.2 (see Plate 1). A metaplastic change and parasite ova are depicted. What is the single most likely tumour type present within the man's cystectomy specimen? ★ ★ ★

A Adenocarcinoma

B Clear cell carcinoma

C Small cell carcinoma

D Squamous cell carcinoma

E Transitional cell carcinoma

16. Following an abnormal cervical smear which showed larger and more irregular nuclei, a 37-year-old woman has a cervical biopsy which shows hyperchromatic and pleomorphic nuclei with no inflammatory cells (see Fig. 1.3). Which single type of pathological tissue alteration is shown here? ★

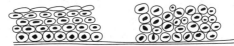

Normal   Biopsy

Fig. 1.3

A Anaplasia

B Dysplasia

C Hyperplasia

D Metaplasia

E Neoplasia

17. The normal adult cell contains two copies of each chromosome, one copy inherited from each parent. To produce oocytes or sperm a reduction to one copy per cell is required. This reduction in the number of chromosome copies per cell in gametogenesis is achieved by meiosis. Which is the single most likely point in the process of meiosis where an error can lead to trisomy? ★

A Bivalents lining up on the mitotic spindle

B DNA replication to produce sister chromatids

C Formation of bivalents

D Genetic recombination

E Separation of bivalents or chromatids

18. As part of treatment of type I diabetes mellitus, patients are required to take exogenous insulin to mimic their normal insulin secretion. Which is the single most appropriate route of administration for insulin in a patient with type I diabetes mellitus? ★

A Inhaled

B Intravenous

C Oral

D Subcutaneous

E Transdermal

19. Once in the body, most drugs undergo metabolism in order to facilitate their eventual elimination from the body. The kinetics of drug elimination are typically either zero-order or first-order. Which single therapeutic advantage is a benefit of drugs with first-order elimination kinetics? ★ ★

A 75% of an intravenous dose will be eliminated in three half-lives

B Steady state plasma concentrations can be reached during multiple dosing

C The drug is excreted unchanged

D The rate of drug elimination is constant

E The rate of drug elimination is independent of the plasma concentration of the drug

20. Salicylate, the active principle of aspirin, is one of a small number of drugs with so-called 'zero-order' elimination kinetics. The majority of drugs have first-order kinetics. Which single property of salicylate best characterizes drugs with zero-order kinetics? ★ ★

A It is a weak acid compound

B It is easy to maintain a constant plasma concentration of the drug.

C Its elimination rate is proportional to the current plasma concentration

D Its elimination half-life is constant

E Its elimination occurs at a constant rate

21. A 34-year-old man is investigated for repeated sudden increases in his blood pressure. He had initially consulted his GP for repeated nosebleeds and headaches, which happened suddenly and without warning. His GP referred him for continuous ambulatory monitoring of his blood pressure. In one 24-hour period his blood pressure rose suddenly from 124/85mmHg to 170/100mmHg. As a result he was given intravenous clevidipine, a calcium channel blocker. While his blood pressure fell (and even went below his normal resting blood pressure to 110/70mmHg), it was noted that his heart rate increased. Which single mechanism accounts best for the increased heart rate in this patient? ★

A Adaptive loss of receptors

B Exhaustion of second messengers

C Exhaustion of essential metabolites

D Physiological adaptation

E Receptor desensitization

EXTENDED MATCHING QUESTIONS

Structure and function of subcellular organelles

For each of the following, select the single organelle which best fits the description given in the statement. Each option may be used once, more than once, or not at all.

A Golgi apparatus

B Lysosome

C Mitochondrion

D Nucleus

E Peroxisome

F Ribosome

G Rough endoplasmic reticulum

H Secretory vesicle

I Smooth endoplasmic reticulum

1. This organelle is present in both bacterial and human cells. ★

2. This organelle, well developed in human macrophages, contains hydrolytic enzymes with an acidic pH optimum. ★

3. This organelle, which contains DNA and RNA, has a double membrane, the inner one of which is highly folded. ★

4. This organelle, with its stack of membranous cisternae, is especially active in processing glycoproteins in salivary cells. ★

5. This organelle, active in liver cells (hepatocytes), degrades very long chain fatty acids via reactions that generate a product broken down by catalase. ★ ★

Pharmacology: agonists and antagonists

Which single option best describes how each of the following drugs exerts its effects? Each option may be used once, more than once, or not at all.

A Chemical antagonist

B Competitive antagonist

C Full agonist

D Inverse agonist

E Non-competitive antagonist

F Partial agonist

G Pharmacokinetic antagonist

H Physiological antagonist

I Superagonist

J Uncompetitive antagonist

K Zero antagonist

6. Dimercaprol (a chelator of toxic heavy metals such as lead, arsenic, and mercury). Desferrioxamine acts in a similar way to remove free iron from the bloodstream. ★ ★

7. Memantine, which acts on NMDA receptors. The same concentration of this drug produces greater effects in reducing the effects of high concentrations of glutamate than with lower concentrations of glutamate. ★ ★

8. Naloxone, which forms covalent bonds with the active site of the mu-opioid receptor. The effects last until the receptors are resynthesized. ★ ★

9. Salbutamol, which causes short-action relaxation of bronchiolar smooth muscle by acting specifically on the β_2 adrenoceptor. ★

10. Statins, which act to reduce cholesterol biosynthesis. The statin binds to the active site on HMG CoA reductase. No covalent bonds are formed between the statin and the enzyme. ★

ANSWERS

Single Best Answers

1. B ★ OHMS 2nd edn → p8

Hydrogen bonds are non-covalent forces that form between electronegative atoms (N or O) and an electropositive hydrogen atom (e.g. >C=O ⋯ H–N<). This arrangement defines the peptide bond. In secondary structures, such as the α-helix (found in keratin) or β-pleated sheets (as in amyloid), the polypeptide chain folds so as to maximize hydrogen bonding between the atoms of the peptide bonds. The other forces mentioned as options also stabilize folded protein structures, but these are associated mainly with tertiary structures.

2. B ★ OHMS 2nd edn → pp8, 10

Haemoglobin consists of more than one polypeptide chain. The key property of haemoglobin is its ability to bind oxygen reversibly over the physiological range of oxygen concentration. It is able to do so by virtue of the cooperative interactions of the 4 polypeptide subunits (cooperativity is a form of allostery). This is an example of the physiological benefits of quaternary protein structure. The myoglobin molecule consists of a single polypeptide chain. Both proteins are water-soluble and globular in shape (E), with each polypeptide chain binding the prosthetic group, haem, with its Fe^{2+} ion (A). All water-soluble proteins shield their non-polar amino acid side-chains from the aqueous environment by means of hydrophobic interactions (D). In both haemoglobin and myoglobin most of the polypeptide chains are arranged as α-helices (C).

3. D ★ OHMS 2nd edn → p12, Fig. 1.5; OHCM → pp55, 143

Collagen is stabilized by covalent cross-links. The triple helical structure of collagen is characterized by the repeating amino acid sequence–Gly–X–Pro–(where Gly is glycine, X is any amino acid, and Pro is proline or its derivative, hydroxyproline). The presence of proline means that each polypeptide chain cannot fold into an α-helix. Some proline residues in the newly synthesized polypeptide chain undergo hydroxylation in a reaction that requires vitamin C as an enzyme cofactor. Once secreted into the extra cellular medium, the immature collagen undergoes several covalent changes, one of which is the formation of cross-links between adjacent triple helices, thereby enhancing the stability of the collagen fibre.

Absence of cross-linking can result from genetic conditions such as Ehlers–Danlos Syndrome (EDS) in which weakened collagen may produce hypermobility of joints (with high risk of dislocation), skin hyperelasticity, and cardiovascular and other problems, reflecting the wide body distribution of collagen. EDS occurs in a variety of genetic forms and inheritance patterns with varying signs and symptoms.

4. A ★ OHMS 2nd edn → p22

The single defining property of the V_{max} value is that it increases with increasing enzyme concentration. The higher the enzyme concentration, the more active sites there are at which the reaction can occur (provided there is adequate substrate). This is the basis of an assay of enzyme activity. A competitive inhibitor (B) has no effect on V_{max}, whereas a non-competitive inhibitor (D) reduces it. The K_m is a measure of the affinity of enzyme active sites for the substrate and has units of concentration (mmol/L). The concentration at which V_{max} occurs is not twice the K_m (C), but rather, K_m is the substrate concentration at $\frac{1}{2}V_{max}$. The units of V_{max} are those of a rate, not a concentration (E).

5. D ★ ★ OHMS 2nd edn → p22

Only option D applies to the mode of action of a non-competitive inhibitor because it forms a covalent complex with the enzyme. The other statements typify competitive inhibitors, which form the other class of inhibitors of enzyme-catalysed reactions. By reacting with the enzyme for an extended or indefinite period of time, a non-competitive inhibitor irreversibly reduces the activity of the enzyme. Penicillin is a good example, inhibiting a critical enzyme (transpeptidase) required for bacterial cell wall synthesis; the action of aspirin on the enzyme cyclo-oxygenase to reduce inflammation is another.

6. C ★ ★ OHMS 2nd edn → pp30–1, 40; OHCM → p426

Complex oligosaccharides are covalently linked to the sphingolipid component of gangliosides. Cerebrosides (A) are also glycosphingolipids, but they have only a simple sugar (glucose or galactose). Phosphatidylinositol (D) contains the simple carbohydrate inositol. Sphingomyelin (E) is a membrane lipid that contains no carbohydrate; nor does cholesterol (B).

Cholera toxins bind to gangliosides in the cell membrane of the intestinal epithelium. Toxins then enter the cell, causing the secretion of anions (notably chloride) into the intestinal lumen. Water then follows the anions into the intestinal lumen by osmosis leading to the profound secretory diarrhoea that characterizes cholera infection.

7. E ★   OHMS 2nd edn → p34 and Fig. 1.20

Glycogen is sparingly soluble in aqueous solution. The branched (and therefore not linear) polysaccharide structure of glycogen means that it is only sparingly soluble in water. This is an important property, as it means that glycogen makes little contribution to the

(a) Glucose

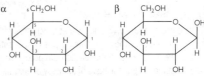

(b) 1–4 glycosidic bond

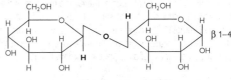

(c) Glycogen (or starch)

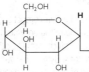

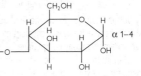
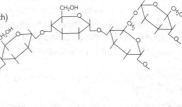

(d) Cellulose

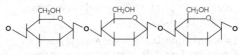

Fig. 1.4

osmotic potential of the cytosol, where it is made and degraded, and hence does not disrupt the osmotic balance of the intracellular milieu. Its glucose residues are linked by α-glycosidic bonds; β-glycosidic bonds are characteristic of the plant polysaccharide cellulose. The reducing properties of glucose are associated with a free aldehyde group on carbon-1; in glycogen, all but one of the carbon-1 groups are a component of a glycosidic bond. Fig. 1.4 shows differences between the two forms of α- and β-glycosidic bonds and the branched nature of glycogen or starch.

8. A ★   OHMS 2nd edn → pp44, 45

Membrane lipids such as phospholipids are amphipathic, with a polar region and a non-polar region; they associate to form a bilayer, with the hydrophobic fatty acid tails in the interior, shielded from the aqueous environment. This arrangement of lipid creates a stable but fluid structure with some of the characteristic permeability properties of biological membranes. Singer and Nicolson first proposed the fluid mosaic model for the cell membrane, in which proteins float in a phospholipid bilayer, in 1972. It has become accepted as the best description for the arrangement of the phospholipid, protein, and other components of the cell membrane. This model displaced earlier models, notably that of Davson and Danielli who, in 1935, correctly proposed the bilayer arrangement of lipid but were wrong in proposing that the proteins formed an extended outer coating of a protein–lipid sandwich.

Another membrane lipid, cholesterol, tends to reduce the fluidity of the bilayer. Protein associates with the lipid bilayer in two ways:

(a) Integral membrane proteins have some of the polypeptide chain embedded in the lipid bilayer,

(b) Peripheral membrane proteins bind loosely to the surface, either to integral membrane proteins or to the charged groups of phospholipids.

9. E ★   OHMS 2nd edn → pp50–3

Only E is a correct statement in relation to cAMP, which stimulates breakdown of hepatic glycogen when blood glucose is low. cAMP is synthesized from ATP, not degraded, by adenylate cyclase and it is degraded, not synthesized, by phosphodiesterase. The latter enzyme is inhibited by caffeine, which thus brings about an increase in intracellular cAMP concentration.

10. C ★   OHMS 2nd edn → pp50, 51, Fig. 1.30

Binding of the ligand, acetylcholine, to the nicotinic receptor at the neuromuscular junction (NMJ) opens a channel that allows the passage of cations (sodium and potassium ions) across the plasma membrane. Potassium leaves the cell and sodium enters, both moving along their respective concentration gradients. The result is depolarization of the membrane of the skeletal muscle fibre, producing an end-plate potential, as the membrane voltage moves to a value halfway between the sodium and potassium equilibrium potentials. This depolarization leads in turn to Ca^{2+} release (D) from the sarcoplasmic reticulum followed by muscle fibre contraction. The opening of the ion channels is extremely rapid, faster than could be achieved by an enzyme-dependent process (e.g. protein kinase as in A), by protein synthesis involving gene transcription (B) or by synthesis of a second messenger (E).

11. C ★   OHMS 2nd edn → pp50, 51, Figs. 1.30, 1.31

Once activated, some G-proteins stimulate the next step in the cell signalling pathway, whereas others inhibit it. Activation of G-proteins is brought about by the binding of a signalling molecule to its specific receptor, not to the G-proteins directly. Thus G-proteins themselves are not ligand-gated ion channels (A), nor are they receptors for hormones and neurotransmitters (E). In the active form the G-protein binds guanosine triphosphate, GTP (not GDP, as suggested in B) and slowly hydrolyses it. G-proteins are integral membrane proteins, at least partially embedded within the lipid bilayer, and on activation they affect the activity of another membrane-bound protein, usually an enzyme or an ion channel. Peripheral membrane proteins (D) are attached to the outer part of the bilayer. See Fig. 1.5 which shows how chemical signals can affect their target cells via indirect coupling (R = receptor, G = G-protein, E = enzyme).

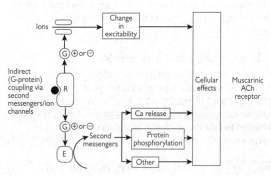

Fig. 1.5

12. E ★   OHMS 2nd edn → pp54, 55

Tight junctions (zonula occludens) are rows of proteins, mainly the claudins and the occludins, which are both embedded in plasma membranes of, and anchor to the cytoskeletons of, adjacent endothelial cells. They form a virtually impermeable barrier to the movement of solutes. The clinical features of the scenario point to a diagnosis of meningitis, where inflammation of the meninges surrounding the central nervous system has altered the permeability of the blood–brain barrier, contributing to the abnormalities of the CSF.

Adherens junctions (A) often form bands around epithelial cells, linking cells together structurally, with each junction connected to the actin of the cell cytoskeleton. The basal lamina (B) is an extracellular matrix that lies beneath all endothelial and epithelial cells. Gap junctions (C) form connections between the cytoplasm of two cells allowing ions and molecules to pass from cell to cell. They provide electrical continuity between cardiac muscle cells. Podocytes (D) are found in Bowman's capsule of the nephron. The long processes of these cells (foot processes, as the name implies) wrap around capillaries forming the slit pores that are important for the special filtration properties of the glomerular tuft capillaries.

13. E ★   OHMS 2nd edn → pp70, 71, Fig. 1.36; OHCM → p440. For details of DMARDs and methotrexate see OHCM → pp548–9

Methotrexate is a cell cycle specific agent that interferes with the S phase. It acts specifically during DNA and RNA synthesis, and so interferes with the Synthesis phase (S phase) of the cell cycle. It therefore has no actions in: G_0, the resting, or Gap nought phase; phase G_1, the Gap 1 phase; the G_2 Gap 2 phase; or M, the Mitosis phase.

Methotrexate was originally devised as an anti-cancer agent, intended to interfere with malignant cell division. It is now used as a disease modifying anti-rheumatic drug (DMARD) in the treatment of rheumatoid arthritis.

14. A ★   OHMS 2nd edn → pp74, 794

Apoptosis is a process of controlled cell death. During embryonic development, limb buds are formed, and at the tip of each limb bud digital rays start to develop. The spaces between the rays are made up of mesenchyme. At about week 7 of development apoptosis occurs in the inter-digital regions and, as the cells break down, differentiation of individual digits is seen. The mediators are unknown, but a blocking of the process of apoptosis would account for the fusion of the digits seen in cutaneous syndactyly.

Atrophy (B) is tissue-wasting following, for example, tissue denervation or lack of normal hormonal supply. Oncosis (C) is abnormal cell death resulting from swelling of tissues and cells. Pyroptosis (D) is a form of cell death associated with antimicrobial inflammatory responses. Necrosis (E) is premature cell death and has many causes including infection, trauma, infarction, toxins, and tissue hypoxia.

15. D ★ ★ ★   OHMS 2nd edn → p75; OHCM → p648

Squamous cell carcinoma is the most likely tumour type present. The photomicrographs show keratinizing squamous metaplasia (left) and eosinophilic and granulomatous inflammation in response to schistosomal ova (right). Areas that have a high prevalence of schistosomal parasitic infestation (such as Egypt) have a correspondingly high incidence of squamous cell carcinoma (SCC) of the bladder, the most common subtype associated with this infection. SCC arising in this context is usually associated with keratinizing squamous metaplasia in the adjacent urothelium. Metaplasia refers to the replacement of one differentiated cell type by another differentiated cell type—in this case, surface urothelium is replaced by keratinizing squamous epithelium.

Primary adenocarcinoma (A) of the bladder is uncommon, and usually associated with urachal remnants (a remnant of the allantois), diverticula, or bladder extrophy. Clear cell carcinoma (B) is seen mainly in either the female genital tract or in the kidney (clear cell renal cell carcinoma). Small cell carcinoma (C) is an uncommon high-grade carcinoma arising from neuroendocrine cells (not squamous metaplasia) and is seen more often in the lung. Transitional cell (urothelial) carcinoma (E) is the commonest type of bladder cancer, and may also be seen in association with schistosomiasis, but with a lower frequency compared to SCC.

Mostafa, M.H. *et al.* (1999). Relationship between schistosomiasis and bladder cancer. *Clinical Microbiology Reviews*, **12** (1): 97–111.

16. B ★   OHMS 2nd edn → pp75, 872–3

Dysplasia is abnormal tissue growth and represents a premalignant condition. Note that the epithelial cells are becoming disorganized with more deeply staining (hyperchromatic) and irregularly shaped (pleomorphic) nuclei. At this stage the cells have not yet breached the basement membrane.

Anaplasia (A) is a loss of cellular differentiation; hyperplasia (C) is an abnormal increase in cell number; metaplasia (D) is transformation of one tissue type into the appearance of another; neoplasia (E) is formation of new cells that may produce a cancer.

17. E ★ OHMS 2nd edn → pp76–7

In the process of meiosis the non-separation of bivalents or chromatids can lead to trisomy. In meiosis each chromosome replicates to produce two sister chromatids (B) which are closely bound to each other along their length. Each duplicated chromosome then pairs up with the equivalent chromosome to form bivalents (C). Even the sex chromosomes pair up as there is some homology between regions of the X and Y chromosomes. The close contact between chromatids allows for an exchange (or crossing over) of genetic material between the homologous chromosomes, known as genetic recombination (D). This is important for mixing of the maternal and paternal genetic material. After this exchange the bivalents line up on the mitotic spindle (A) and the first meiotic division takes place with the separation of bivalents, therefore separating each member of an homologous chromosome pair into a separate cell. The simpler second meiotic division, in which sister chromatids separate to produce haploid cells, follows these events.

In trisomy, the zygote resulting from fusion of oocyte and sperm contains three, not two, copies of a chromosome. This happens because of imperfect separation (non-disjunction) either of bivalents in the first meiotic division, or of chromatids in the second, leading to a gamete with two copies of a chromosome (or with none) rather than the normal single copy. Non-disjunction occurs in up to 10% of meiotic divisions. The embryos that develop from these gametes are usually non-viable and account for most of the first trimester miscarriages. Some, though, are viable and produce recognizable syndromes such as trisomy of chromosome 21 in Down's syndrome or trisomy of chromosome 18 in Edwards' syndrome.

18. D ★ OHMS 2nd edn → pp84–5

Diabetes mellitus type I usually starts in childhood and is the result of an autoimmune destruction of the patient's pancreatic B-cells. Type I diabetes requires treatment with insulin. The standard mode of delivery is subcutaneous via either single-use syringes or insulin pens. Inhaled insulin (A) has been tried but all forms have now been withdrawn. Intravenous administration (B) requires close supervision because of the risk of sudden hypoglycaemia, and is used on inpatients with difficult-to-manage diabetes mellitus (e.g. those with diabetic ketoacidosis). Oral insulin (C) is not effective since it is a polypeptide hormone and will be digested in the bowel and will not reach the liver intact. Transdermal administration (E) is feasible, but is currently rarely used.

19. B ★ ★ OHMS 2nd edn → pp88–9, Fig. 1.47

After a single oral dose, the plasma concentration of any drug increases until further absorption is balanced by metabolism and/or excretion; it then falls. A drug with first-order elimination kinetics is removed from the plasma (and the body) at a rate proportional to its plasma concentration. In consequence the half-life of such a drug is constant regardless of plasma concentration. This constancy of the half-life means that, with multiple dosing, a reasonably steady-state plasma concentration can be attained—an important aid to consistent dosing and treatment.

First-order elimination kinetics are characterized by enzyme-catalysed reactions, where the rate of elimination is proportional to the drug's plasma concentration. These enzymes are not readily saturated and therefore increasing plasma concentration is matched by increased drug metabolism. After three half-lives, 12.5% of the initial dose would survive; hence 87.5% has been eliminated (not 75% as in A). Drugs with first-order kinetics do not have a constant rate of elimination (D); the rate is not independent of plasma concentration (E).

20. E ★ ★ OHMS 2nd edn → pp90–1

While salicylate is acidic (A), it is the fact that elimination occurs at a constant rate, independent of plasma concentration, that classifies it as having zero-order kinetics. This constancy occurs because elimination depends on enzyme action, but unlike the enzymes of first-order elimination kinetics, there is a limit to their capacity to eliminate the drug. With increasing plasma concentration, the enzymes will become saturated, giving an upper limit to drug elimination. Drug elimination then occurs at a constant rate. Of course, over time it may be possible for enzyme induction to occur to increase the rate of elimination, but elimination will still have an (increased) upper limit and elimination will again become constant and independent of plasma concentration of the drug.

Unlike salicylate, drugs with first-order kinetics are eliminated from the body at a rate proportional to their current plasma concentration (C), since in first-order kinetics there is effectively no upper limit to the rate at which enzymes can metabolize the drug. This means that for any drug with first-order kinetics, the half-life of elimination is a constant (D) and this makes it relatively easy to set up a dosing regimen that provides a constant plasma concentration of drug (B). For zero-order kinetics, since elimination occurs at a constant rate, the half-life of the drug in the body is variable, not constant, and depends on the initial plasma concentration.

21. D ★   OHMS 2nd edn → p92

Physiological adaptation accounts best for the increased heart rate in this patient. Clevidipine is a member of the dihydropyridine group of drugs that selectively antagonizes L-type (voltage-dependent) calcium channels in vascular smooth muscle. Clevidipine therefore relaxes the smooth muscle of arterioles to lower the total peripheral resistance (TPR) of the vasculature. Since mean arterial pressure is the product of cardiac output (CO) and TPR, this drug will reduce arterial pressure but will not affect cardiac output. The arterial baroreceptors will sense the fall in blood pressure and this would normally produce a reflex increase in both CO (stroke volume times heart rate) and TPR. Since, in this patient, clevidipine is blocking the TPR response, only cardiac output will respond and this is seen as the increase in heart rate. This is an example of physiological adaptation to a drug-induced alteration of function.

Drug resistance—the loss of agonist effect—can have various causes. Adaptive loss of receptors (A) is a cellular response to continuous stimulation that reduces the efficacy of the drug and can be reversed by removal of the stimulus. The continual stimulation by a drug and activation of its receptors leads to the use of metabolically expensive second messengers (B); exhaustion of these or of essential metabolites (C) can reduce the efficacy of a drug.

Receptor desensitization (E) is usually rapid and caused by phosphorylation of G-proteins or a conformational change in ion channels. It is reversed as new receptors are synthesized.

Note that another class of calcium channel antagonists (the phenylalkylamine calcium channel blockers) have selective actions on L-type calcium channels in cardiac muscle and will reduce cardiac output while having little effect on vascular smooth muscle. Verapamil is an example.

Extended Matching Questions

1. F ★

Proteins are synthesized on ribosomes in both bacterial and human cells. The other organelles in the options list are only present in eukaryotic cells.

2. B ★

Lysosomes are concerned with the selective degradation of a wide range of biomolecules in eukaryotic cells, especially phagocytic ones.

The enzymes concerned are enclosed by the lysosomal membrane and have an acidic pH optimum (about pH5). Both these features help to protect the cell's contents from unwanted degradation by the lysosome's acid hydrolases.

3. C ★

Both the mitochondrion and the nucleus contain DNA and RNA and are enclosed within an organelle bound by a double membrane. However, the inner membrane of the nucleus is smooth, whereas that of the mitochondrion is highly folded in the form of cristae.

4. A ★

The Golgi apparatus consists of a stack of flattened membranous cisternae, which form a polarized structure. Newly synthesized glycoproteins enter at one face, and after covalent modifications by Golgi enzymes, leave the opposite face, where they are sorted into the appropriate vesicle. The endoplasmic reticulum has stacked membranes but does not process glycoproteins.

5. E ★★

The peroxisome is an organelle with a limited distribution in human tissues, but is active in the liver. There, it has several functions, one of which is the breakdown of very long-chain fatty acids. The peroxisomal pathway differs from the similar mitochondrial one in generating hydrogen peroxide, a potentially harmful reaction product that is degraded by catalase to water and oxygen.

General feedback on 1–5: OHMS 2nd edn → pp60–3, 158–62

6. A ★★

A chemical antagonist interacts directly with a drug to prevent it from reaching its target. A chemical antagonist does not depend on the interaction with the agonist's receptor (although that can happen). A chelator binds to the metal and prevents it reaching the target tissues and thus prevents its toxic effects.

7. J ★★

Uncompetitive antagonists differ from non-competitive antagonists in that they require receptor activation by an agonist before they can bind to a separate allosteric binding site. This requirement for prior binding of agonist means that in uncompetitive antagonism, the effects of higher concentrations of agonist are inhibited to a greater extent than lower concentrations at the same concentration of antagonist. The agonist for the NMDA receptor is glutamate so in this case memantine acts as a low-affinity, voltage-dependent, uncompetitive antagonist at glutamate NMDA receptors. Memantine is used in the treatment of Alzheimer's disease.

8. E ★★

A non-competitive antagonist binds to the same receptor as the agonist and, once bound, dissociates very slowly or, as in the case of naloxone, not at all. This means that there is no change in the occupancy of the receptor in the presence of the agonist.

9. C ★

An agonist is a molecule that binds to a receptor. A full agonist binds and has a high affinity for, and can activate, the receptor with the same efficacy as the endogenous agonist. Salbutamol mimics the action of adrenaline (noradrenaline) on the β_2 adrenergic receptor, relaxing bronchiolar smooth muscle, and is used in the treatment of asthma.

10. B ★

A competitive antagonist binds reversibly to the active site of a receptor but does not activate the receptor and thus blocks the actions. This decreases the potency of the agonist but if the agonist concentration increases it can compete successfully for the receptor and displaces the competitive antagonist.

General feedback on 6–10: OHMS 2nd edn → pp80–3

CHAPTER 2

CELLULAR METABOLISM

Cellular metabolism is divided into catabolism— responsible for converting nutrients into the energy sources and smaller molecules required for the chemical reactions of the body—and anabolism, which is the interconversion and synthesis of the molecules that maintain the body's structure and function.

This chapter examines the control of metabolism and the central metabolic pathways. Such control includes compartmentalization of metabolic processes and the cooperation between the metabolic activities of different organs. Metabolic control is important because metabolism must match the availability of nutrients to the demand for the products of the metabolic processes and both will vary over time. The synthesis of adenosine triphosphate (ATP), with its high-energy phosphate bond, lies at the heart of these central metabolic pathways. Most of the ATP is produced by oxidative phosphorylation in the mitochondria, but glycolysis and the tricarboxylic acid cycle (also known as the citric acid cycle or Krebs cycle) provide additional amounts.

Of the nutrients entering the body from the diet, fat, glucose, and amino acids are the main fuels for cellular metabolism. The utilization of lipids, fatty acids, and ketone bodies is important in metabolism in addition to the key role played by glucose. Glucose is the fuel for energy production in glycolysis. It is also manufactured by gluconeogenesis and stored as glycogen by glycogenesis. It is important to know how different organs utilize different fuels and how energy production alters between the fed state and starvation. Amino-acid metabolism and coenzymes in amino acid oxidation are also important although some details, including the urea cycle, have not been covered here. Energy balance and the relationship between food intake and energy expenditure lead to the concept of body mass index (BMI). The BMI offers a quick method of quantifying the nutritional status of a person, and BMI values may be helpful in

7. The predominant ketone bodies are acetoacetate and β-hydroxybutyrate and they increase in plasma concentration when acetyl-CoA in cells rises as a result of reduced plasma glucose and greater dependence on fatty acids and proteins as sources of metabolic energy. Ketone bodies can be utilized by many tissues and become important additional sources of energy when plasma glucose concentration falls and ketosis develops in fasting and starvation. Which single organ is unable to metabolize ketone bodies? ★

A Adrenal glands

B Brain

C Heart

D Kidney

E Liver

8. Organs such as the brain rely heavily on glucose as their main source of energy in the well-fed state, while many other tissues can utilize other substrates in addition to glucose, depending on their relative abundance. Which single cell type relies exclusively on glucose as its only source of energy? ★

A Cardiac muscle cells

B Neurones

C Red blood cells

D Retinal cells

E Skeletal muscle cells

9. Glycolysis brings about the breakdown of the 6-carbon sugar glucose to the 3-carbon intermediate pyruvate. The rate of the glycolytic pathway is matched to the cell's demand for energy by controlling the activity of the key regulatory enzyme phosphofructokinase-1 (PFK-1). Which single metabolite contributes most to the activation of PFK-1 in liver cells? ★

A AMP

B ATP

C Citrate

D Cyclic AMP

E Fructose-1,6-bisphosphate

10. The pentose phosphate pathway has an important role in supplying 5-carbon sugars for nucleotide biosynthesis, but it also has one other key metabolic function. Which single process is the other main metabolic role of the pentose phosphate pathway? ★ ★

A Interconversion of monosaccharides, such as glucose and galactose

B Synthesis of 2,3-diphosphoglycerate in the red blood cell

C Synthesis of fructose-2,6-bisphosphate for metabolic control of glycolysis

D Synthesis of NADH for oxidative phosphorylation to make ATP

E Synthesis of NADPH for anabolism (metabolic biosynthesis)

11. Hormones play key roles in regulating and integrating metabolism when physiological circumstances change. Many hormones bring about their effects through second messengers, while others stimulate gene expression. Cells in the target organs have specific hormone receptors. For example, blood glucose concentration is maintained during the early stages of the unfed or fasting state by the actions of specific hormones on specific organs. Which single combination of hormone and organ is responsible for maintaining plasma glucose concentration in the early stages of fasting? ★ ★

A Adrenaline and skeletal muscle

B Corticosteroid and adipose tissue

C Glucagon and liver

D Insulin and pancreas

E Thyroxine and cardiac muscle

12. In the fed state, glucose is the primary fuel for many tissues, but in fasting, starvation, and even in prolonged aerobic exercise circulating glucose and that from glycogen stores become depleted. Plasma glucose concentration must then be maintained by gluco-neogenesis. Apart from the liver, which single other tissue is also able to contribute significantly to overall gluconeogenesis? ★ ★

A Brain

B Cardiac muscle

C Pancreas

D Renal cortex

E Skeletal muscle

13. In order to avoid self-digestion, pancreatic acinar cells secrete proteases as inactive precursors. These precursors are activated on entering the duodenum. Which single protease precursor is most important in activating all other protease precursors found in pancreatic exocrine secretion? ★ ★

A Chymotrypsinogen

B Procarboxypeptidase A

C Procarboxypeptidase B

D Proelastase

E Trypsinogen

14. Many metabolically important coenzymes are derivatives of vitamins of the B group. Dietary deficiency of such vitamins causes metabolic disease. Which single coenzyme, derived from Vitamin B, is essential in most metabolic reactions of amino acids? ★ ★

A Biotin

B Flavin adenine dinucleotide (FAD)

C Nicotinamide adenine dinucleotide (NAD)

D Pyridoxal phosphate

E Thiamine pyrophosphate

15. A metabolic pathway is most efficient when all the enzymes involved are located within one confined area of the cell. Each subcellular organelle is invariably characterized by a distinctive set of enzymes appropriate to the metabolic functions of that compartment. Which single metabolic pathway is localized to the mitochondrion? ★

A Fatty acid synthesis

B Glycogen breakdown

C Glycolysis

D Pentose phosphate pathway

E Tricarboxylic acid cycle

16. Different parts of the cell are functionally specialized, and the distribution of metabolic enzymes in the various organelles or subcellular sites reflects this fact. This co-localization of metabolically related enzymes to specific organelles enhances efficiency. For example, in the liver the cytochrome P450 enzyme complex plays an important role in detoxification of compounds. Which single organelle is the main location for the cytochrome P450 enzyme complex in hepatocytes? ★

A Endoplasmic reticulum

B Golgi apparatus

C Lysosome

D Mitochondrion

E Peroxisome

17. The body's energy requirements are met by the intake of food. The main requirements to be met by the diet in energy terms are: basal metabolism (for the basic maintenance of the body), meeting the energy requirements of actually digesting and absorbing food, and physical activity. What is the single best estimate of the percentage of total daily energy requirement used by basal metabolism on a normal diet and average physical activity levels? ★

A 10%

B 20%

C 40%

D 60%

E 80%

18. The term 'vitamin' is a contraction of 'vital amine' and vitamins play essential roles in cell metabolism and in maintaining normal tissue integrity. For many vitamins a lack of dietary intake can lead to a characteristic deficiency disease of that vitamin. Such deficiency diseases can also arise when vitamins ingested in the diet fail to be absorbed in the gut, often because of loss of functional tissue as a result of surgery or disease processes, particularly in the small intestine. Apart from the B vitamins, which single vitamin is not transported by chylomicrons? ★

A Vitamin A

B Vitamin C

C Vitamin D

D Vitamin E

E Vitamin K

19. A 68-year-old man attends his GP for an annual health check. His height is measured as 160 cm and his weight is 83kg and the GP calculates the patient's body mass index (BMI). Which single category of body weight descriptors best describes his BMI value? ★

A Underweight

B Normal weight

C Overweight

D Obese

E Severely obese

EXTENDED MATCHING QUESTIONS

Important biochemical metabolites

For each of the following statements, choose the single metabolite that best matches the description given. Each option may be used once, more than once, or not at all.

A Acetoacetate

B Acetyl-CoA

C Alanine

D Cholesterol

E Citrate

F Glucose

G Glucose-6-phosphate

H Glutamate

I Glycogen

J Lactate

K Oxaloacetate

L Palmitate

M Pyruvate

N Urate

O Urea

1. This metabolite is the major end-product of glycolysis in the red blood cell. ★

2. This metabolite, synthesized from fatty acids in the liver, is exported in the blood to other tissues as a source of energy. ★ ★

3. This metabolite constitutes 10% of the tissue mass of liver and 2% of skeletal muscle. ★ ★

4. Particularly in starvation, this metabolite is exported from skeletal muscle to the liver for glucose synthesis. ★ ★

5. This metabolite makes a substantial contribution to fatty acid synthesis, by activating the rate-limiting enzyme in the pathway and providing that enzyme with one of its substrates. ★ ★

ANSWERS

Single Best Answers

1. D ★   OHMS 2nd edn → pp98–9, 127, 166, 168

Glucose is synthesized largely by the liver in the process of gluconeogenesis, starting from non-carbohydrate precursors such as lactate, glycerol and certain amino acids. Lactate is generated continuously by erythrocytes and by skeletal muscle during severe, anaerobic exercise. Lactate is transferred via the blood to the liver for gluconeogenesis, so that during severe and prolonged exercise the supply of glucose to the contracting muscle is maintained. This metabolic cycle of glucose into lactate in muscle and lactate back to glucose in liver is named after the two scientists Carl and Gerti Cori who first described it.

This cycling does not occur between the other pairs of organs or tissues in the option list.

2. B ★ ★   OHMS 2nd edn → pp104–5, 136

Stimulation of PDH activity would be consistent with an increased demand for cellular energy as ATP. During muscle contraction the increased intracellular Ca^{2+} concentration directly stimulates PDH.

A fall in plasma adrenaline concentration (A) tends to lower Ca^{2+} levels. Active breakdown of fatty acids (C) generates large amounts of acetyl-CoA, which inhibits PDH allosterically. The enzyme phosphoprotein phosphatase removes the phosphate group from inactive PDH, hence inhibition of the phosphatase (E) renders PDH less active. Decreasing the activity of the TCA cycle (D), which oxidizes acetyl-CoA, would have the same effect.

3. C ★   OHMS 2nd edn → pp108–11

Excessive heat production arises as follows: oxidative metabolism generates reduced coenzymes in the mitochondrion, where the electron transport chain re-oxidizes them. In the process of re-oxidation of reduced coenzymes a gradient of hydrogen ions is established across the inner mitochondrial membrane (more protons outside), and the energy of the proton gradient drives ATP synthesis.

This production of ATP is called oxidative phosphorylation. Weak acids, like uncouplers, transfer protons through the lipid bilayer of the inner membrane, thereby abolishing the proton gradient and making ATP synthesis impossible. The energy of oxidative metabolism is thus lost as heat, and in the process weight gain is minimized.

Uncouplers do not interfere directly with the accumulation of reduced coenzymes (A) and do not affect the structural integrity of mitochondrial membranes (B). Uncouplers reduce, and do not increase, ATP synthesis (D) and uncouplers do not inhibit the electron transport chain (E), responsible for pumping protons out of the mitochondrion.

Physiologically, the controlled uncoupling of mitochondria occurs in the cells of brown adipose tissue in neonates, in order to generate heat for the maintenance of body temperature.

4. E ★   OHMS 2nd edn → pp104–12

The maximum total is 38: 2 from glycolysis, 2 from the Krebs cycle, and 34 from oxidative phosphorylation in the mitochondria.

5. B ★   OHMS 2nd edn → pp113, 127

About 85% of the energy requirement of resting skeletal muscle comes from fatty acid metabolism. Although the skeletal muscle has considerable stores of glycogen, these are not utilized until the muscle begins to exercise, when energy production switches to utilizing glucose-6-phosphate produced from glycogenolysis. The glucose-6-phosphate enters directly into glycolysis. Glucose cannot leave skeletal muscle fibres—they lack the glucose-6-phosphatase to enable this to happen. Glucose from gluconeogenesis in the liver, including that produced from skeletal muscle lactate by the Cori cycle, can enter the muscle fibres to be used during exercise.

6. A ★ ★ ★   OHMS 2nd edn → pp113, 116

β-Oxidation of the 16-carbon fatty acid generates 8 acetyl-CoA, each with two carbons in the acetyl group, by means of 7 'turns' of the spiral pathway (not 8, since the last turn forms 2 acetyl-CoA). Hence 7 NADH and 7 FADH$_2$ are also generated. Complete oxidation of 8 acetyl-CoA yields a nominal 96 ATP; re-oxidation of 7 NADH forms 21 ATP; re-oxidation of 7 FADH$_2$ gives 14 ATP. Thus the total yield of ATP is 131 molecules per molecule of palmitic acid. Remember though that the fatty acid must first be converted to its acyl-CoA derivative in a reaction that uses the equivalent of 2 ATP (since ATP becomes AMP, not ADP). So the net (overall) yield is 129 ATP. This high value accounts for why dietary fat yields more than twice the energy of carbohydrate, gram for gram.

7. E ★ OHMS 2nd edn → p124

During starvation the liver maintains blood glucose levels by gluconeogenesis which leads to increased production of ketone bodies in mitochondria. The liver cannot metabolize ketone bodies as it lacks the enzyme β-ketoacyl-CoA transferase. Ketone bodies enter the bloodstream and can be metabolized by all the tissues, other than liver, mentioned in the option list.

In severe hypoglycaemia, as can occur in diabetes mellitus, concentrations of ketone bodies can be very high, leading to ketoacidosis. Acetoacetate spontaneously converts to acetone, a volatile compound that can often be smelled on the breath of ketoacidotic patients.

8. C ★ OHMS 2nd edn → p127

Red blood cells do not contain mitochondria and therefore rely on glucose and glycolysis as their only source of energy. Note that normally the brain uses only glucose as an energy source, consuming each day some 75% of the available glucose. However, in starvation the brain can adapt to utilize ketone bodies (e.g. acetoacetate) and so is not exclusively dependent on glucose. All of the other cell types (A, B, D, and E) on the option list contain mitochondria and can utilize a variety of substrates for energy production.

9. A ★ OHMS 2nd edn → pp132–3

AMP acts as a signal to the cell that ATP levels are depleted (since ATP breakdown forms ADP and AMP). Activation of PFK-1 by AMP will activate glycolysis as a way of restoring intracellular ATP levels. As expected, ATP itself (B) inhibits PFK-1 activity. Citrate (C), formed during the rapid breakdown of fatty acids via acetyl-CoA, also inhibits PFK-1, in part so that the liver can conserve glucose during starvation.

Fructose-1,6-bisphosphate (E) is an intermediate in glycolysis; its isomer, fructose-2,6-bisphosphate, stimulates PFK-1. Cyclic AMP (D) has an inhibitory effect on glycolysis by inhibiting the activity of the enzyme PFK-2, which synthesizes fructose-2,6-bisphosphate.

10. E ★ ★ OHMS 2nd edn → pp128–30, 138–9

The pentose phosphate pathway has two oxidative steps which bring about synthesis of metabolic reducing power in the form of NADPH, required for anabolic metabolism and membrane stabilization. It is a branch off the glycolytic pathway at the level of glucose-6-phosphate. A genetic deficiency of the first enzyme in the pathway, glucose-6-phosphate dehydrogenase, causes one form of haemolytic anaemia.

Interconversion of monosaccharides (A) is not performed by the pentose phosphate pathway. 2,3-diphosphoglycerate (B) and fructose-2,6-bisphosphate (C) are also made by side-reactions of glycolysis but are not involved in the pentose phosphate pathway. NADH (D) is generated by glycolysis itself (and other metabolic pathways); do not confuse NADH and NADPH, as these reduced coenzymes have very different metabolic functions.

Cellular metabolism

11. C ★★   OHMS 2nd edn → pp96, 108–9, 142

At the onset of fasting, the initial fall in blood glucose concentration is counteracted by the breakdown of hepatic glycogen, stimulated by glucagons released from the pancreatic islets.

Degradation of glycogen stores in skeletal muscle, activated by adrenaline (A), cannot generate free glucose, since muscle lacks the key enzyme glucose-6-phosphatase. Corticosteroids (B) and thyroxine (E) can both mobilize glucose leading to maintenance of plasma glucose, but not in combination with the organs with which they are paired. More importantly, these hormones operate through nuclear receptors which up-regulate gene expression, a process whose maximal effects will take days to attain. So any effects of gene expression are unsuited to the early phases of fasting. Insulin (D) is, of course, released by the pancreatic islets in response to a *rise* in blood glucose.

12. D ★★   OHMS 2nd edn → pp127, 156

The renal cortex is the only tissue other than the liver that can perform gluconeogenesis. It can be responsible for up to 10% of total glucose generation by gluconeogenesis.

The brain (A) is highly dependent on glucose as an energy source, consuming about 75% of glucose production each day. In starvation the brain is also able to metabolize significant quantities of ketone bodies. Cardiac muscle (B) is able to utilize a wide range of substrates for energy production, but does not perform gluconeogenesis. Little or no gluconeogenesis occurs in the pancreas (C). Skeletal muscle (E) utilizes primarily glucose, and muscle fibres store glucose as glycogen. Skeletal muscle does not release glucose into the blood, but lactate produced by exercising muscle does pass into the blood and can be converted to glucose in the liver by the Cori cycle.

13. E ★★   OHMS 2nd edn → p150

Duodenal epithelial cells (enterocytes) secrete enteropeptidase. This activates pancreatic trypsinogen when panceatic secretion enters the duodenum, and active trypsin then activates the other pancreatic proteases. Trypsin can also activate trypsinogen. Trypsin breaks down proteins and peptide chains by hydrolysing peptide bonds of lysine and arginine.

Chymotrypsinogen (A) is activated by trypsin and can also be activated by enteropeptidase. Chymotrypsin breaks down proteins by cleaving peptide bonds of aromatic amino acids such as tryptophan, tyrosine, and phenylalanine. Procarboxypeptidase A (B) and procarboxypeptidase B (C), once activated by trypsin, cleave terminal amino groups from proteins by hydrolysing the peptide bonds at the C-terminal. Proelastase (D) is similarly activated by enteropeptidase and trypsin to produce elastase, which selectively digests the protein elastin.

14. D ★★   OHMS 2nd edn → pp20, 100–1, 136, 152

Many reactions of amino acids entail the transfer of their α-amino group, leaving behind their carbon skeleton. Such amino group transfer requires the coenzyme pyridoxal phosphate, derived from dietary vitamin B$_6$.

Biotin (A) is essential for carboxylation reactions. Riboflavin and niacin give rise to redox coenzymes such as FAD (B) and NAD (C), respectively. Thiamine (E) in its pyrophosphate form is an important coenzyme in reactions involving acyl group transfer.

15. E ★   OHMS 2nd edn → pp102–3, 120–1, 128–30, 138–9, 140

The mitochondrion is responsible for the complete oxidation of the breakdown products of carbohydrate, fat, and protein catabolism. The acetyl-CoA generated by this metabolism feeds into the tricarboxylic acid (TCA) cycle within the mitochondrion. Fatty acid synthesis (A) occurs in the cytosol of the cell, as do glycogen breakdown (B), glycolysis (C), and the pentose phosphate pathway (D).

16. A ★   OHMS 2nd edn → p159

Within liver cells the smooth endoplasmic reticulum (ER) is the main subcellular site for detoxification, and the cytochrome P450 enzyme complex located there plays an active role in this process. The other organelles mentioned as options are also functionally specialized, but not with respect to detoxification. Some therapeutic drugs induce the synthesis of cytochrome P450 enzymes, a fact of clinical significance, since, over time, the presence of increasing amounts of these enzymes will lead to more rapid inactivation of the drug and hence lower the drug's efficacy.

17. D ★   OHMS 2nd edn → p172

In a normal day, without a large amount of physical exercise, the basal metabolism will be about 60% of the total energy requirement of the body. The basal metabolic rate (BMR) is the energy required to sustain life and can be estimated from the oxygen consumption of an awake person at complete mental and physical rest, in the post-absorptive state. Basal metabolic rate correlates with the lean body mass and varies with age, gender, height, pregnancy, and other factors. A BMR value for a 70kg male, aged 30 and 6 feet tall (183cm), might be around 1,700 kilocalories per day. On a normal light to medium activity pattern the total daily energy requirement might therefore be about 2,900 kilocalories per day.

Obesity can be described as the commonest form of malnutrition in the Western world and usually arises when food calorie intake exceeds the daily energy requirements of the body, so that excess calories are stored as fat. It is obviously important for good health to match food intake to metabolic requirements.

18. B ★   OHMS 2nd edn → pp114, 175

Chylomicrons are large (75–1,200 nm diameter) lipoprotein particles that are manufactured in epithelial cells of the small intestine. These lipoproteins transport dietary lipids from the intestine to other parts of the body. They enable fats, normally insoluble in water, to be transported in the bloodstream. Thus, part of the role of chylomicrons is to transport the fat-soluble vitamins A, D, E, and K, which are absorbed into the body in the same way as fats. Of those vitamins on the option list, vitamin C is the only vitamin that is not fat-soluble. Vitamin C and vitamins of the B complex (B_1, thiamine; B_2, riboflavin; B_3, niacin; B_5, pantothenic acid; B_6, pyridoxine; B_7, biotin; B_9, folic acid; and B_{12}, cyanocobalamin) are water-soluble and are also mostly absorbed in the small intestine but do not pass into chylomicrons.

19. D ★   OHMS 2nd edn → p180

BMI is calculated thus:

BMI = Weight in kilograms / (height in metres)^2

This gives a value for this man's BMI of $83/(1.6)^2$ or 32.4 kilograms per square metre. Note that the units of BMI are not usually given. The values of BMI that can be obtained are classified as follows:

Underweight	less than 20
Normal weight	20 to 25
Overweight	25 to 30
Obese	31 to 40
Severely obese	greater than 40

The man is therefore obese. Note that there are different systems for classifying BMI, some identifying severely underweight as well as subdivisions of the obese categories. The risks to health associated with obesity are numerous and include type II diabetes, coronary heart disease, hypertension, osteoarthritis, and some cancers. This makes the problem of obesity a major challenge for public health and other physicians.

Extended Matching Questions

1. J ★

Since erythrocytes lack mitochondria, they derive all their metabolic energy (ATP) from glycolysis. The glycolytic end-product in most cells is pyruvate. However, in order to regenerate NAD for continued glycolysis, the red cell must reduce pyruvate to lactate.

2. A ★★

The 'ketone bodies', of which acetoacetate is one, are a water-soluble form of fatty acid. They are made only by the liver, which secretes them into the blood plasma. Many tissues, especially cardiac muscle, use ketone bodies as a source of ATP. Liver also exports glucose, but this metabolic fuel cannot be made from the fatty acids commonly found in the human body.

3. I ★★

Glycogen is a store of glucose units and is present in high concentrations in liver and muscle. In liver, its breakdown helps to maintain the blood glucose concentration. Skeletal muscle breaks down glycogen to glucose as a source of metabolic energy during exercise.

4. C ★★

During starvation, muscle protein is degraded to amino acids as a source of energy. The amino acid alanine is exported to the liver for gluconeogenesis in order to maintain the blood glucose concentration in a situation of inadequate food intake. Lactate is also used for the same purpose, but at all times.

5. E ★★

The starting point for synthesis of fatty acid is acetyl-CoA in the cytosol. The main source of acetyl-CoA is citrate, exported from the mitochondrion. Citrate is also an allosteric activator of the rate-limiting enzyme in the pathway, acetyl-CoA carboxylase.

General feedback on 1–5: OHMS 2nd edn → pp102, 120–1, 124–5, 127, 156

CHAPTER 3

MOLECULAR AND MEDICAL GENETICS

Genetics has come a long way since the pioneering work on plant inheritance patterns by the Augustinian monk, Gregor Mendel, in the mid-nineteenth century. In the first decades of the twentieth century, Archibald Garrod, a London physician, was studying a class of diseases which came to be called 'inborn errors of metabolism'. As a result of studies on conditions such as alkaptonuria (a rare disease involving altered phenylalanine and tyrosine metabolism, with production of dark urine and a rare form of arthritis), Garrod postulated the 'one gene–one enzyme' hypothesis, namely that most inborn errors of metabolism result from errors in single genes that code for enzymes. This showed remarkable foresight, since the actual nature of DNA and the way genes are transcribed and translated was not fully established until the work of Watson and Crick and others in the 1950s and beyond. One gene–one enzyme (or one protein) has now been modified to become one gene–one peptide, but the principle holds. As more has been learned about human genetics and genetic mutation, especially following the Human Genome Project, the number of genetic defects known to underpin diseases and predisposition to disease has burgeoned. All this new knowledge is adding to earlier knowledge of diseases that were detected by studying chromosome number (cytogenetics) or by examining family pedigrees for the patterns of disease inheritance. Studies of family pedigrees exposed the genetic nature of diseases as diverse as cystic fibrosis, haemophilia, sickle-cell disease, and Huntington's disease.

Nowadays, a doctor's training in medical genetics will cover the genetic code, gene expression, gene regulation and mutation, cancer genetics, chromosomal abnormalities, abnormalities at the gene level, genetic polymorphism, the principles of gene therapy, and the emerging science of pharmacogenetics. As it has become evident not only that diseases are a direct expression of particular genes or mutations, but that genetic predisposition can be identified for a great number of diseases, both ethical and therapeutic questions arise. For example, will every healthy person want or need to have knowledge of his or her own future risk for specific diseases? To what extent will gene therapies or pharmaco-genetics have to be tailored to an individual's genetic constitution, and at what financial cost? ■

SINGLE BEST ANSWERS

1. 'Deoxyribonucleic acid (DNA) makes ribonucleic acid (RNA) makes protein' is the central dogma of molecular biology, whereby the cell's genetic information is converted into proteins with specific functions. The processes involved are catalysed by enzymes, which are active either throughout the cell cycle or preferentially at a certain phase of it. Which single enzyme is most active during the S phase of the cell cycle? ★

A DNA polymerase

B Peptidyl transferase

C Poly (A) polymerase

D Reverse transcriptase

E RNA polymerase

2. A DNA sequence coding for a peptide consisting of 80 amino acids undergoes a mutation. Amino acid analysis of the mutated peptide shows that it has only 30 amino acids. The first fourteen amino acids are identical to the normal peptide, but amino acids 15 to 30 differ from the original peptide. Which single type of mutation is most likely to have occurred? ★

A Nucleotide deletion in the codon for amino acid 15

B Nucleotide deletion in the codon for amino acid 30

C Nucleotide deletion in the intron

D Nucleotide substitution in the codon for amino acid 15

E Nucleotide substitution in the codon for amino acid 30

3. The ENCODE consortium has recently completed its characterization of 1% of the human genome by various high-throughput techniques. One of its findings highlighted the number and complexity of the RNA transcripts that the genome produces. Which single term best describes genomic components that are derived from functional genes that have lost the original functions of their parental genes? ★ ★ ★ ★

A Alternative splicing

B Constrained elements

C Intergenic transcription

D Non-coding RNA (ncRNA) genes

E Pseudogenes

4. RNA is a biologically important type of molecule that is central to gene regulation and expression. The diversity of RNA molecules is reflected by the variety of functions they perform. From a clinical point of view, mutational changes affecting some types of RNA have been linked to pathological processes, such as cancer. Which type of RNA negatively regulates gene expression at the post-transcriptional level and has been implicated in cancer pathogenesis? ★ ★

A Messenger RNA (mRNA)

B MicroRNA

C Ribosomal RNA (rRNA)

D Small nucleolar RNA (snoRNA)

E Transfer RNA (tRNA)

5. The messenger RNA (mRNA) for a dementia-associated gene is found to be about 500 nucleotides longer when isolated from neurones than when isolated from glial cells. The nucleotide sequence of genomic DNAs isolated from the two cell types is identical. Which single mechanism best accounts for the difference in the sizes of the mRNAs? ★ ★

A Alternative splicing

B Capping

C Polyadenylation

D Post-translational modification

E Site-specific recombination

6. Duchenne muscular dystrophy (DMD) is an X-linked genetic mutation that causes the complete loss of the dystrophin protein in 1:3,500 boys each year in the UK. Many different strategies have been suggested for treating DMD. The dystrophin gene is very large. It is 79 exons long and covers 2.6 million base pairs. This large size has been a challenge for gene therapy. Utrophin is expressed during development and performs a similar function to dystrophin but is down-regulated after birth. However, its genome is smaller, and potentially it could substitute for dystrophin. Many of the mutations in the dystrophin gene are large deletions or nonsense mutations that could, in principle, be treated by a 'molecular patch' that creates a smaller but functional dystrophin protein as result of exon skipping across the altered DNA. A clinical trial run in association with Great Ormond Street Hospital, London has demonstrated restoration of some muscle function using one particular approach. Which single gene therapy method is most likely to have been used by the Great Ormond Street group? ★ ★ ★ ★

A Adenoviral-mediated dystrophin mini-gene

B Anti-sense oligonucleotides

C Full-length dystrophin DNA plasmid vector

D Recombinant adeno-associated viral vector (rAAV)-mediated dystrophin mini-gene

E Utrophin up-regulation

7. A 1-year-old boy developed bilateral retinoblastoma. There is a history of this tumour in his family. Genetic testing reveals a mutation in a gene on chromosome 13 called the RB1 gene. Which single alteration of function is the most likely consequence of the mutation to chromosome 13? ★ ★ ★

A Proto-oncogene activation

C Proto-oncogene amplification

B Proto-oncogene loss

D Tumour suppressor gene activation

E Tumour suppressor gene loss

8. A 25-year-old pregnant woman attends a prenatal ultrasound scan at 20 weeks. The scan shows that her fetus has a rocker-bottom foot. Which single genetic error is most likely to have caused this fetus's condition? ★ ★

A Amplification of a specific trinucleotide sequence in a gene

B Deletion of bases within a coding region of a gene

C Gain of one homologous chromosome

D Loss of a portion of a chromosome

E Point mutation of a base within a coding region of a gene

9. Leber's optic neuropathy is a genetic condition that causes blindness in young adults. When an affected woman has children, all of them inherit the disease. When an affected man has children, none of them does. Which single term describes best the mode of inheritance of Leber's optic neuropathy? ★ ★

A Autosomal dominant

B Autosomal recessive

C Mitochondrial

D X-linked

E Y-linked

10. A genetic polymorphism is said to occur when a particular gene is present in different forms (alleles) in a population. Typically, such alleles produce slightly different but non-deleterious phenotypes. Such genetic polymorphism is responsible for much of human diversity and also for variations in susceptibility to disease. DNA polymorphisms can be classified by the genetic analysis technique by which they have been detected. Which single type of polymorphism, also called 'structural variation', has recently been characterized by assay-based comparative genomic hybridization (CGH)? ★ ★ ★

A Copy number variants (CNVs)

B Restriction fragment length polymorphisms (RFLPs)

C Simple sequence repeats (SSRs)

D Single nucleotide polymorphisms (SNPs)

E Variable number of tandem repeats (VNTRs)

11. A 60-year-old man is diagnosed with a metastatic gastrointestinal stromal tumour (GIST). Immunohistochemistry performed on his tissue sample reveals that he is a good candidate for treatment with imatinib—a drug designed to bind a particular molecular target. Name the single gene product whose mutation is specifically targeted by imatinib in GIST patients? ★ ★ ★ ★

A c-Kit (Cytokine receptor CD20)

B CD20 (Cluster of differentiation 20)

C EGFR (Epidermal growth factor receptor)

D HER2 (Human epidermal growth factor receptor 2)

E VEGF (Vascular endothelial growth factor)

EXTENDED MATCHING QUESTIONS

Types of genetic mutation, and how they cause disease

For each of the following genetic diseases, select the single option that best defines the nature of the underlying mutation. Each option may be used once, more than once, or not at all.

A Deletion

B Fusion

C Insertion

D Inversion

E Monosomy

F Nonsense

G Substitution

H Translocation

I Trinucleotide repeat

J Triploidy

K Trisomy

1. In sickle-cell anaemia, this mutation causes the replacement of glutamic acid by valine on the surface of the HbS protein. ★

2. In Huntington's disease (chorea), this mutation leads to the phenomenon of anticipation, whereby the disease becomes more severe in successive generations. ★

3. In one type of leukaemia, this mutation generates the Philadelphia chromosome, which contains reciprocally exchanged genetic material. ★

4. In cystic fibrosis, this mutation causes the loss of a phenylalanine amino acid residue, resulting in improper folding of the cystic fibrosis transmembrane regulator (CFTR) polypeptide chain. ★

5. In Edwards' syndrome, this mutation occurs when a pair of homologous chromosomes fails to separate at meiosis. ★

ANSWERS

Single Best Answers

1. A ★   OHMS 2nd edn → pp64–5, 192–4, 196

The S phase of the cell cycle refers to the synthesis of DNA, catalysed by DNA polymerase; this enzyme would thus be expected to be most active during this phase.

Poly (A) polymerase (C) and RNA polymerase (E) both participate in RNA synthesis, which is active throughout the cell cycle. The former adds the poly (A) tail that protects the 3' end of most messenger RNA molecules. The latter catalyses the process of chain elongation for all species of RNA. Peptidyl transferase (B) catalyses the formation of the peptide bond in protein synthesis, a process that likewise is not restricted to any one phase of the cell cycle. Reverse transcriptase (D) only occurs in cells infected with the HIV virus.

2. A ★   OHMS 2nd edn → pp184–5

A truncated protein occurred following a nucleotide deletion in codon 15, resulting in a premature stop codon being introduced after codon 30. The deletion of codon 15 produced a frame shift in translation of the DNA triplets so that amino acids 15 to 30 differ from the original coded peptide and codon 31 now becomes a stop codon. Deletion of three consecutive base pairs spanning two codons and the consequent frame shift is found in many patients suffering from cystic fibrosis.

Introns (C) are not translated into proteins.

A single nucleotide substitution (D, E) may lead to no change in peptide sequence because the genetic code is redundant. For example, many amino acids are coded by four triplets in which the first two base pairs are the same, but the third nucleotide can be any of the four possible base pairings. In this example substitution of a third nucleotide would produce a triplet that still coded for the original amino acid. In other cases a single base-pair substitution can produce a missense codon. This occurs in sickle-cell disease where, in consequence, valine replaces glutamic acid in β-haemoglobin.

The mutation has become conserved in the population because is also confers a degree of resistance to malarial infection. This is an example of balancing selection where a harmful gene remains in a population because in the heterozygote (normal allele with sickle-cell allele) the benefits for survival outweigh the ill-effects.

3. E ★★★★ OHMS 2nd edn → p205

Pseudogenes are often found in introns of genes and can influence the structure and function of the human genome.

Alternative splicing (A) means that one transcript can generate multiple mRNAs, resulting in multiple proteins. However, it implies that information in DNA is not linearly related to that of protein. Since only 40% of the evolutionarily constrained bases were found within protein-coding exons, it was suggested that 'protein coding loci can be seen as a cluster of small constrained elements (B) dispersed in a sea of unconstrained sequences' (Gerstein et al. 2007). Non-coding RNA (D) genes lack open reading frames and are hard to identify, but take part in gene regulation, RNA processing and protein synthesis. Genes appear to extend into intergenic regions (C). For example, there are pseudogenes and ncRNA genes, which are located within introns of protein-coding genes.

Gerstein, M, Bruce, C, & Rozowsky, J (2007). What is a gene, post-ENCODE? History and updated definition. *Genome Research*, **17**: 669–81.

4. B ★★ OHMS 2nd edn → p192

Micro-RNAs are complementary to part of the messenger RNA molecule and can block the mRNA from being translated, or accelerate its degradation and therefore have a regulatory function.

Messenger RNA (A) is made up of a series of codons that specify the precise sequence of amino acids in a peptide or protein. Messenger RNA is transcribed from DNA in the nucleus and then moves to the cytoplasm, where it interacts with the ribosomal RNA (C) of the ribosomes in the process of translation that forms proteins. Transfer RNA (E) identifies individual amino acids in the cytoplasm and brings these to interact with mRNA and ribosomal RNA in the translation process.

Small nucleolar RNA (snoRNAs) as in option D, are involved in modification of other RNAs, such as rRNAs or tRNAs. SnoRNAs associate with enzymes and guide them to a specific target on an RNA by base-pairing to that RNA and then performing the nucleotide modification. Although there is evidence to suggest that some snoRNAs might have microRNA-like activity, they are not, as yet, implicated in the development of cancer.

Esquela-Kercher, A, & Slack, FJ (2006). Oncomirs—microRNAs with a role in cancer. *Nature Reviews Cancer*, **6**(4): 259–69.

Mattick, JS, Taft, RJ, & Faulkner, GJ (2010). A global view of genomic information—moving beyond the gene and the master regulator. *Trends in Genetics*, **26**(1): 21–8.

5. A ★★   OHMS 2nd edn → pp194–5

Before the RNA is translated, the precursor messenger RNA (pre-mRNA) molecule undergoes three main modifications: 5′ capping (B), 3′ polyadenylation (C), and then RNA splicing. Alternative splicing of pre-mRNA refers to differential inclusion and exclusion of exon sequences, which accounts for the difference in sizes of the mRNAs. This process is also responsible for doubling the number of proteins encoded by the genes.

Post-translational modification (D) is the chemical modification of a protein after its translation. Site-specific recombination (E) is a process of DNA breakage and reunion that requires no DNA synthesis, but changes nucleotide sequence.

6. B ★★★★   OHMS 2nd edn → pp198, 206

Exon skipping uses short strands of DNA known as 'anti-sense oligonucleotides' (AOs). These act as molecular patches, which are able to restore production of the protein dystrophin. As the name suggests, the exon skipping encourages the cellular machinery to 'skip over' an exon. Small pieces of DNA (the AOs) are used to mask the exon that carries the mutation so that it is ignored during the protein production. The exon-skipping AOs need to be tailored for each mutation; while there are 'hot spots' along the gene, not everyone can be treated by this method.

Normal adenoviral vectors cannot fit the whole dystrophin genome. Newer gutless vectors exist and have a large capacity of up to 28kb. However, the use of adenoviral vectors has problems, as they are too large to cross the extracellular matrix that surrounds the skeletal muscle fibres. The size of the dystrophin gene can be overcome by using 'mini-genes' that fit easily into the adenoviral vectors (A) and generate a milder form of DMD called Becker muscular dystrophy. The full-length dystrophin cDNA does not present a problem for plasmid vectors (C). However, delivery of these plasmids is inefficient in muscle tissue. The rAAV vectors (D) seem promising for gene delivery to muscle despite their limited insert capacity of only 5kb. The rAAV particle is small and can penetrate the extracellular matrix.

AOs and rAAVs look to have the best prospects for gene therapy for DMD. Utrophin (E) is a homologue of dystrophin. Activation of the promoters of the utrophin gene can up-regulate utrophin expression and lead to the less severe phenotype. Several strategies are aimed at investigating stimulation of the expression of utrophin.

van Deutekom, JCT, & van Ommen, G-J B (2003). Advances in Duchenne Muscular Dystrophy gene therapy. *Nature Reviews Genetics*, **4**: 774–83.

→ http://www.musculardystrophy.org/about_muscular_dystrophy/ research_faqs/612_what_is_exon_skipping_and_how_does_it_work

7. E ★★★   OHMS 2nd edn → pp876–7

Retinoblastoma is a rare childhood tumour of the eye. Most cases present within the first 3 years of life and are sporadic. The condition may affect one or both eyes. About 20% of unilateral cases and all bilateral tumours are believed to be hereditary. The hereditary form of retinoblastoma tends to present earlier than the sporadic disease. Retinoblastoma is caused by a mutation in a tumour suppressor gene that prevents its normal expression. Such 'loss of function' mutations contribute to the development of cancer by inactivating the normal inhibition of cell growth provided by tumour suppressor gene proteins.

Oncogenes encode proteins that control cell proliferation, apoptosis, or both. Activation or amplification of oncogenes by mutations, gene amplification, or chromosomal rearrangements can therefore lead to increased cell proliferation or increased cell survival of cells carrying such alterations. The activation leads to either a structural alteration in the oncogene or an increase in, or deregulation of, its expression.

Many cancers are caused by alterations in oncogenes. For example, activating point mutations occur in a substantial proportion of melanomas. Amplification of *MYC* has been found in small cell lung cancer, breast cancer, oesophageal cancer, and many others. Chromosomal rearrangements leading to oncogenic activity are common in prostate cancer.

Croce, C (2008). Oncogenes and cancer. *New England Journal of Medicine* **358**: 502–11.

8. C ★★   OHMS 2nd edn → pp206–7

Rocker-bottom foot is highly suggestive of Edwards' syndrome. This syndrome results from the presence of the usual two copies of chromosome 18 plus an additional copy, a condition known as trisomy 18. Chromosomal abnormalities can be broadly divided into numerical (e.g. aneuploidy—such as trisomy 21, known as Down's syndrome—or polyploidy) and structural (translocations, deletions, as in option D, or insertions).

Single-gene abnormalities due to a mutation in a gene which codes for a specific protein may arise due to deletion of bases (B) as in Duchenne muscular dystrophy. A mutation in a gene may also cause insertion of bases (as in haemophilia A), or substitution of one base for a different base (E) as occurs in sickle-cell anaemia. Trinucleotide repeat diseases, such as Fragile X syndrome or Huntington's disease (chorea), are characterized by amplification (that is repeated copies) of a specific trinucleotide sequence (A) in a gene.

9. C ★★   OHMS 2nd edn → pp158, 206

A woman's ovum contributes all the mitochondria of the zygote at fertilization; the man's sperm makes no such contribution. Hence any gene on the mitochondrial DNA is inherited from the mother (maternal inheritance), and all the children of an affected woman will themselves inherit the condition. For genes on the nuclear DNA, no such pattern of inheritance is expected. A man with an autosomal dominant (A) condition will (on average) pass on the mutant gene, and hence the disease, to half his children. A woman with an autosomal recessive (B) disease will most likely have all heterozygous children who are clinically normal. Most X-linked (D) genetic disorders are inherited in a recessive manner, with a female carrier passing on the mutant gene, and hence the disease, to half her sons. The rare Y-linked (E) genetic conditions are only transmitted from father to son.

10. A ★★★   OHMS 2nd edn → pp208–9

'Structural variation' is characterized by copy number variants (CNVs). Until recently, the differences observed in human genetic composition were mainly rare changes in the quantity and structure of chromosomes. However, the introduction of genome scanning array technologies and comparative DNA sequence analyses has uncovered the large amount of 'structural variation' that exists in the human genome. This comprises microscopic and submicroscopic forms, which include deletions, duplications, and large-scale copy number variants.

It is believed that these structural variants contribute millions of nucleotides of heterogeneity to every genome, and are likely to make an important contribution to human diversity and disease susceptibility. Array-CGH approaches use labelled fragments from a genome competitively hybridized with a second differentially labelled genome to arrays that are spotted with cloned DNA fragments. This reveals copy number variations between the two genomes. VNTRs (E), RFLPs (B), and SSRs (C) result in variations in the fragment length pattern produced after digestion of DNA with restriction enzymes or PCR amplification of a specific DNA fragment. As the name implies, SNPs (D) occur when one nucleotide (A, T, C, or G) is replaced by another nucleotide in a DNA sequence.

Feuk, L, Carson, AR, & Scherer, SW (2006). Structural variation in the human genome. *Nature Reviews Genetics*, **7**(2): 85–97.

11. A ★ ★ ★ ★ OHMS 2nd edn → p210

Patients with GIST can be treated with imatinib—a specific inhibitor of several tyrosine kinase enzymes—if their cancer cells bear a c-Kit gene mutation. Imatinib is just one example of an 'individualized medicine' that is tailored to a particular patient's genetic make-up. Another example of a tyrosine kinase inhibitor (TKI) is gefitinib for mutations in EGFR (C). Increases in EGFR due to mutation are seen in lung cancers as well as other cancers. Other targeted molecular approaches introduced in cancer therapy include rituximab for CD20 (B) mutations in haematological cancers; humanized monoclonal antibodies, such as trastuzumab for HER2 (D) mutations in breast cancer; or bevacizumab for VEGF (E) mutations in metastatic colon cancer.

Extended Matching Questions

1. G ★

Exchange of one amino acid for another in a mutant protein is often the result of a single base substitution, causing the change of that codon to one for a different amino acid. The presence of a non-polar amino acid (valine) on the surface of HbS causes the mutant haemoglobin molecules to aggregate, thereby distorting the red blood cell and causing anaemia.

2. I ★

The Huntington protein in Huntington's disease contains a repeated sequence of glutamine residues, brought about by expansion of a trinucleotide repeat in the coding region of the gene. The mutation is caused by chromosomal misalignment in the region of the Huntington gene at meiosis. The more the 3-base sequence is repeated, the more likely chromosomal misalignment becomes. Hence, in successive generations of an affected family, one sees the phenomenon of anticipation, whereby the disease becomes clinically more severe or has an earlier age of onset.

3. H ★

The reciprocal exchange of DNA between non-homologous chromosomes is a not uncommon mutation. The outcome of such a translocation is one chromosome with an abnormally long arm, and one with a shorter arm. In this Philadelphia chromosome, a lymphocyte growth factor gene is transferred downstream from an active promoter sequence. The ensuing excessive cell division gives rise to chronic myeloid leukaemia.

4. A ★

The most common mutation in British patients with cystic fibrosis is the deletion of 3 consecutive bases, causing the loss of a critical phenylalanine residue at position 508 in the CFTR protein. The mutant polypeptide chain does not fold properly. As a result, the newly synthesized protein is not inserted into its correct location in the apical membrane of epithelial cells of exocrine pancreas, respiratory airways, and other tissues.

5. K ★

If a pair of homologous chromosomes fails to separate at meiosis, one of the resulting gametes will have two copies of that chromosome, instead of one (and one gamete will have none). If a male gamete with the two copies fuses with a female gamete at fertilization, then the resulting zygote will contain 3 copies of the affected chromosome, instead of two—trisomy. Edward's syndrome (trisomy of chromosome 18) is an example, but Down's syndrome (trisomy 21) is a better known one. Be careful to distinguish trisomy from triploidy (3 copies of the full set of chromosomes).

General feedback for 1–5: OHMS 2nd edn → pp184–5, 206, 207

CHAPTER 4

NERVE AND MUSCLE

Higher animals have four basic tissue types: epithelial tissue, connective tissue, nervous tissue, and muscle. Of these, nerve and muscle are grouped together as 'excitable cells' because the cell membrane has the ability to vary membrane ion conductance and membrane voltage so as to transmit meaningful signals within and between cells. Within excitable cells information is transmitted using either an amplitude-modulated (AM) code using slow, electrotonic potentials, or a frequency-modulated (FM) code when signalling is by action potentials.

Much of the signalling between excitable cells occurs at chemical synapses where a chemical neurotransmitter is released from presynaptic cells and then interacts with postsynaptic membrane receptors. Clinical symptoms can arise when the release of chemical neurotransmitters is disturbed, or when availability of postsynaptic receptors is altered. Thus, a reduction in dopamine release from basal ganglia substantia nigra cells is found in Parkinson's disease, while myasthenia gravis results from loss of nicotinic acetylcholine receptors at the neuromuscular junction of skeletal muscle. Sometimes transmission from cell to cell is not by chemical neurotransmitter but by electrical synapses, where gap-junctions provide direct electrical connectivity. Transmission between cardiac muscle cells occurs in this way. Some cardiac arrhythmias, such as Wolff–Parkinson–White syndrome, are a consequence of an abnormal path of electrical conduction between cardiac muscle fibres.

Sensory cells on and within the body pass information via afferent pathways from the peripheral nervous system into the central nervous system (CNS). CNS processes and sensory information are integrated to produce outputs from the CNS. These outputs pass by various efferent routes to the effector organs: skeletal muscle, cardiac muscle, smooth muscle, and glands. It is through these effectors that the CNS is able to exert control over the body and to interact with the environment. Alterations of function anywhere in the afferent, integrative, or efferent aspects of the system, as well as defects in the effectors themselves, are likely to lead to significant clinical symptoms and signs.

The efferent outflow from the CNS has two major components. One, the somatic nervous system, innervates only skeletal muscle. The other is the autonomic nervous system (ANS), which innervates cardiac muscle, smooth muscle, and the glands of the viscera and skin. The ANS is further subdivided into a sympathetic system (with thoracolumbar outflow) and a parasympathetic system (with craniosacral outflow). These two outflows differ significantly in anatomical arrangement, neurotransmitters, and function.

Detailed knowledge of the ANS becomes important in interpreting abnormal visceral function and in understanding the therapeutic rationale for drugs which inhibit or mimic ANS transmitters. ∎

SINGLE BEST ANSWERS

1. A 78-year-old woman presents to her GP complaining of neck pain and inability to move her arm properly. Her right arm biceps and supinator tendon reflexes are absent but the triceps reflex is normal compared to her left arm. Two-point discrimination, joint position sense, and vibration and pinprick sensations are all normal. Sensory nerve conduction and electromyogram (EMG) tests reveal that the nerve conduction velocity appears normal but the compound muscle action potential size is decreased on the right. Which is the single most likely location for the underlying pathology in this patient? ★ ★ ★

A Dorsal root

B Neuromuscular junction

C Peripheral nerve

D Spinal nerve

E Ventral root

2. Fig. 4.1 is a diagrammatic representation of the spinal cord, the sympathetic chain, and the paravertebral ganglia, as well as some related structures. Which single, labelled structure in the diagram contains only unmyelinated, postganglionic sympathetic fibres? ★ ★

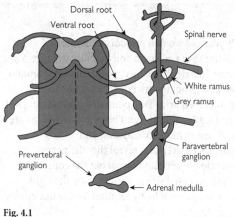

Dorsal root

Ventral root

Spinal nerve

White ramus

Grey ramus

Paravertebral ganglion

Prevertebral ganglion

Adrenal medulla

Fig. 4.1

A Dorsal root

B Grey ramus

C Sympathetic chain

D Ventral root

E White ramus

3. All living cells show a transmembrane voltage, called the resting membrane potential. In excitable cells this potential is typically around −70mV. Which single ionic movement is primarily responsible for the production of the resting membrane potential (RMP)? ★

A Active pumping of sodium ions out of the cell

B Chloride ions entering the cell along a concentration gradient

C Potassium ions entering the cell by electrochemical attraction

D Potassium ions leaving the cell along a concentration gradient

E Sodium ions entering the cell along a concentration gradient

4. During the production of an action potential in a nerve axon the membrane potential moves very rapidly (in about a millisecond) from close to E_K, the Potassium Equilibrium Potential, to a peak just below the Sodium Equilibrium Potential, E_{Na}. The voltage returns quickly towards the resting value, undershoots it slightly, and then returns to the resting membrane potential (Fig. 4.2). Which single process must occur at the peak of the action potential before the membrane voltage can move towards E_K? ★ ★

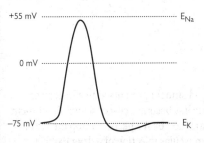

Fig. 4.2

A Active pumping of sodium ions out of the axon

B Efflux of potassium out of the axon

C Hyperpolarization of the axon membrane

D Inactivation of the voltage-dependent sodium channels

E Influx of sodium into the axon

5. A 12-year-old child attends a paediatric liver clinic. A blood test is required, but the child is very anxious. Which single type of anaesthesia would be most appropriate in this case? ★

A Inhaled nitrous oxide (N_2O)

B Intravenous thiopental

C Local injection of lidocaine

D Oral diazepam

E Topical EMLA®

6. When a local anaesthetic is applied to a peripheral nerve, it is possible for conduction to be blocked in all fibre types in the nerve. Depending on their diameter, some fibres succumb more slowly to, and recover more quickly from, local anaesthetics. Which single nerve axon type is the first to recover function after a local anaesthetic? ★

A Aα axon

B Aβ axon

C Aδ axon

D Aγ axon

E C axon

7. A 21-year-old student presents with a history of facial tics. He has become self-conscious about them and fears stigmatization by his peers. To stop the tics, he is given an intramuscular injection of a drug that acts presynaptically at the neuromuscular junction to prevent neurotransmitter release. Which single drug is most likely to be injected in this patient? ★ ★

A Botulinum toxin

B Edrophonium

C Rocuronium

D Suxamethonium

E Tubocurarine

8. A 75-year-old man suffers from heart failure. Once he has established that there are no contra-indications, his doctor prescribes a non-selective ß-adrenoceptor antagonist (bisoprolol) together with an angiotensin-converting enzyme (ACE) inhibitor. Which is the single most important effect of a non-selective ß-adrenoceptor antagonist (a beta blocker) on heart rate? ★

A Negative chronotropic effect

B Negative inotropic effect

C Positive chronotropic effect

D Positive inotropic effect

E Negative dromotropic effect

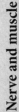

9. A 75-year-old diabetic woman goes to her GP for an eye examination. He applies eye drops to dilate her pupils. Which is the single most likely pharmacologically active compound to be present in the eye drops? ★ ★

A Atropine

B Chloramphenicol

C Dexamethasone

D Pilocarpine

E Tetracaine

10. Fig. 4.3 shows a schematic diagram and an electron micrograph of a sarcomere. What is the single name given to the region of the sarcomere labelled IV? ★

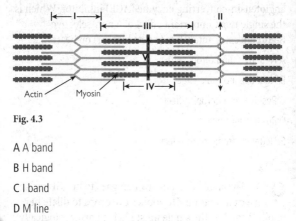

Fig. 4.3

A A band

B H band

C I band

D M line

E Z line

11. Skeletal muscle contraction is monitored by a variety of sensory receptors in joints, ligaments, tendons, and the muscle itself. These receptors measure the speed, extent, and strength of muscle contraction and joint movement. One set of receptors senses tension produced by contraction of the muscle and feeds this information back to the spinal cord where an inhibitory interneurone can be activated to reduce alpha motor neurone input to the muscle. Therefore the reflex can reduce the tension developed by muscle contraction. Which single sensory receptor type detects muscle tension? ★

A Free nerve ending

B Golgi tendon organ

C Joint afferent

D Muscle spindle

E Pacinian corpuscle

12. A 70-year-old man comes into A&E with a 48-hour history of palpitations and is diagnosed with atrial fibrillation (AF). He has no symptoms of heart failure and his electrolytes are normal. He is given anticoagulants and then given an infusion of amiodarone for cardioversion. An hour later his ECG shows sinus rhythm. The cardiac action potential can be divided into 5 phases (Fig. 4.4). Which single phase of the action potential does amiodarone affect? ★ ★

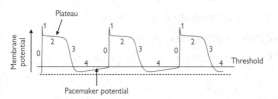

Fig. 4.4

A Phase 0

B Phase 1

C Phase 2

D Phase 3

E Phase 4

13. A 25-year-old woman presents with sudden visual problems and slightly slurred speech. She had a history of muscle weakness and changes in sensation that have resolved. She is diagnosed with a demyelinating disease, multiple sclerosis. Which single myelin-producing cell type of the central nervous system is primarily affected in multiple sclerosis? ★

A Astrocytes

B Ependymal cells

C Microglia

D Oligodendrocytes

E Schwann cells

14. A 25-year-old woman presents with ptosis (drooping eyelids), double vision, and generalized muscle weakness. She says that her muscles get fatigued very quickly, for example when she is brushing her hair. High levels of serum autoantibodies confirm a diagnosis of myasthenia gravis. Which single step in neuromuscular transmission is impaired in myasthenia gravis? ★

A Acetylcholine vesicle exocytosis into synaptic cleft

B Postsynaptic acetylcholine deactivation

C Postsynaptic acetylcholine receptor binding

D Presynaptic acetylcholine synthesis

E Presynaptic acetylcholine vesicle formation

15. In motor neurone disease (MND) cell damage occurs as a result of several mechanisms that are thought ultimately to lead to cell death of motor neurones. What is the single most likely final common pathway leading to cell death in MND? ★ ★

A Apoptosis

B Glutamateric excitotoxicity

C Necrosis

D Oxidative stress

E Protein aggregation

16. A 30-year-old man presents with decreased pain and temperature sensation over the lateral aspects of both arms. His light touch, vibration, and joint position sensation are preserved. MRI shows a malformation of the base of the brain and enlargement of the central canal of the spinal cord. Which single part of the spinal cord is most likely to be affected in this patient? ★ ★ ★

A Anterior horns of spinal grey matter

B Crossing anterior spinal commissural fibres

C Dorsal (posterior) columns and dorsal roots

D Dorsal (posterior) columns, lateral corticospinal tracts, and spinocerebellar tracts

E White matter

EXTENDED MATCHING QUESTIONS

Neurotransmitters

From the list below, choose the single most appropriate neurotransmitter described in each of the following statements. Each option may be used once, more than once, or not at all.

A Acetylcholine

B ATP (adenosine triphosphate)

C GABA (γ-aminobutyric acid)

D Glutamate

E Glycine

F Nitric oxide

G Noradrenaline

H Serotonin

I Substance P

J Neuropeptide Y

K Vasoactive intestinal polypeptide

1. The neurotransmitter used by all preganglionic autonomic neurones and all somatic motor neurones. ★

2. This neurotransmitter is synthesized from tyrosine and is deactivated by monoamine oxidase (MAO) and catechol-O-methyl transferase (COMT). ★

3. α-amino-3-hydroxy-5-methyl-4-isoxazolepropionic acid (AMPA) and N-methyl-D-aspartic acid (NMDA) are receptors activated by this neurotransmitter. ★

4. This neurotransmitter acts by volume transmission and does not activate a specific receptor. ★

5. Clonidine inhibits the release of this neurotransmitter by activation of a negative feedback pathway. ★ ★

ANSWERS

Single Best Answers

1. E ★ ★ ★   OHMS 2nd edn → pp216, 252

The patient presents with no sensory disability but only motor symptoms. This indicates that the sensory input is intact and therefore rules out the dorsal root (A), peripheral nerves (C), and spinal nerves (D) as possible sites of injury. Since an electromyogram (EMG) can be recorded, both nerve conduction and muscle contraction are present and the neuromuscular junctions (B) are functioning, although the compound muscle action potential (CMAP) is reduced in size. The most likely explanation is a problem in a ventral root on the right side of the body causing selective loss of motor axons which results in a smaller EMG. Loss of some motor axons does not affect the conduction velocity of the nerve, just the size of CMAP.

2. B ★ ★   OHMS 2nd edn → pp218–19

Sympathetic autonomic neurones have cell bodies in the lateral horn of the spinal cord grey matter and their myelinated axons pass out of the cord via the ventral root (D) of the spinal nerve and through the white ramus (E) to the paravertebral ganglia. Many preganglionic fibres synapse here with postsynaptic unmyelinated fibres, while other preganglionic sympathetic fibres pass directly through the paravertebral ganglia and synapse in the prevertebral ganglia (the superior mesenteric, inferior mesenteric, and coeliac ganglia) or the adrenal medulla. The sympathetic chain (C) contains a mixture of preganglionic and postganglionic axons. The dorsal root (A) is sensory and contains both myelinated and unmyelinated fibres entering the spinal cord.

The grey ramus contains only unmyelinated postganglionic axons. These pass from the paravertebral ganglion through the white ramus before joining other myelinated and unmyelinated fibres in the spinal nerve. Sympathetic postganglionic fibres taking this route innervate blood vessels of skin and muscle, sweat glands, and the pilomotor muscles of hair.

3. D ★ OHMS 2nd edn → pp220–1

At rest the cell has a much higher permeability to potassium ions than to sodium ions. Potassium leaves the cell, driven down a concentration gradient. The efflux of positively charged potassium ions, due to the potassium permeability of the resting membrane, leaves the cell with a negative internal charge: the resting membrane potential.

The active pumping of sodium ions out of the cell (A) in exchange for potassium ions creates the high internal potassium concentration and low internal sodium concentration typical of all living cells. The internal negativity and low membrane permeability to chloride tends to keep negatively charged chloride ions out of the cell and they do not enter along a concentration gradient (B). Although the efflux of potassium down a concentration gradient is the primary cause of the resting membrane potential, once the negative internal potential is established, potassium ions can be pulled back into the cell by electrochemical attraction (C). The resting membrane potential in fact occurs close to the equilibrium potential for potassium, when potassium efflux due to concentration is just balanced by influx due to electrochemical attraction. Although, at the resting potential, sodium entry into cells is also favoured by concentration (E) and electrochemical gradients, the sodium permeability is of the order of 5% of that for potassium and the small inward leakage of sodium ions is promptly corrected by the sodium–potassium exchange pump. The equilibrium potential for each ion species can be calculated from its concentration gradient using the Nernst equation.

4. D ★ ★ OHMS 2nd edn → pp222–3

When an axon is depolarized to the threshold voltage there is a dramatic increase in the sodium permeability of the membrane, allowing sodium influx (E) along both concentration (high external sodium) and electrochemical attraction (cell inside negative) gradients. In one of the few positive feedback processes known in cells, this sodium influx causes further depolarization, leading to greater sodium permeability, and yet more sodium entry. The change in membrane voltage rapidly accelerates to a point close to the sodium equilibrium potential (E_{Na}).

Before the resting membrane potential can be restored, the high sodium permeability must be switched off and the membrane potential must be moved back towards E_K. The voltage-dependent sodium channels activated at threshold show spontaneous closure once they have been depolarized for a millisecond or so. This inactivation of the sodium channels occurs at the peak of the action potential. By this time the depolarization of the membrane has also brought about opening of voltage-dependent potassium channels

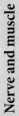

Nerve and muscle

which now allow an efflux of positively charged potassium ions (B), again driven by electochemical and concentration gradients. This efflux moves membrane voltage in a negative direction towards the resting membrane potential. The higher-than-normal potassium permeability causes an undershoot (hyperpolarization) of the membrane voltage (C). The negative membrane voltage now closes the voltage-dependent potassium channels and the resting potassium permeability is restored producing the resting membrane potential once again.

Active sodium pumping (A) maintains the low internal sodium and high internal potassium concentrations required for the above processes, but does not contribute directly to each action potential.

5. E ★   OHMS 2nd edn → pp224–6

Local anaesthetics can be administered topically, intravenously, subcutaneously, and directly into the CNS (epidural and spinal). An eutectic mixture of local anaesthetic (EMLA®) is a commonly used topical local anaesthetic for children prior to intravenous cannulation. Obviously it does not require needles and it is painless, although it does take time to act because it must first diffuse through the skin.

Nitrous oxide (A) is a volatile anaesthetic, commonly used in combination with oxygen as Entonox®, for pain relief during labour or with other volatile agents to maintain general anaesthesia. Thiopental (B) is an intravenous thiobarbiturate used as an induction agent for general anaesthesia.

Lidocaine injection (C) is commonly used for local anaesthesia, particularly in dentistry, and is used in obstetric practice for spinal and epidural anaesthesia. Oral diazepam (D) is a long-acting benzodiazepine producing anxiolysis. It also lowers epileptic threshold. In the past it used to be a common form of premedication given to children and anxious adults before surgery.

6. A ★   OHMS 2nd edn → pp224–5, 742

In a mixed peripheral nerve the large myelinated Aα axons recover first and the small unmyelinated C fibres are the last to recover. The largest fibres are also the last to succumb to the anaesthetic. Aα axons supply skeletal muscle and emerge from muscle spindles and Golgi tendon organs.

Aβ axons (B) come from cutaneous mechanoreceptors and muscle spindle secondary receptors, while Aδ axons (C) convey information about crude touch, pressure, cold temperature, and discriminating pain. Aγ axons (D) supply the intrafusal fibres of muscle spindles, and

C axons (E) transmit information about poorly localized pain and warm-temperature sensation.

Local anaesthetics therefore have their quickest and longest lasting effects on the smaller fibres that transmit pain, temperature, and crude touch sensation, and these effects are valuable in managing pain. In principle, motor control and discriminating touch sensation carried by the larger fibres is less affected, or affected for a shorter period. Anecdotally, anyone who has had a local anaesthetic at the dentist's will be familiar with these effects.

7. A ★★ OHMS 2nd edn → pp230–1; OHCM → p591

Botulinum toxin (Botox®) is commonly used temporarily to paralyse muscles to reduce spasms and tics. It does this by inhibiting presynaptic SNARE proteins and preventing release of acetylcholine at the neuromuscular junction of skeletal muscle. SNARE stands for **s**oluble **N**SF **a**ttachment protein **re**ceptor. So called 'NSF proteins' are N-ethylmaleimide-sensitive fusion proteins and they are important in the fusion of vesicles to the cell membrane, causing the release of neurotransmitters that is an essential part of chemical synaptic transmission.

Edrophonium (B) is a reversible anticholinesterase inhibitor used in the diagnosis of myasthenia gravis. Its administration temporarily increases the amount of acetylcholine at the neuromuscular junction, which compensates for weakness and fatiguability of contraction seen in myasthenia. Rocuronium (C), suxamethonium (D), and tubocurarine (E) act at the postsynaptic site to block nicotinic acetylcholine receptors.

8. A ★ OHMS 2nd edn → pp219, 242–5

Changes in heart rate are known as chronotropic effects. Changes in force of contraction are referred to as inotropic effects. Stimulation of the sympathetic nerves increases heart rate (positive chronotropy), while stimulation of the parasympathetic fibres from the vagus nerve slows the heart rate (negative chronotropy). Beta blockers inhibit the sympathetic innervation by blocking cardiac ß-adrenoceptors, particularly at the sino-atrial node, to produce a negative chronotropic effect.

Increased sympathetic activity increases not only the heart rate, but also the force of contraction (positive inotropic effect) in both the atria and the ventricles. However, as there is virtually no parasympathetic innervation in the human ventricles, parasympathetic nerve stimulation has no direct effect on the inotropic state of the ventricles. Dromotropic effects are alterations to conduction velocity in the heart. Sympathetic activity enhances the speed of conduction giving a positive dromotropic effect, particularly at the atrio-ventricular node. Parasympathetic innervation slows conduction velocity.

Beta blockers not only slow the heart rate and reduce cardiac work in patients with heart failure, but also reduce renin production by the kidney, which, by reducing salt and water retention, reduces plasma volume. This also helps to reduce cardiac work and the oxygen demand of the heart.

9. A ★★   OHMS 2nd edn → p238

This question tests knowledge about the clinical use of agonists and antagonists of muscarinic acetylcholine receptors. Pupil constriction is produced by the release of acetylcholine by the parasympathetic autonomic fibres on to the circular smooth muscle of the iris. The correct answer is atropine—a muscarinic receptor antagonist, which inhibits iris circular muscle contraction and therefore dilates the pupil. The drops are also given to relax the ciliary muscle of the eye, again by inhibiting parasympathetic activation. The lens of the eye then accommodates for distance vision and does not change focal length during the examination. Regular eye examinations, including fundoscopy—visual examination of the retina—are part of the management of patients with diabetes mellitus to check for the all-too-common complication of diabetic retinopathy.

Chloramphenicol (B) is a topical antibiotic that can be used to treat eye infection. Dexamethasone (C) eye drops can be used as a topical steroid for local treatment of inflammation. Pilocarpine (D) is a muscarinic receptor agonist, which mimics parasympathetic contraction of the ciliary muscle and causes contraction of iris circular muscle. It is used to constrict the pupil and allow drainage of aqueous humour through the canal of Schlemm. This can reduce the raised intraocular pressure of glaucoma. Tetracaine (E) is a short-acting anaesthetic used before procedures on the eye.

10. B ★   OHMS 2nd edn → p249

The area labelled IV on the diagram is the H-band (option B) where only myosin filaments are found.

Option A (III on the diagram) is the A band, a wide, dark band where thick myosin filaments overlap with thin actin filaments. Option C (I on the diagram) is the I band, where actin filaments do not overlap with myosin filaments. Option D (V on the diagram) is the M line, where myosin filaments are anchored. Option E (II on the diagram) is the Z line where actin filaments are anchored; the distance between two Z lines is equal to one sarcomere.

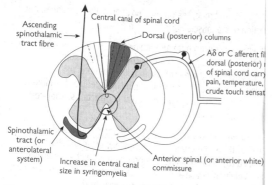

Ascending spinothalamic tract fibre

Central canal of spinal cord

Dorsal (posterior) columns

Aδ or C afferent fil dorsal (posterior) of spinal cord carr pain, temperature, crude touch sensat

Spinothalamic tract (or anterolateral system)

Increase in central canal size in syringomyelia

Anterior spinal (or anterior white) commissure

Fig. 4.6

fibres enter the spinal cord they branch to ascend and descend one two spinal segments in Lissauer's tract (not shown) before synapsing with second-order neurones. These neurones decussate, passing through the anterior spinal commissure, before ascending to the thalamus in the contralateral spinothalamic tract (anterolateral syste

Damage to anterior spinal commissural fibres prevents the upwar transmission of pain, temperature, and crude touch sensation in t contralateral spinothalamic tract, but touch sensation can still rea the cortex via the ipsilateral dorsal columns. In this way pain and temperature sensation become 'dissociated' from touch sensation for the affected dermatomes. This can lead to skin burns and injur because of incomplete sensory information.

Spinal cord lesions present in a variety of clinical scenarios. For example, poliomyelitis and Werding–Hoffman disease cause flacci paralysis due to destruction of anterior horns (A). Tabes dorsalis (a tertiary syphilis) presents with impaired proprioception and omotor ataxia due to damage to dorsal roots and columns (C). amin B₁₂ neuropathy and Friedreich's ataxia present with ataxi, hyperreflexia and impaired position and vibration sense, due age to dorsal columns and lateral corticospinal and cerebellar tracts (D). Random white matter (E) lesions occur ir le sclerosis due to demyelination. Symptoms may include mus, intention tremor, and scanning speech.

ded Matching Questions

motor neurones and preganglionic autonomic fibres with cell e central nervous system use acetylcholine as neurotransmitter

11. B ★ OHMS 2nd edn → p252

Golgi tendon organs are, as the name implies, located in the tendons that attach muscles to the skeleton. These receptors are therefore ideally placed to measure the tension developed by muscular contraction, especially if the load is high and muscle contraction causes tension to rise rather than the load to be moved, as in isometric contraction. The inhibitory reflex to which they contribute is therefore designed to match contraction to load and to prevent over-contraction and possible injury to muscles.

Free nerve endings (A) innervate muscle nociceptors found in the muscle sheath that detect noxious stimuli and muscle damage. Muscle spindles (D) detect changes in muscle length rather than tension and they feed back on to alpha motor neurones to match muscle contraction to the length required for a particular movement to occur. If the load on the muscle is increased and the muscle is stretched, then muscle spindles increase their rate of firing and this raises the rate of firing of alpha motor neurones so that proper muscle length is restored. The sensitivity of muscle spindles can be controlled by their own gamma motor neurones. Joint afferents (C) innervate ligaments and bone rather than muscle and provide information about joint movements and joint position. Pacinian corpuscles (E) are found in the skin and detect high frequency vibration.

12. D ★ ★ OHMS 2nd edn → pp254–6, 426–31

The action potential of the cardiac myocyte is divided into five phases. The correct answer is phase 3: rapid repolarization due to potassium efflux via open voltage-gated slow K+ channels. Amiodarone blocks the voltage-gated K+ channels which results in slowing of the potassium efflux. This prolongs the repolarization phase leading to an increased duration for the cardiac action potential. This is associated with an increased effective refractory period (ERP), which 'steadies the heartbeat' and helps to suppress dysrhythmias, such as in atrial fibrillation.

13. D ★ OHMS 2nd edn → pp212–15, 262

There are two basic cell types in the nervous system: neurones and glial cells. The neurones are the excitable cells, which transmit electrical impulses. The glial cells are non-neural but provide both mechanical and physiological support for the nervous system. Only two glial cell types produce myelin: oligodendrocytes in the central nervous system (CNS) and Schwann cells in the peripheral nervous system (PNS). The correct answer is therefore D (oligodendrocytes). In multiple sclerosis the myelin sheaths around the axons within the CNS are damaged, leading to a demyelination and a broad spectrum of signs and symptoms resulting from impaired neural transmission, as seen in this patient. It usually occurs in young adults. Women are affected twice as often as are men.

Astrocytes (A) are responsible for formation of the blood–brain barrier. Ependymal cells (B) line cavities within the CNS and secrete cerebrospinal fluid. Microglia (C) are CNS phagocytes. An example of Schwann cell (E) damage within the PNS is Guillain–Barré syndrome.

14. C ★   OHMS 2nd edn → pp228–31, 264

Neuromuscular transmission takes place at the neuromuscular junction (Fig. 4.5). An action potential in the motor nerve depolarizes the presynaptic terminal, called the motor endplate, causing calcium entry and exocytosis of acetylcholine from vesicles into the synaptic cleft (A). The acetylcholine binds to nicotinic acetylcholine receptors on the postsynaptic (muscle fibre) membrane. The receptors are a part of ligand-gated ion channels and binding causes sodium and potassium membrane conductance to increase in the muscle fibre membrane. This causes a depolarization of the

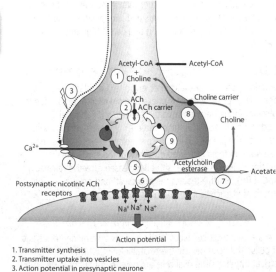

1. Transmitter synthesis
2. Transmitter uptake into vesicles
3. Action potential in presynaptic neurone
4. Voltage-gated Ca²⁺ channel activation
5. Exocytosis
6. Receptor activation in postsynaptic neurone
7. Transmitter deactivation
8. Precursor recycling
9. Vesicular recycling

Fig. 4.5

muscle fibre membrane, the production of an action potential, and contraction of the muscle fibre.

Myasthenia gravis is an autoimmune disease where autoantibodies may either impair the ability of acetylcholine to bind to nicotinic receptors or destroy the receptors. In both situations the effectiveness of overall acetylcholine binding is reduced leading to weaker, more rapidly fatiguing, muscular contractions. Therefore, option C is the correct answer.

Once released from the postsynaptic receptors, acetylcholine is deactivated (B) by the enzyme acetylcholinesterase. Acetylcholine is synthesized (D) from choline in the presynaptic cell by the enzyme choline acetyltransferase and this is not affected in myasthenia, nor is the incorporation of acetylcholine into vesicles (E).

15. A ★★   OHMS 2nd edn → p265

Cell death may occur as a result of necrosis or apoptosis. In MND apoptosis is the final common pathway leading to cell death. Apoptosis, also called programmed cell death, is often a part of the normal development and modelling of tissues. Normally it is triggered by the appropriate extracellular signals, but in many neurodegenerative disorders it is triggered pathologically. Necr... (C) is the more common type of cell death and always represe... pathological process resulting from, for example, tissue dam...

The triggers for cell apoptosis in MND are thought to incl... that can cause cells to become stressed. Such factors inc... glutamateric excitotoxicity (B), in which glutamate rece... over-stimulated; oxidative stress (D) resulting from mu... gene for superoxide dismutase—an enzyme that nor... levels of free radicals in cells; or protein aggregates... from abnormal folding of large proteins. All are th... role in motor neurone injury and many feature in... neurodegenerative diseases. The eventual demi... neurones, however, occurs by programmed ce...

16. B ★★★   OHMS 2nd edn → p2...

This question focuses on the clinical pres... damage. This patient has developed a c... syringomyelia associated with a conge... malformation. The correct answer is '... usually arising by enlargement of th... canal, creates pressure which caus... spinal commissural fibres. This g... presentation of 'dissociated sen...

Fig. 4.6 shows a cross-section of sp... pain, temperature, and crude touch sensa...

Exten...

1. A

All somatic... bodies in th...

2. G ★

Fig. 4.7 describes the various mechanisms of noradrenaline biosynthesis and reuptake.

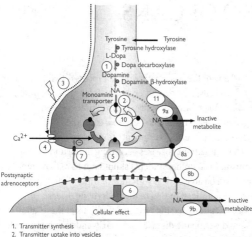

1. Transmitter synthesis
2. Transmitter uptake into vesicles
3. Action potential in presynaptic neurone
4. Voltage-gated Ca^{2+} channel activation
5. Exocytosis
6. Receptor activation in postsynaptic neurone
7. Feedback inhibition of Ca^{2+} channels (α_2 receptors)
8. (a) Uptake 1 and (b) uptake 2
9. Transmitter deactivation by (a) MAO and (b) COMT
10. Vesicular recycling
11. Transmitter recycling

Fig. 4.7

3. D ★

These are the ionotropic receptors for glutamate. Metabatrophic receptors for glutamate are also found. These activate ion channels indirectly via G-proteins.

4. F ★

Nitric oxide is a gas. It is synthesized on demand and does not act via receptors but activates second messenger systems.

5. G ★★

Clonidine is an α_2 adrenoreceptor agonist that acts presynaptically to inhibit the release of noradrenaline.

General feedback on 1–5: OHMS 2nd edn → pp228–30, 241, 246.

CHAPTER 5

GROWTH OF TISSUES AND ORGANS

Many of the basic pathological processes that take place in cells, tissues, and organs are common, regardless of tissue types. These are due to aetiologies and pathogenetic mechanisms that lead to a common fate. Understanding these allows students to develop a logical approach to classifying diseases according to the underlying mechanism. In so doing, students should not have to memorize lists, and will be able to deal with new or unfamiliar clinical scenarios. An understanding of the underlying disease processes, including having precise definitions of these, allows doctors to describe the diseases accurately and to communicate more clearly.

Unfortunately, many of the terms sound like each other, but fortunately, there are not too many terms.

In recent years, the molecular mechanisms underlying many disease processes that may have been known for decades have been uncovered. It is important to know these as they may have implications for management, for example genetic counselling, or may lead to development of new therapies. ■

SINGLE BEST ANSWERS

1. A 42-year-old man has had his left lower leg in plaster for 6 weeks to treat a fractured tibia and fibula. On removal of the plaster, he noticed that his left thigh and calf had smaller diameters compared with the right. What is the single best name for the process that explains the appearance of the left leg? ★

A Apoptosis

B Atrophy

C Dysplasia

D Hypertrophy

E Necrosis

2. A 58-year-old man has a chest X-ray examination to investigate a dry cough that has persisted for 4 weeks. He has taken medication for hypertension for the last 10 years, but is otherwise in good health. The lung fields are clear radiologically, but the cardiac shadow appears enlarged, and the cardiac : thoracic ratio is increased. What is the single most likely mechanism by which the cardiac abnormality has occurred? ★ ★

A Dysplasia

B Hyperplasia

C Hypertrophy

D Metaplasia

E Neoplasia

3. A 63-year-old man has a small papule removed from the right side of his nose. The sample is sent for pathological examination. The microscopic section of the pathology report reads 'The piece of skin shows increased numbers of mature sebaceous glands present in the dermis. These are connected to the epidermis, and associated with follicular plugging and surrounding inflammation'. What is the single best term to describe the process that underlies the histological description given? ★

A Dysplasia

B Hyperplasia

C Hypertrophy

D Metaplasia

E Regeneration

4. In cigarette smokers, cells of the bronchial epithelium may change from ciliated columnar to stratified squamous epithelium in histological appearance. What is the single best term for the process that is described? ★

A Dysplasia

B Hyperplasia

C Hypertrophy

D Metaplasia

E Neoplasia

5. A 65-year-old man has a 10-year history of gastro-oesophageal reflux disease related to alcohol use and obesity. He has had previous endoscopic examinations with biopsy, which showed 'Barrett's oesophagus'. He now complains of weight loss and dysphagia for solids and liquids, and an ulcerated malignant stricture is seen on endoscopy and biopsied. Which is the single most likely diagnosis? ★ ★

A Adenocarcinoma

B Gastrointestinal stromal tumour

C Leiomyoma

D Small cell carcinoma

E Squamous cell carcinoma

6. A 72-year-old man undergoes a right upper lobectomy for squamous cell carcinoma of the lung. Fig. 5.1 (see Plate 2) shows a photomicrograph taken from a section close to the bronchial resection margin. What single most important feature indicating malignant behaviour is shown? ★ ★

A Invasion of lamina propria

B Invasion of lymphovascular space

C Invasion of thick-walled blood vessel

D Squamous cell carcinoma *in situ*

E Ulceration of surface epithelium

7. A 68-year-old man was referred to a gastroenterologist following a positive faecal occult blood test. On investigation, he was found to have a 5cm polypoid mass in his descending colon and several large nodules within his liver. Biopsy and analysis of the colonic mass confirmed an adenocarcinoma. Which is the single most likely explanatory link between the masses in the colon and liver? ★ ★

A Adenocarcinoma of colon and cirrhosis of liver

B Direct spread of adenocarcinoma

C Incidental finding of liver nodules

D Metastases of adenocarcinoma via bloodstream

E Metastases of adenocarcinoma via lymphatics

8. A 44-year-old man has an obstructing tumour in the proximal ascending colon and undergoes a hemicolectomy. Fig. 5.2 (see Plate 3) shows the microscopic appearances of the tumour. A hereditary abnormality is suspected and he undergoes genetic testing. Which is the single most likely genetic abnormality one would expect to find in this patient? ★ ★ ★ ★

A APC gene mutation

B DNA mismatch repair gene mutation

C Rb gene mutation

D STK11 gene mutation

E VHL gene mutation

9. A 26-year-old woman presents with headaches, ataxia and visual disturbance. On fundoscopy, she is found to have a retinal tumour (Fig. 5.3, see Plate 4) A hereditary syndrome is suspected and imaging of the kidneys and brain is undertaken, revealing a cystic cerebellar lesion with a small mural nodule, and cystic lesions in both kidneys. Which of the following tumour suppressor genes is the single one most likely to be mutated? ★ ★ ★

A APC gene on chromosome 5

B p53 gene on chromosome 17

C Rb gene on chromosome 13

D VHL gene on chromosome 3

E WT1 gene on chromosome 11

EXTENDED MATCHING QUESTIONS

Neoplasms

From the options listed below, choose the term that best applies to the neoplasms described overleaf. Each option may be used once, more than once, or not at all.

A Adenoma

B Adenocarcinoma

C Cystadenoma

D Cystadenocarcinoma

E Cystadenofibroma

F Leiomyoma

G Leiomyosarcoma

H Lipoma

I Liposarcoma

J Lymphoma

K Malignant melanoma

L Neurofibroma

M Rhabdomyoma

N Rhabdomyosarcoma

O Squamous papilloma

P Squamous cell carcinoma

1. A 64-year-old man has a nephrectomy performed for an 8cm mass in the upper pole of his right kidney. The sample is sent for pathological examination. The microscopic section of the report reads 'The tumour consists of sheets of clear cells with bland nuclei. No necrosis is seen and mitoses are scanty. The tumour infiltrates the renal sinus'. ★ ★

2. A 28-year-old man has a lump removed from his left forearm. The sample is sent for pathological examination. The microscopic section of the report reads 'There is a circumscribed nodule composed of mature adipose fat'. ★

3. A 72-year-old man has a warty lesion biopsied from skin in front of his ear. The sample is sent for pathological examination. The microscopic section of the report reads 'There are fragments of skin exhibiting papillomatosis. There are irregular islands of atypical squamous epithelium seen in the superficial and deep dermis. Numerous mitoses, including atypical mitotic figures, are noted'. ★ ★

4. A 72-year-old man has had several needle core biopsies taken from his prostate during investigation for urinary obstruction. The samples are sent for pathological examination. The microscopic section of the report reads 'The prostatic tissue shows numerous small uniform glands lined by a single layer of cuboidal epithelium. Focally, there is diffuse infiltration by single cells. In addition, prostatic glands are seen around nerves'. ★ ★ ★

5. A 38-year-old woman has an ovarian mass excised. The sample is sent for pathological examination. The microscopic section of the report reads 'There are multiple cysts mainly lined by a single layer of columnar cells containing abundant intracellular mucin. Some cysts are

focally lined by stratified columnar epithelium, exhibiting nuclear pleomorphism. The tumour is surrounded by a thin fibrous capsule, which is intact for most part. On examination of multiple sections, small nests of bland mucin-secreting epithelium are seen outside the capsule, along with lakes of extravasated mucin and surrounding fibroblastic proliferation.' ★ ★ ★

ANSWERS

Single Best Answers

1. B ★   OHMS 2nd edn → pp868–9

The skeletal muscles of the left thigh and lower leg have undergone atrophy from immobilization and disuse. This is due to decrease in the size of the individual muscle fibres. They eventually assume normal size when normal activity is resumed. Apoptosis or programmed cell death would lead to a small decrease in number of cells (A). Dysplasia is disordered maturation of tissue (C). Hypertrophy is the opposite of atrophy, and denotes an increase in the size of cells (D).

2. C ★ ★   OHMS 2nd edn → pp451, 868–9

The heart has to pump harder against outflow resistance raising systemic blood pressure. To achieve this, the cardiomyocytes of the left ventricle undergo enlargement or hypertrophy. This is distinct from hyperplasia which means that the number of cells is increased (B). Hyperplasia cannot take place since cardiomyocytes are end cells, incapable of cell division. Metaplasia (D) is the name given to the process by which one type of mature tissue is transformed to another type of mature tissue, not normally native for that site.

3. B ★   OHMS 2nd edn → p869

Hyperplasia of sebaceous glands is due to increase in number of cells, in turn causing an increase in number of glands. This results in an increase in tissue mass, hence the papule. Regeneration (E) can sometimes lead to an increase in number of cells, e.g. in liver, but the process is preceded by loss of cells, either through necrosis, apoptosis, or surgical excision.

4. D ★   OHMS 2nd edn → pp868–9, 872

This question tests basic knowledge of the terms used to classify abnormal tissue growth. The correct answer is metaplasia because the changes described are from one fully differentiated tissue type to another fully differentiated type. Note that these changes may not necessarily be precancerous, but do have a strong association with cigarette smoking, which has a well-established relationship with carcinoma of the lung.

5. A ★★ OHMS 2nd edn → pp870–1; OHCM → pp620–1

Barrett's mucosa or Barrett's oesophagus is an important risk factor for the development of adenocarcinoma of the distal oesophagus (44 x increased risk). Gastrointestinal stromal tumours and leiomyomas (B and C) are mesenchymal neoplasms that are not associated with Barrett's oesophagus and would usually have a different appearance endoscopically (e.g. smooth submucosal mass). Small cell carcinoma is a tumour exhibiting neuroendocrine differentiation (D). This is a rare tumour of the oesophagus, and is not associated with Barrett's oesophagus, nor is squamous cell carcinoma (E) which is the commonest variety of malignancy of the oesophagus.

6. B ★★ OHMS 2nd edn → pp872–4

The photomicrograph (Fig.5.1, see Plate 2) shows carcinoma *in situ* undermining and replacing the surface respiratory epithelium as well as a nest of invasive carcinoma lying within a lymphatic vessel beneath the epithelium (bottom centre of field of picture). The latter indicates that a tumour is capable of metastasis.

7. D ★★ OHMS 2nd edn → pp874–5

The correct answer is metastases of adenocarcinoma via the hepato-portal system which drains blood from the bowel to the liver. Cirrhosis is a diffuse process affecting the whole liver, although several large nodules may be present (A). There is no aetiological relationship between cirrhosis and adenocarcinoma and if the two conditions coexisted, it would be entirely incidental. Direct spread of the tumour may affect the paracolic tissues or left kidney (B). Small liver nodules are a common incidental finding on radiological examination (C). These are generally solitary, and may be a haematoma or benign tumour, for example of blood vessels (haemangioma); these are generally of small sizes, less than 1cm. Metastases via the lymphatics would drain to regional lymph nodes (E).

8. B ★★★★ OHMS 2nd edn → pp876–8; OHCM → p524

Hereditary non-polyposis colon cancer (HNPPCC) is the most likely expected genetic abnormality (young age, right-sided cancer with mucinous phenotype) and is due to mutation in one of five DNA mismatch repair genes. Two other genetic abnormalities from the options that may specifically be associated with colonic cancer are

APC gene mutations (A) (familial polyposis coli) and STK11 gene mutation (D) (Peutz–Jeghers syndrome).

9. D ★★★ OHMS 2nd edn → pp876–8; OHCM → pp726–7

Von Hippel–Lindau syndrome is an autosomal dominant condition caused by a mutation in the VHL gene on chromosome 3, characterized by predisposition to development of retinal angiomas, CNS haemangioblastomas, renal cell carcinoma, and phaeochromocytoma. Mutations in WT1 (E) may be associated with paediatric Wilms' tumour (nephroblastoma) and Ewing's sarcoma while children with Rb gene mutations (C) may develop retinoblastoma. APC gene mutations (A) are not associated with renal tumours and mutations are present in many different kinds of tumours, including tumours of breast, lung, and colon.

Extended Matching Questions

1. B ★★

This is a clear cell carcinoma of the kidney or renal cell carcinoma. Although the description does not mention glands, renal cell carcinomas are thought be derived from renal tubular epithelium which is both an absorbing and a secretory epithelium, and malignant tumours derived from glandular epithelium are termed adenocarcinoma. Renal cell carcinomas typically have bland nuclei. Invasion of the renal sinus implies that this is a malignant tumour and hence an adenocarcinoma rather than an adenoma, which is a benign tumour.

2. H ★

A lipoma is a benign tumour derived from adipose tissue. A liposarcoma is the malignant counterpart, and there are no features to support malignant transformation.

3. P ★★

Squamous cell carcinomas sometimes resemble warts clinically, and the term 'papillomatosis' ('finger-like projections') is a microscopic correlate of a macroscopic warty appearance. The features of malignancy are the architecture of glands (irregular) and atypical cytomorphology, including presence of atypical mitotic figures. On the other hand, squamous cell papillomas may have a papillomatous configuration but lack the histological features of malignancy.

4. B ★★★

The name can be deduced from the tissue of origin of the tumour, and from salient features observed. Prostate comprises glandular epithelium and as such, most tumours show glandular differentiation. The glandular differentiation is shown by the glands seen. This is an adenocarcinoma and there are three features that point to malignancy. Firstly, normal prostate glands have 2 cell layers, an inner mucin-secreting layer and an outer basal cell layer. Proliferation of the glandular component alone signifies malignancy, as do the presence of single cells which imply loss of differentiation and infiltration. Lastly, perineural invasion is a feature of several types of carcinomas, and is not uncommonly found in prostatic carcinoma.

5. D ★★★

The name can be logically deduced from components of the tumour, which can be ascertained from reading the description provided. The prefix cyst- denotes the presence of cysts, adeno- suggests glandular differentiation, and carcinoma suggests that the tumour is malignant. Mucin secretion is a function of glandular epithelium; in turn, tumours derived from glandular epithelium contain the prefix 'adeno'. The tumour has invaded the capsule; capsular invasion or invasion of adjacent structures is a feature of malignancy. The fibroblastic proliferation is a reaction to tumour invasion and not an intrinsic part of the tumour. If fibrous tissue were an intrinsic part of the tumour, it would contain the prefix 'fibro-' within the tumour name.

General feedback on 1–5: OHMS 2nd edn → pp870–1

CHAPTER 6

TECHNIQUES OF
MEDICAL SCIENCES

There are a limited number of laboratory techniques that underlie the large number of clinical investigations that are used routinely. Knowing and understanding the basis for these tests is essential in appreciating the clinical application of the various tests. Important parameters of clinical diagnostic tests are test sensitivity—how well are those with a condition correctly identified by the test and how low is the rate of false positives; and test specificity—how well does the test correctly identify those without the condition and what is the rate of false negatives. The cost-effectiveness of a test is also an important consideration. Familiarity with the underlying mechanisms will also help students and doctors to determine when to use the tests, to realize their value and limitations, and hence to exercise caution in interpretation.

This chapter has questions that test knowledge of the mechanisms underlying a variety of techniques. Their application in clinical use is tested using a number of clinical scenarios. ■

TECHNIQUES OF MEDICAL SCIENCES
SINGLE BEST ANSWERS

1. This method involves cutting DNA with restriction enzymes, separating the fragments by electrophoresis on an agarose gel, and then probing with complementary DNA to identify a gene of interest. What is the single best term to describe this technique? ★

A Gene chip microarray assay

B Northern blot

C RT-PCR (reverse transcriptase polymerase chain reaction)

D Southern blot

E Western blot

2. This method can be used to isolate a specific protein by passing an extract of interest through a gel matrix; it is most often used to purify recombinant proteins or antibodies. What is the single best term to describe this technique? ★ ★

A Affinity chromatography

B Electrophoresis

C Fluorescence resonance energy transfer (FRET)

D Mass spectrometry

E Yeast 2-hybrid assay

3. Cytology is the method used to screen for cervical carcinoma and pre-cancer. It may also detect many other pathological conditions. Other than cervical carcinoma, which is the single condition that is most likely to be picked up by cervical cytology? ★ ★

A Adenocarcinoma of the endometrium

B Brenner tumour

C Mucinous cystadenocarcinoma of the ovary

D Serous cystadenocarcinoma of the ovary

E Uterine leiomyoma

4. A 45-year-old man complains of weight loss over the last 6 months associated with intermittent central abdominal pain and diarrhoea. He was on holiday in India a month ago and his symptoms have worsened since his return. On examination, generalized lymphadenopathy is found. A penile ulcer and a few nodules are noted on his lower legs. A number of investigations are performed. Which single finding would most likely prompt you to perform an HIV test as the next test? ★ ★ ★ ★

A Antigen positivity for *Giardia lamblia* after testing of faeces

B Colonic biopsy showing ulceration of the colonic mucosa and scattered granulomas in the submucosa

C Fine needle aspiration cytology of axillary lymph node showing a mixture of lymphoid cells

D Serology positive for herpesvirus type 2 (HSV-2)

E Skin biopsy showing vascular proliferation in the dermis, and immunoreactivity for human herpesvirus 8

5. During investigation of a 36-year-old man for weight loss, a single nodule in the right lobe of liver is found on ultrasound of the abdomen. A liver biopsy is performed, and the histological examination shows an adenocarcinoma. Positive immunochemical staining for which single antibody is most likely to confirm that this is a primary tumour of the liver? ★ ★ ★

A α-Fetoprotein

B β-HCG

C CA 99

D CA 125

E Melan-A

6. A dorsal root ganglion is removed from a patient with a complete brachial plexus avulsion during motor nerve reconstruction. The academic neurologist wants to know if there has been a change in the distribution of a particular sodium channel protein subunit in sensory afferents. Which method is the single most appropriate investigation to answer this question? ★ ★

A Enzyme-linked immunosorbent assay (ELISA)

B Immunocytochemistry

C *In situ* hybridization (ISH)

D Polymerase chain reaction (PCR)

E Western blot

7. A 9-month-old baby is brought into the A&E department with a 24-hour history of high fever, vomiting, and lethargy. Meningitis is suspected. A number of investigations are performed. What is the single fastest way to identify the causative agent? ★

A Blood culture

B Brain MRI

C Gram stain of cerebral spinal fluid (CSF)

D PCR (polymerase chain reaction)

E Serology

8. A randomized, double-blind, placebo-controlled multi-centre trial is performed with 2,000 patients to test the effects of a new drug for use in diabetes. As well as looking for improvements in the condition, other outcome measures are adverse effects. What type of clinical trial is this most likely to be? ★

A Phase 0

B Phase I

C Phase II

D Phase III

E Phase IV

Single Best Answers

1. D ★   OHMS 2nd edn → pp898–9

Southern blot is the correct answer. A northern blot (B) is similar to a southern blot except that the starting material is RNA, not DNA; therefore, northern blot measures the amount of mRNA in a sample, whereas a southern blot measures DNA levels. A western blot is used to detect specific proteins in a given sample of tissue homogenate (E). Gene chip microarray (A) measures changes in the levels of mRNA in tissues. Each consists of an arrayed series of thousands of spots of DNA oligonucleotides each containing tiny amounts of specific DNA sequences. Two sets of differentially labelled cDNAs are prepared and hybridized to the gene chip, and computer analysis allows determination of which genes are up- or down-regulated. In reverse transcription polymerase chain reactions (C), an RNA strand is reverse transcribed into complementary DNA (cDNA) using reverse transcriptase, and the resulting cDNA is then amplified using real-time PCR to see if the gene is expressed in a specific tissue or cell type.

2. A ★★   OHMS 2nd edn → pp908, 910–13

In affinity chromatography—the correct answer—the protein to be purified is passed through a column coated with a specific ligand or competitive inhibitor to which the protein will attach. Proteins not exhibiting appreciable affinity for the ligand will pass through the column, whereas those which recognize the inhibitor will be captured to an extent related to the affinity constant under the experimental conditions. The trapped protein is then eluted from the column and further purified. FRET is a method whereby presumed interacting proteins are labelled with different fluorophores and then expressed in the same cell (C). If the proteins interact they produce energy transfer which is detected by confocal microscopy. Mass spectrometry measures the mass-to-charge ratio of charged particles and is used for determining masses of particles, for the determination of the elemental composition of a sample (D). It can provide molecular fingerprints of proteins by the analysis of the peptide fragments. Yeast 2-hybrid assay is a technique used to discover protein–protein interactions and protein–DNA interactions by testing for physical interactions (E). Bait and prey cDNAs are introduced into mutant yeast strains. If the bait (known protein) and prey (unknown protein) interact, gene transcription occurs and a reporter gene is switched on.

3. A ★★   OHMS 2nd edn → p917

Cervical cytology is aimed at detecting dyskeratotic cells exfoliated or scraped by the cytobrush. These are usually squamous cells denoting cervical intraepithelial neoplasia (CIN) or cervical carcinoma. More unusual tumours, located higher up in the endocervical canal or indeed the endometrium (A) may also shed neoplastic cells which are seen on cervical cytology. Brenner tumours (B) occur in the ovary, as do mucinous (C) and serous (D) cystadenocarcinomas of the ovary. The cystadenocarcinomas may exfoliate cells into the peritoneal cavity (E); these may be found in ascitic fluid, but will not be picked up by cervical cytological examination. Mesenchymal tumours such as a leiomyoma will not exfoliate.

4. E ★★★★   OHMS 2nd edn → pp917–25

A vascular proliferation of the skin which expresses HHV-8 is diagnostic of Kaposi's sarcoma, which in turn is almost pathognomonic of HIV infection. A and B would account for the diarrhoea and abdominal pain. Colonic submucosal granulomas on histology suggest that the patient has Crohn's disease, and this may have been exacerbated by a giardial infection. The mixture of lymphoid cells on FNAC reflects a reactive lymphadenopathy, which may be observed in HIV infection, but is not specific (C). Serum positivity for HSV-2 provides the cause for the penile ulcer (D).

5. A ★★★   OHMS 2nd edn → pp920–1

Primary liver cancer or hepatocellular carcinoma expresses α-fetoprotein on the cell surface detectable by immunohistochemical staining (A); it also produces α-fetoprotein which is highly elevated in serum. α-fetoprotein may also be expressed by some testicular and ovarian tumours, but these do not have the morphological appearances of an adenocarcinoma. In a young person, the tumour is almost invariably caused by hepatitis B infection, and this may also be detected by immunohistochemistry.

CA 99 and CA 125 may be expressed by a variety of epithelial tumours and therefore are not specific; they are not expressed by hepatocellular carcinoma (C and D). Melan-A is used to confirm melanoma (E).

6. B ★★   OHMS 2nd edn → pp902–5, 920–1, 924–5, 930–1

Whilst all methods are possible correct answers, only immunocytochemistry has the resolution to identify the individual subtypes of afferents that express the protein. This would be achieved using double-labelling methods with specific markers. ELISA is a popular method to detect proteins, usually by using specific kits (96-well plates) coated with antibodies to the antigen of interest (A). This method would not be appropriate here. ISH and PCR detect mRNA levels rather than protein, and an increase in mRNA may not always lead to increased protein expression (C and D). Western blot would detect a general increase in protein level but does not have the resolution for localization within the dorsal root ganglion (E). The clinical importance of determining whether the nerves are sensory or not is that whilst motor efferent nerves regenerate, in this case, sensory afferents cannot.

7. D ★   OHMS 2nd edn → pp923–6;
OHCM → pp834–5

All of the answers are tests for meningitis but PCR is the fastest. PCR allows isolation of DNA fragments from bacterial or viral genomic DNA by selective amplification of a specific region of DNA. PCR also permits identification of non-cultivable or slow-growing microorganisms from tissue culture assays. Its diagnostic value is the detection of infectious agents and the discrimination of non-pathogenic from pathogenic strains by virtue of specific genes. The high sensitivity of PCR permits virus detection soon after infection and even before the onset of disease. Blood and throat swab cultures are used to grow bacteria, viruses, and fungi but these take time (days) to grow before identification of the causative agent can be confirmed. In early cases of infection (A), a brain MRI may be normal but it is important in ruling out other potential diagnoses such as stroke or brain abscesses (B). Often, CT or MRI scans are performed at a later stage to assess for complications of meningitis. A Gram stain will identify bacteria, but does not give a specific identity (C). Moreover, it will not detect viruses. Serology involves the identification of antibodies when an infection is suspected. This is often done with ELISA methodology (E) to identify the specific antibodies and therefore the pathogen responsible for the infection.

8. D ★   OHMS 2nd edn → p940

Phase 0 is a 'first-in-human' trial. Phase 0 trials are designed to speed up the development of promising drugs by establishing very early on whether the drug behaves in humans as was expected from preclinical studies. Phase 0 trials include the administration of a single sub-therapeutic dose to 10–15 healthy subjects to gather preliminary data on the agent's pharmacokinetic and pharmacodynamic properties. A phase 0 study gives no data on safety or efficacy since the dose is too low to have therapeutic effect.

In phase I trials a small (20–80) group of healthy volunteers are selected to assess the safety, pharmacokinetics, and pharmaco-dynamics of a drug. Phase I trials also normally include dose escalation studies so that the appropriate dose for therapeutic use can be found.

Phase II trials are performed on larger groups (20–300) and are designed to assess how well the drug works. Phase II studies are sometimes divided into phase IIA (specifically designed to assess dosing requirements) and phase IIB (specifically designed to study efficacy).

Phase III studies are randomized controlled multi-centre trials on large patient groups (300–3,000) and are the definitive assessment of how effective the drug is, in comparison with the effectiveness of a current 'gold standard' treatment compared to a placebo. Side-effects are closely monitored and information collected about the safety of the drug before marketing. Phase III trials are the most expensive, time consuming and difficult trials to design and run because of their size and comparatively long duration, especially in chronic medical conditions.

A phase IV trial is a post-marketing surveillance trial clarifying the risks, benefits, and optimal doses of a drug after it receives permission to be sold.

THE BIOMEDICAL SYSTEMS

CHAPTER 7

MUSCULOSKELETAL SYSTEM

The functions of the musculoskeletal system are to protect internal organs, to provide support, and to enable locomotion and movement. In addition, bone is the store of calcium in the body, and thereby plays a role in calcium homeostasis. Muscles, through contractions and their origins from, and insertions on to, specific points of bony surfaces, exert particular actions. In turn, each muscle has its own innervation by specific nerves and its own blood supply. Understanding the actions of muscles depends on knowing the names of muscles and their locations, origins, and insertions. Knowing the nerve and blood supply of the muscles helps one work out logically the effect of weakness or lack of action of the muscles following damage to their innervation or blood supply.

Knowing the names of muscles, nerves, and blood vessels allows one to communicate effectively with other healthcare colleagues. But such knowledge in itself is insufficient, and learning the function of specific muscles is important, as is familiarity with the causes and consequences of their lack of function.

The questions in this chapter start with basic knowledge that provides the groundwork of future learning, and then progress to test applied knowledge using clinical scenarios. We hope that this approach will not only emphasize the structure–function relationship of the complex components of the musculoskeletal system, but will also help students realize the clinical importance of learning seemingly long and tedious names and make the learning more interesting. It is customary to include the skin with the musculoskeletal system because of its close association with muscles, bones, and joints which together produce the surface landmarks of the body. The skin's functions include protection, prevention of water loss, and thermoregulation. ∎

1. A 36-year-old man has a mole biopsied by his GP. This is diagnosed as a melanoma and is then treated by wide local excision 3 weeks later. The skin re-excision specimen is sent to the laboratory for examination. What is the single most abundant cell type in the scar tissue? ★

A Adipocyte

B Endothelial cell

C Fibroblast

D Macrophage

E Neutrophil

2. There are several types of cartilage which are modified by the constituents of their matrix, which in turn confer mechanical properties suited to function in their locations. Elastic cartilage contains elastic fibres within the extracellular matrix. Which is the single most likely location for elastic cartilage? ★

A Articular surface of femur

B Intervertebral discs

C Larynx

D Pubic symphysis

E Trachea

3. In bone remodelling, reabsorption is initiated and undertaken by osteoclasts; the cavity formed is filled in by formation of osteoid by osteoblasts, which is subsequently mineralized. Name the cell that is indicated by the arrow in Fig. 7.1 (see Plate 5). ★

A Erythroblast

B Myeloblast

C Osteoblast

D Osteoclast

E Osteocyte

4. Although the components of skin are similar throughout the body, anatomical and regional variation occurs. Fig. 7.2 is a photomicrograph taken from the sole of the foot. It shows structures that are abundant in this site. Name the structure that is indicated by the arrow in Fig. 7.2a (see Plate 6). ★

A Eccrine gland

B Erector pili muscle

C Pacinian corpuscle

D Sebaceous gland

E Stratum spinosum

119

5. A 20-year-old man presents to A&E having fallen with an outstretched hand. His right wrist is very swollen and he has a dinner fork deformity (a dorsal displacement of the hand in relation to the forearm). Radiography demonstrates a fracture across a bone in the forearm. Which is the single most likely bone to be fractured? ★

A Distal radius

B Distal ulna

C Hamate

D Lunate

E Scaphoid

6. Following a slip whilst rock-climbing, a 37-year-old man complains of a painful, weak shoulder. He is unable to rotate or lift his arm properly and the pain radiates down his arm, particularly at night. Physical examination reveals that he has a limited range of movement, particularly between 0° and 30° abduction. MRI detects a full-thickness tear in a muscle inferior to the acromion of the scapula. Which muscle is the single most likely muscle to be injured? ★

A Deltoid

B Infraspinatus

C Long head of biceps

D Subscapularis

E Supraspinatus

7. A 28-year-old man falls off his motorbike on to his neck and shoulder. He damages the anterior rami (roots) of spinal nerves C5 and C6. Which movements are the most likely to be significantly reduced at the elbow? ★ ★

A Extension and pronation

B Extension and supination

C Flexion only

D Flexion and pronation

E Flexion and supination

8. A patient has come into A&E following an RTA (road traffic accident) and has a deep cut in his wrist. On examination he cannot flex the distal interphalangeal joints of his hand. Which is the single most likely muscle whose tendons have been damaged? ★

A Flexor carpi radialis (FCR)

B Flexor carpi ulnaris (FCU)

C Flexor digitorum profundus (FDP)

D Flexor digitorum superficialis (FDS)

E Flexor pollicis longus (FPL)

9. A 60-year-old woman falls heavily, which results in a mid-shaft fracture of the humerus. Which single nerve is most likely to be affected by this injury? ★ ★

A Axillary nerve

B Median nerve

C Musculocutaneous nerve

D Radial nerve

E Ulnar nerve

10. Following a fracture of the medial epicondyle of the left humerus, a 42-year-old man develops hypothenar wasting, and the metacarpophalangeal (MCP) joints of the 4th and 5th digits of the left hand are extended. Which nerve is the single most likely to be damaged? ★

A Deep branch of the radial nerve

B Median nerve

C Musculocutaneous nerve

D Superficial branch of the radial nerve

E Ulnar nerve

11. During a routine breast examination, a lump is identified in the right breast of a 43-year-old woman, and small lumps are felt on the anterior wall of the axilla. Which lymph nodes are found on the anterior wall of the axilla and are the single most likely first site of breast cancer metastasis? ★

A Apical lymph nodes

B Brachial lymph nodes

C Infraclavicular lymph nodes

D Pectoral lymph nodes

E Subscapular lymph nodes

12. A 23-year-old woman who is a competitive rower complains of numbness and tingling over her thumb and first two digits which is worse at night. Which single finding on a motor test would confirm a diagnosis of carpal tunnel syndrome? ★

A Inability to abduct all fingers

B Inability to adduct all fingers

C Inability to extend the wrist and all fingers

D Inability to flex the wrist and all fingers

E Inability to oppose the thumb

13. A 21-year-old man takes part in a charity parachute jump. He lands awkwardly, his right ankle becomes swollen and tender within a few minutes, and he is unable to stand. He is sent for a radiograph, which shows no fracture of the tibia and fibula, but does show that the tarsal bone that articulates with them is fractured. Which single tarsal bone is the most likely to have been fractured in this patient? ★

A Calcaneus

B Cuboid

C Medial cuneiform

D Navicular

E Talus

14. There are three structural classifications for joints: synovial, cartilaginous, and fibrous. Examples of all three are found in the lower limb. Which single synovial hinge joint in the lower limb is the most likely to allow flexion and extension, and also allows rotation? ★

A Ankle (talocrural)

B Hip

C Inferior tibiofibular

D Knee

E Pubic symphysis

15. A 45-year-old man is recovering from a surgical operation but has contracted a hospital-acquired infection that is treated via intramuscular antibiotic injections into the buttock region. After one of these injections, the physiotherapist notes that he has developed a positive Trendelenberg's sign with the pelvis dropping towards the left when he stands on the right leg. Which single muscle group is the most likely to have become paralysed by an inappropriate intramuscular injection? ★ ★

A Left hip abductors

B Right hip abductors

C Left hip adductors

D Right hip adductors

E Left gluteus maximus

16. The muscles of the lower limb are found in groups and compartments where the muscles all have similar actions. Which leg muscle is the single most likely to dorsiflex the ankle and invert the foot? ★

A Gastrocnemius

B Peroneus longus

C Plantaris

D Tibialis anterior

E Tibialis posterior

17 The majority of the blood supply to the lower limb is derived from the terminal branches of the external iliac artery. Which lower limb artery is the single most likely to begin at the posterior side of the adductor hiatus? ★

A Anterior tibial

B Femoral

C Popliteal

D Posterior tibial

E Profunda femoris

18 A 24-year-old woman goes to her GP with a 1-week history of mild right leg pain. The pain is confined to the right calf and seems to get worse when she walks but is also present when she rests. She describes the pain as a dull ache. There is no back pain and no history of trauma. On examination, the right calf feels slightly warmer than the left and there is mild swelling, but no discoloration. Dorsiflexion of the right foot increases the calf pain and on palpation there is a tender area in the middle of the gastrocnemius muscle. All peripheral pulses are present. She smokes about 15 cigarettes a day and is taking the contraceptive pill. Which blood vessel is the single most likely to be affected in this case? ★ ★

A Anterior tibial vein

B Greater saphenous vein

C Lesser (small) saphenous vein

D Posterior tibial vein

E Profunda femoris vein

19. Venous return from the lower limb to the heart is via a network of superficial and deep veins and connecting perforating veins. Blood flows from the superficial veins into the deep veins. Which is the single most important mechanism for venous return from the lower limb when standing? ★

A Gravity

B Muscle pump

C Respiratory pump

D Smooth muscle contraction

E Vena cava compression

20. True leg length is measured between two bony features; one is on the pelvis and the other is on the medial malleolus of the tibia. What is the name of the single osteological feature on the pelvis used for measuring true leg length? ★

A Anterior inferior iliac spine

B Anterior superior iliac spine

C Iliac crest

D Ischial tuberosity

E Pubic tubercle

21. A 21-year-old woman has suspected meningitis. A lumbar puncture is ordered to take a sample of the cerebrospinal fluid for analysis. Which are the two vertebrae between which a lumbar puncture is normally performed? ★

A T11–T12

B T12–L1

C L1–L2

D L2–L3

E L3–L4

22. Most vertebrae have typical features, which include a vertebral body, a neural arch, and seven processes for articulating with adjacent vertebra and muscle/ligament attachment points. However, the vertebrae in each region have distinctive features that allow them to be distinguished from each other. Which is the single most characteristic feature of lumbar vertebrae? ★

A Bifid spinous processes

B Circular vertebral foramen

C Heart-shaped vertebral body

D Kidney-shaped vertebral body

E Transverse foramen

23. A lesion affecting the long thoracic nerve leads to a 'winged' scapula and difficulty in abducting the arm past horizontal. Which single muscle is the most likely to be paralysed? ★

A Deltoid

B Levator scapulae

C Rhomboids

D Serratus anterior

E Supraspinatus

24. A 48-year-old man has suffered from low back pain for a number of years. An epidural injection of steroids is recommended. What are the two layers that define the epidural space? ★

A Arachnoid mater and dura mater

B Arachnoid mater and pia mater

C Dura mater and pia mater

D Dura mater and the bony walls of the spinal canal

E Pia mater and spinal cord

25. A 68-year-old woman complains of left hip pain, which is worse on walking upstairs. She has had this for 6 months, but it is gradually getting worse. Her GP arranges for an X-ray examination of the hip. Which radiological feature shown in the X-ray in Fig. 7.3 is the single most helpful diagnostic clue that makes osteoarthritis the likely diagnosis? ★ ★

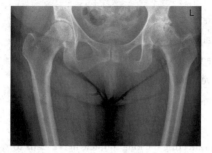

Fig. 7.3

A Narrowing of joint space

B Osteopenia

C Osteophyte formation

D Radio-opaque round bodies in joint space

E Sub-chondral cyst

EXTENDED MATCHING QUESTIONS

Muscles

Which muscle(s) are the most likely to be paralysed and the cause of the problems described in each of these cases? Each option may be used once, more than once, or not at all.

Options:

A Adductor pollicis

B Abductor pollicis brevis

C Biceps brachii

D Deltoid

E Flexor digitorum profundus (medial)

F Flexor digitorum superficialis

G Latissimus dorsi

H Rhomboids

I Palmar interossei

J Serratus anterior

K Supraspinatus

L Trapezius

M Triceps brachii

N 3rd and 4th lumbricals

O 1st and 2nd lumbricals

1. A 34-year-old woman undergoes a radical mastectomy for breast cancer in her left breast. A week later, the medial border of her left scapula is displaced laterally and posteriorly away from the thoracic wall. This becomes more evident when she pushes with her left hand on a wall. She is also unable to abduct the arm above the horizontal plane. ★ ★

2. A 32-year-old woman is diagnosed with rheumatoid arthritis. This affects her carpal bones in both hands and there is swelling in the carpal tunnel area. Her thumb movements are weak. ★ ★

3. A 54-year-old woman who works as a secretary has a 6-month history of right little finger weakness and difficulty with adduction of all her fingers. ★

4. A 27-year-old man is involved in a knife attack and suffers a deep penetrating knife wound to his right anterior arm. He notices that he is only able to weakly flex his right shoulder, and flexion of his right elbow and supination of the forearm are greatly weakened. ★

5. A 73-year-old man has nasal cavity cancer with metastases identified in the cervical lymph nodes on both sides. He undergoes surgery to remove the lymph nodes. Two weeks later, he notices that he has difficulty elevating and retracting his right shoulder. When the surgeon examines him, he finds that the right shoulder droops, with problems elevating the right arm above the horizontal. ★ ★

Nerves

Select the nerve that is most likely to have been damaged in each of the following scenarios. Each option may be used once, more than once, or not at all.

A Common peroneal nerve

B Femoral nerve

C Inferior gluteal nerve

D Lateral plantar nerve

E Medial plantar nerve

F Obturator nerve

G Pudendal nerve

H Saphenous nerve

I Sciatic nerve

J Superior gluteal nerve

K Sural nerve

L Tibial nerve

6. A 24-year-old man who has fractured the neck of the fibula of his left leg finds that when the cast is removed he is unable to dorsiflex his left foot. ★

7. A 15-year-old male is involved in a knife attack. He has a laceration on the anterior lateral side of his right leg. When he walks, he has to lean forward and has to push back with his hand on his right thigh to extend and lock his knee. ★

8. An 18-year-old man is knocked off his motorbike and suffers a pelvic fracture of the rami of the pubis and ischium on the left side. He is unable to adduct his left thigh and there is diminished sensation along the medial thigh. ★

9. A 55-year-old woman has a Baker's cyst in her right leg that has increased in size over the last 3 months. She goes to her GP reporting that she has burning, tingling sensations in the sole of her right foot. The symptoms get worse when she stands or walks. She reports that she does not seem able to push off as well with her right leg when she walks. ★

10. A 34-year-old man is involved in a road traffic accident and suffers severe internal injuries. The doctors perform a saphenous cutdown to insert a cannula for prolonged administration of fluids. When the patient recovers, he complains of pain along the medial border of his foot. ★

Single Best Answers

1. C ★   OHMS 2nd edn → pp268–9

The scar tissue is rather mature by 3 weeks, and composed of fibroblasts with intervening collagenous matrix. Within days of the initial incision or biopsy, acute inflammatory cells (E) and macrophages (D) migrate to the area, followed by granulation tissue which is rich in capillary-type blood vessels (B), but these are gradually replaced by fibroblasts. Note that the question refers to the scar tissue and not the melanoma.

2. C ★   OHMS 2nd edn → p270

Elastic cartilage is found in the larynx. Articular cartilage of the femur (A) and the trachea (E) contains hyaline cartilage, which is the most abundant form of cartilage. The pubic symphysis (D) and intervertebral discs (B) contain fibroelastic cartilage.

3. D ★   OHMS 2nd edn → pp271–3

The multinucleate cell responsible for bone resorption is the osteoclast. Osteoblasts (C) synthesize and secrete type I collagen, which is the main constituent of bone matrix, along with other non-collagenous proteins, and is also responsible for mineralization. Osteocytes (E) are terminally differentiated osteoblasts which are entombed in lacunae within bone matrix. Erythroblasts (A) and myeloblasts (B) are haemopoietic cells present in the marrow cavity, and are not directly involved in bone remodelling.

4. A ★   OHMS 2nd edn → pp274–7

Acral skin, present in the hands and feet, is characterized by thick or hyperplastic epidermis and dermal tissue that contains abundant collagen. Blood vessels are plentiful, as are the eccrine glands indicated in Fig. 7.2 (Plate 6). These produce sweat and account for 'sweaty hands and feet', especially when stimulated by the sympathetic cholinergic branch of the autonomic nervous system. Sebacous glands (D) are found in association with hair, and are unlikely to be the structure shown as the soles of the feet are hairless.

5. A ★   OHMS 2nd edn → pp278-9

Fracture of the distal radius is the most common fracture in adults under the age of 45. It is commonly known as a Colles' fracture, and typically occurs with a fall on an outstretched hand. The ulna (B), which lies alongside the radius, is unaffected. Hamate (C), lunate (D), and scaphoid are small bones of the hand found in the wrist. Although a scaphoid (E) fracture may also occur following a fall on an outstretched arm, especially if the force is on the palm, this answer (E) is incorrect as the scenario reads 'bone in the forearm'. This is an example of how students may be caught out if they do not read the question carefully.

6. E ★   OHMS 2nd edn → p290 and Fig. 5.16

The supraspinatus muscle forms the superior portion of the rotator cuff and passes underneath the acromion of the scapula and so is prone to injury and tendonitis in this area.

7. E ★★   OHMS 2nd edn → pp294, 296-9

The biceps brachii muscle (a flexor and supinator) and brachialis muscle (a flexor) are innervated by the musculocutaneous nerve (C5,6). C5 and C6 can be clinically tested both by the biceps and by the supinator (brachioradialis) reflexes.

8. C ★   OHMS 2nd edn → pp292, 294

The tendon of the flexor digitorum superficialis muscle (D) splits and inserts into the middle phalange and acts on the proximal interphalangeal joint. The tendon of the deep flexor (FDP) (C) continues to the distal phalange and acts on the distal interphalangeal joint of the digit and so is the correct answer here. The FCR (A) and FCU (B) muscles insert on to the flexor retinaculum in the wrist. The FPL muscle (E) inserts on the distal phalange of the thumb and flexes the interphalangeal joint of the thumb.

9. D ★★   OHMS 2nd edn → pp296-9

The radial nerve descends in the spiral groove between the lateral and the medial head of triceps and is prone to injury in a mid-shaft fracture of the humerus. The musculocutaneous nerve (C) is separated from the humerus at this level by the brachialis muscle. The median (B) and ulnar (E) nerves are separated from the humerus at this level by the medial head of the triceps brachii muscle.

A lesion of the radial nerve would cause wrist drop (the radial nerve supplies the extensors) and sensory loss would occur over the first interosseal web.

The ulnar nerve descends into the forearm posterior to the medial epicondyle of the humerus. This nerve supplies the hypothenar muscles and the medial two lumbricals that flex the metacarpal (MCP) joints and extend the proximal interphalangeal joints (PIP). A lesion in the ulnar nerve will result in unopposed extension of the MCP joint. There is no flexion of the proximal and distal interphalangeal joints in this patient because the flexor digitorum profundus muscle is also denervated. A more distal lesion of the ulnar nerve (for example at Guyon's canal in the wrist) would result in flexion of these distal joints resulting in the classic claw hand.

11. D ★   OHMS 2nd edn → p302, Fig. 5.30

70% of breast lymphatics drain through the axilla via the pectoral lymph nodes. Whilst the lymph also drains through the apical (A) and infraclavicular (C) nodes, the first location that metastasis spreads to is usually the pectoral lymph nodes. Therefore, during routine breast examination, it is important to feel the anterior wall of the axilla i.e. the posterior surface of pectoralis major. Lymphatics from the arm drain through the brachial nodes (B) which are on the lateral wall of the axilla.

12. E ★   OHMS 2nd edn → p305, Fig. 5.31

Carpal tunnel syndrome describes pathology of the wrist that affects the median nerve; this innervates the opponens pollicis which moves the thumb to touch the little finger. Abduction (A) and adduction (B) of the fingers is performed by the dorsal and the palmar interossei muscles which are innervated by the ulnar nerve. The extensors of the hand and wrist (C) are innervated by the radial nerve. Most flexors of the forearm (D) are innervated by the median nerve but in this case the lesion is distal to the supply.

13. E ★   OHMS 2nd edn → pp310–11

3–5% of foot fractures are to the talus, but are probably under-reported. The talus articulates with the tibia and fibula bones to form the ankle joint proper. The calcaneus (A) forms the heel bone and articulates with the talus, which sits on top of it. The other tarsal bones: navicular (D), cuboid (B) and three cuneiforms (medial (C), intermediate, and lateral) fit together closely, forming the transverse arch and the medial and lateral longitudinal arches. The arches act as shock absorbers and energy storage mechanisms for the foot. During jumping and landing, the arches can compress whereas the talus is sandwiched between the calcaneus and tibia and fibula above. The mechanism of injury is that the talus is compressed by the calcaneus below and the tibia and fibula above.

14. D ★   OHMS 2nd edn → pp312–17

The knee joint (medial and lateral femoral condyles with the corresponding menisci and tibial plateau along with the posterior patella) is primarily a hinge joint that allows flexion and extension, but for full extension, there is rotation of the medial femoral condyle which passively locks the knee when it is fully extended. The unlocking of the knee is active and done by the popliteus muscle at the back of the knee. The hip joint (B) is a synovial ball and socket and thus allows flexion, extension, abduction and adduction, and medial and lateral rotation. The ankle (A) is a pure hinge synovial joint and undergoes just flexion and extension. The pubic symphysis (E) is a cartilaginous joint made of fibrocartilage and is relatively immoveable. The inferior tibiofibular joint (C) is a fibrous joint, where fibrous tissue attaches between the tibia and fibula. There is little movement between the bones and the sheet acts as more of an attachment site for muscles.

15. B ★ ★   OHMS 2nd edn → p318

The hip abductors are gluteus medius, gluteus minimus, and tensor fasciae latae; all are innervated by the superior gluteal nerve. The hip abductors help to shift the weight of the body over the supporting leg when going from a double to a single support. Therefore the muscles that are affected involve the right hip abductors, since when the patient stands on his right leg the pelvis drops to the left, indicating that the muscles on the right are not working. The superolateral quadrant of the buttock is relatively free of nerves and vessels and is frequently used for intramuscular injections in order to avoid the sciatic nerve and other important structures. An alternative site is over the gluteus medius in a triangular area bounded by the anterior superior iliac spine, the tubercle of the iliac crest, and the greater trochanter. The hip abductors are innervated by the superior gluteal nerve, which has been injured by the injection.

16. D ★   OHMS 2nd edn → pp322–3

The tibialis anterior (TA) is the only muscle on the list that is found in the anterior compartment of the leg and therefore is the only dorsiflexor. The TA is anterior and on the lateral side of the tibia; the other lateral compartment muscles evert the foot as their tendons pass over the ankle on the lateral side, whereas the TA tendon passes over the anterior of the ankle and inserts into the top of the medial arch of the foot. Therefore its actions are to invert the foot. The peroneus longus muscle (B) everts the foot. Gastrocnemius (A) and plantaris (C) muscles plantarflex the ankle. Finally, the tibialis posterior muscle plantar muscle (E) flexes and inverts the foot.

Moore, K, Dalley, A, & Agur, A, (2009). *Clinically Oriented Anatomy*, pp589–600. London: Lippincott Williams & Wilkins.

17. C ★   OHMS 2nd edn → pp330–1, 334

The femoral artery (B) is the main blood supply of the lower limb and is a continuation of the external iliac artery. It becomes the femoral artery as it passes under the inguinal ligament and enters the femoral triangle. The largest branch of the femoral artery is profunda femoris (E) (the deep artery of the thigh) which starts approximately 1–5cm inferior to the inguinal ligament. It passes deep to pectineus and adductor longus muscles. The femoral artery descends through the femoral triangle before passing through the adductor canal and terminating as it passes through the adductor hiatus, where it changes its name and becomes the popliteal artery (C). The anterior (A) and posterior (D) tibial arteries arise from the popliteal artery as it enters the lower leg.

Moore, K, Dalley, A, & Agur, A (2009). *Clinically Oriented Anatomy*, Ch. 5. London: Lippincott Williams & Wilkins.

18. D ★ ★   OHMS 2nd edn → p332

The patient is young and the presence of peripheral pulse makes intermittent claudication, and therefore arterial disease, very unlikely. Swelling of the leg and local tenderness with no pain reported in any other part of the leg tend to rule out sciatica. The fact that she is taking the contraceptive pill and smokes makes a deep vein thrombosis (DVT) most likely. Pain, the most common symptom, is typically described as dull and aching, and is aggravated by walking. Homan's sign (increased pain on dorsiflexion) is not very reliable and dorsiflexion of the foot can cause the thrombus to dislodge. As the name suggests, DVTs affect the deep veins rather than the superficial veins that lie outside the fascia. The deep veins take the names of the arteries that they travel alongside. Therefore from the description of the pain being in the middle of the gastrocnemius muscle, the most likely vessel that has the thrombus is the posterior tibial vein (D). The greater (B) and lesser (C) saphenous veins are superficial. The anterior tibial vein (A) is on the anterior side of the leg.

Moore, K, Dalley, A, & Agur, A, (2009). *Clinically Oriented Anatomy*, pp532–40. London: Lippincott Williams & Wilkins.

19. B ★   OHMS 2nd edn → p332

Blood travels from the superficial to the deep veins through perforating veins that pass through the deep fascia. There are one-way pocket valves in these perforating veins that prevent blood going backwards from the deep to the superficial veins. In addition, the perforating veins are at an oblique angle so that when the muscles contract and the pressure increases inside the deep fascia, the perforating veins are compressed. Compression of the veins prevents blood flowing from the deep to the superficial veins.

This pattern is important, as it ensures that the majority of the venous blood will be in the deep veins and this enables the muscular contractions to propel blood towards the heart against gravity (B). During inspiration, the pressure in the thorax falls and this negative pressure is transferred to the great veins causing blood to move along from high pressure regions to low pressure regions, and so upwards towards the heart. At the same time, the downward movement of the diaphragm causes pressure in the abdomen to rise, pushing venous blood back to the heart (C). This becomes more important in exercise when breathing is faster and deeper. When standing, blood tends to pool in the veins of the legs. Gravity helps return blood from the head and upper limbs (A). There is sympathetic activation of the smooth muscle in the walls of the veins (D) but most veins have a thin tunica media and thus the rhythmic contraction and relaxation of the smooth muscle in the walls of the veins, which pushes blood back to the heart, is not a major contributor to the venous return for the lower limb. There is more smooth muscle in the walls of the great saphenous vein as it lies outside of the fascia.

20. B ★   OHMS 2nd edn → pp306–7

The measurement of true leg length is done between the anterior superior iliac spine (ASIS) and the medial malleolus. The ASIS is easier to identify than the inferior spine (A) as it is at the anterior end of the iliac crest and is more prominent. The iliac crest is not used as it curves and therefore is not a fixed point (C). The pubic tubercle is difficult to find (E). The ischial tuberosities are the attachment of the hamstring muscles, and are posterior and have to be palpated deeply (D).

21. E ★   OHMS 2nd edn → pp344–5

In the adult, the spinal cord ends around vertebral level L1-L2 and, below this, the vertebral foramen is taken up with the spinal nerve roots (cauda equina) of the lumbar, sacral, and coccygeal levels. A lumbar puncture is therefore performed inferior to the end of the spinal cord (L3-L4), since the cauda equina nerve roots are displaced by the needle as it is inserted to remove the sample of CSF.

22. D ★   OHMS 2nd edn → p338

Distinguishing features of lumbar vertebrae are: kidney shaped vertebral bodies (D); triangular vertebral foramen smaller than cervical; short blade-like spinous processes that are thick and broad.

Distinguishing features of cervical vertebrae are: oval vertebral bodies; large triangular vertebral foramen; transverse foramen (E) (for the vertebral arteries); and bifid spinous processes (A). Distinguishing features of thoracic vertebrae are: heart-shaped body (C); articulation processes on the body for head of rib; circular vertebral

Musculoskeletal System

foramen (B); long slender transverse process with articulation facet for tubercle of rib; long posteroinferiorly placed spinous processes.

Moore, K, Dalley, A, & Agur, A, (2009). *Clinically Oriented Anatomy*, pp443–50. London: Lippincott Williams & Wilkins.

23. D ★   OHMS 2nd edn → p340

The serratus anterior muscle stabilizes the scapula during abduction between 90° and 180° and maintains its close proximity to the rib-cage. The deltoid muscle (A), an arm abductor, is supplied by the axillary nerve. The supraspinatus muscle (E) abducts the arm from 0° to 30° and is supplied by the suprascapular nerve. The rhomboids (C) are innervated by the dorsal scapular nerve and retract the shoulder blades. The levator scapulae elevates the scapula—it is innervated by the cervical and dorsal scapular nerves.

24. D ★   OHMS 2nd edn → pp344–5

Therapeutic injections directed at spinal nerves should be placed in the epidural (also known as extradural) space. This lies between the dura mater and the bony walls of the spinal canal (D), since this is where the nerve roots traversing from the intervertebral foramina are located. Cerebrospinal fluid lies within the subarachnoid space between arachnoid mater and pia mater (B). If the dura mater and arachnoid mater become separated due to disease or injury a sub-dural space is created (A). The pia mater forms a fine layer covering the spinal cord (E) and brain. Note that option C does not exist in reality since the arachnoid lies between pia and dura—it is a trick distractor!

25. A ★ ★   OHMS 2nd edn → pp346–7

Narrowing of joint space is the earliest radiological feature of osteoarthritis. This is demonstrated by comparing the appearance of the abnormal left side with the normal appearance on the right side. Osteophytes (C) and sub-chondral cysts (E) are late features seen in more advanced disease, and are absent in Fig. 7.3. Osteopenia (B) is seen in inflammatory arthritides such as rheumatoid arthritis. Radio-opaque round bodies in the joint space are seen with synovial chondromatosis (D).

Extended Matching Questions

1. J ★ ★

During axillary node dissection, two nerves are at risk of being damaged; these are the thoracodorsal nerve and the long thoracic nerve. The thoracodorsal nerve innervates the latissimus dorsi muscle, and damage to it causes loss or weakened medial rotation and adduction of the arm. The nerve injured in this case is the long thoracic nerve to the serratus anterior muscle. This causes winging of the scapula. The actions of the serratus anterior muscle are protraction of the scapula and its stabilization against the thoracic wall. The muscle also rotates the scapula as part of the physiological joint that gives the shoulder a greater range of movement. Thus patients are unable to abduct the arm above the horizontal as the scapula will not rotate to give more articulation in the glenoid cavity for the head of the humerus.

2. B ★★

The abductor pollicis brevis muscle is innervated by the median nerve which passes through the carpal tunnel. Compression of the carpal tunnel therefore compresses the median nerve, and muscles supplied by the nerve distal to this point are affected. The median nerve innervates most of the thenar muscles at the base of the thumb, except the adductor pollicis muscle which is innervated by the ulnar nerve. This is carpal tunnel syndrome.

3. I ★

The palmar interossei adduct the 2nd, 4th and 5th digits and assist the lumbricals. The ulnar nerve innervates most of the small muscles in the hand except the 1st two lumbricals and most of the thenar muscles (see question 2). The action of the lumbricals is to flex the metacarpophalangeal joints and extend the interphalangeal joints of the 2nd–5th digits.

4. C ★

The biceps brachii muscle is the most powerful supinator of the forearm when it is supine. It also flexes the forearm, and the short head resists shoulder dislocations anteriorly. It is actually a three-joint muscle, crossing and affecting the glenohumeral, elbow, and proximal radio-ulnar joints.

5. L ★★

An awareness that the CNXI (spinal accessory) is located superficially in the lateral cervical region is important as damage to the CNXI is the most common iatrogenic nerve injury caused by doctors. The CNXI innervates the trapezius muscle which can be divided into ascending and descending, depending on the orientation of the muscle fibres. The descending muscle fibres elevate the scapula, while the ascending fibres depress the scapula. All fibres retract the scapula. The descending and ascending parts act together to rotate the glenoid cavity superiorly which is important for the range of movement and being able to get the arm above the horizontal.

General feedback on 1–5: OHMS 2nd edn → pp290–9

Moore, K, Dalley, A, & Agur, A, (2009). *Clinically Oriented Anatomy*, Ch. 6. London: Lippincott Williams & Wilkins.

6. A ★

The common peroneal nerve is one of the terminal branches of the sciatic and comes around from the posterior side of the leg to the anterior side, winding around the neck of the fibula. Palsy of this nerve is a common cause of foot drop and can even be caused by minor clinical events e.g. crossing legs, bandaging of the knee.

7. B ★

The femoral nerve is the most lateral structure of the femoral triangle and innervates the quadriceps muscle group. These muscles extend the knee and so lacerations that damage the femoral nerve cause these muscles to be denervated. The knee can be locked by using the hand to push the knee into extension.

8. F ★

The obturator nerve enters the thigh through the obturator foramen. It innervates the adductor muscles in the medial thigh as well as giving sensory innervation to the skin in the medial thigh.

9. L ★ ★

Although an uncommon occurrence, the tibial nerve can be compressed by a popliteal aneurysm or haemorrhage, or as in this case a Baker's cyst. Such cysts are abnormal collections of synovial fluid in synovial-membrane-lined sacs in the popliteal fossa. In adults they can get large and extend as far as the mid-calf and may interfere with knee movements or compress the tibial nerve. The tibial nerve innervates the plantarflexors of the leg and is sensory to the sole of the foot.

10. H ★

The saphenous nerve accompanies the great saphenous vein anterior to the medial malleolus. The saphenous nerve can be cut or caught by a ligature during closure of a surgical wound.

General feedback on 6–10: OHMS 2nd edn → pp324–9

Moore, K, Dalley, A, & Agur, A, (2009). *Clinically Oriented Anatomy*, Ch. 5. London: Lippincott Williams & Wilkins.

CHAPTER 8

RESPIRATORY AND CARDIOVASCULAR SYSTEM

Oxidative metabolism is essential for our cellular life. Although tissues such as skeletal muscle can operate for short periods anaerobically, human life does not continue for long in the absence of a ready supply of oxygen. Adequate oxygen delivery to tissues is essential for aerobic metabolism and disorders of delivery ultimately become life-threatening. The factors contributing to oxygen delivery are summarised in the oxygen flux equation:

OXYGEN FLUX = CARDIAC OUTPUT × ARTERIAL OXYGEN CONTENT

The cardiac output is the product of heart rate and stroke volume and amounts to about 5 litres per minute. The arterial oxygen content is the product of the blood's haemoglobin concentration multiplied by the haemoglobin's % saturation. The latter is determined by the partial pressure of oxygen in the blood. This is higher in arterial than in venous blood. A small, additional amount of oxygen is carried dissolved in the blood, the amount again determined by the oxygen partial pressure. The five litres of arterial blood delivered to the tissues each minute contain about 1000ml of oxygen. Only a quarter of this (250ml) is needed to support resting metabolism. There is therefore a large safety factor in oxygen delivery. This can be utilized, in concert with adaptive changes to cardiac output, vascular resistance and pulmonary ventilation, in situations such as muscular exercise, where oxygen demand increases dramatically, or at high altitude where inspired oxygen is low.

Oxygen delivery depends on the cardiovascular system, respiratory system and the blood. In the lungs, blood in the alveoli is brought into close proximity with alveolar air so that oxygen can diffuse easily into the blood and carbon dioxide, a major waste product of metabolism, can diffuse into the alveolar air. Alveolar air is kept refreshed with atmospheric air by pulmonary ventilation which keeps the partial pressures of oxygen and carbon dioxide in alveolar air and pulmonary capillary blood in a constant equilibrium. This process ensures that pulmonary venous blood and systemic arterial blood have high oxygen and low carbon dioxide partial pressures. Once in the blood, almost all of the oxygen combines with haemoglobin and is transported by the cardiovascular system to the tissues. The flow of blood reaching any tissue is determined by the output of the heart and the vascular resistance provided by the tissue's arterioles, much like Ohm's law relates voltage, resistance, and current in electrical circuits. The control of vascular smooth muscle is complex and shows important differences between different vascular beds. It may involve local factors including oxygen and carbon dioxide partial pressures and pH, local temperature, local chemical factors, as well as autonomic neural or hormonal control. Cardiac output and alveolar ventilation are also closely regulated to match oxygen delivery to metabolic requirements. This is achieved by feedback mechanisms which regulate arterial blood pressure and arterial blood gas concentrations.

The carbon dioxide produced by oxidative metabolism reacts with water to generate carbonic acid. This weakly dissociates to form bicarbonate and protons. Carbonic acid and bicarbonate not only contribute to carbon dioxide transport to the lungs but are the body's most important buffer system. The carbonic acid/bicarbonate system is regulated by controlling the excretion of carbon dioxide by the lungs and the renal excretion of protons and bicarbonate. This in turn regulates the other buffer systems to maintain acid–base balance and constant pH.

The interlocking body systems responsible for oxygen delivery are vulnerable to many forms of disorder and disease, from pulmonary disorders such as asthma, COPD and fibrosis which reduce oxygen uptake, or coronary heart disease which impairs the heart and heart failure which reduces cardiac output, or the anaemias which reduce oxygen carriage. It is not surprising that these systems contribute so much to morbidity and mortality, and it is worth remembering that because of the large safety factor built into these systems a significant proportion of normal function is often gone before a person feels unwell at rest or during modest exercise. ■

SINGLE BEST ANSWERS

1. A 64-year-old man presents to A&E with shortness of breath and haemoptysis (coughing up blood). On clinical examination he is found to have finger clubbing and decreased air entry on the left side of the chest. A chest radiograph confirms the presence of a large left-sided pleural effusion. A small bore drain is to be inserted into the 'safe triangle' of the thorax to drain the fluid. Which is the single best location for insertion of the needle? ★

A One rib space below the level of dullness on percussion in the mid-axillary line

B Posteriorly, one rib space below the level of dullness on percussion

C The 2nd intercostal space in the mid-clavicular line

D The 5th intercostal space in the mid-axillary line

E The 9th intercostal space in the mid-axillary line

2. A 20-year-old male presents with right sided pleuritic pain. His chest expansion is reduced and on percussion his chest is hyper-resonant on the right side. His breath sounds, tactile vocal fremitus (TVF), and vocal resonance (VR) are reduced. What is the single most likely diagnosis? ★ ★

A Empyema

B Haemothorax

C Pleural effusion

D Spontaneous pneumothorax

E Tension pneumothorax

3. A 52-year-old woman complains of hoarseness over a period of 4 weeks in the absence of an upper respiratory tract infection. Bronchoscopy reveals a paralysed left vocal fold. Chest radiography reveals a 2cm peripheral lesion in the left lung field and mediastinal adenopathy. Which single nerve is most likely to be involved? ★

A Left accessory nerve

B Left glossopharyngeal nerve

C Left recurrent laryngeal nerve

D Left superior laryngeal nerve

E Left vagus nerve

4. A child inhales a small part of a toy. In which single part of the bronchial tree is the object most likely to lodge?

A Left inferior lobar bronchus

B Left superior lobar bronchus

C Right inferior lobar bronchus

D Right middle lobar bronchus

E Right superior lobar bronchus

5. What is the single best name for the volume of air in the lungs when chest musculature is at rest and lung recoil is just balanced by chest wall recoil? ★

A Expiratory reserve volume

B Functional residual capacity

C Inspiratory reserve volume

D Residual volume

E Vital capacity

147

6. A 60-year-old male shopfitter has a 7-year history of progressive breathlessness on exertion and now reports breathlessness at rest. Although he stopped smoking 3 years ago, he smoked cigarettes heavily for many years (60 pack years). Chest radiography shows large bullae in both lungs, and plasma biochemistry indicates that he has an alpha$_1$-antitrypsin deficiency. On examination the physician observes that the anterior–posterior and lateral diameters of the chest are increased. Which of the following is the single most likely cause of the increase in chest dimensions? ★ ★

A Decreased airway resistance

B Decreased elastic recoil of the chest wall

C Decreased elastic recoil of the lungs

D Decreased gas exchange

E Decreased pulmonary surfactant

7. A lung freshly removed from an animal cadaver is inflated with air and the pressure–volume relationship is measured at different lung volumes under conditions of no airflow (Curve A in Fig. 8.1). The lung is then filled with physiological saline and the process repeated giving Curve B. These two static pressure–volume relationships show the compliance of the lung in different conditions. Which of the following is the single best explanation as to why the lung is more compliant in Curve B than in Curve A? ★

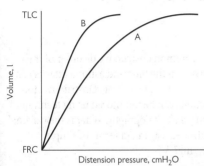

STATIC compliance curves—no airflow
(Functional Residual Capacity to Total Lung Capacity)

Fig. 8.1

A Air is more elastic than saline

B Distension pressure is more effective with water than with air

C Saline dilutes pulmonary surfactant

D Saline reduces airway resistance

E Saline reduces alveolar surface tension

8. Airflow through the airways of a lung is governed by the pressure gradient between the lung and the atmosphere and by the resistance of the airways to air flow. Airway resistance is determined by the Poiseuille equation. Which single element of the Poiseuille equation has the greatest effect on airflow in the normal lung (when breathing room air at sea level)? ★

A Length (of the airway).

B Radius (of the airway)

C The number, 8

D The value of π

E Viscosity (of the air).

9. Asthma is a common obstructive disorder of the smaller airways in the lung and asthma attacks can produce severe difficulty in breathing. Obstructive and other lung conditions can be monitored using techniques such as spirometry and vitalography. What is the cardinal feature of uncontrolled asthma in terms of simple lung-function testing? ★

A Air trapping

B Decreased peak expiratory flow rate

C Decreased vital capacity

D Increased peak expiratory flow rate

E Increased vital capacity

10. Fig. 8.2 shows the static pressure–volume curve for the lung measured with zero airflow, plus the dynamic pressure–volume curves as might be recorded during a single inspiration and expiration of a tidal volume. A vertical dotted line crosses the three curves at points A, B, and C. Which of the following is the single best explanation as to why the lung volume at point B is greater than at point A? ★ ★

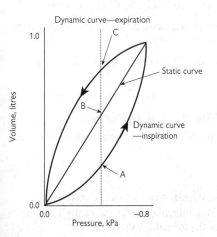

Fig. 8.2

A Airflow resistance is higher at A than at B, and so the volume is reduced.

B Pressure has been applied to the alveoli, but airflow is not yet complete.

C Surfactant effects on surface tension in alveoli vary between inspiration and expiration.

D Volume B is halfway between points A and C.

E Work must be done to overcome static compliance before air can flow.

11. Patients with some forms of pulmonary fibrosis may develop thickening of the alveolar septa. This increases the diffusion distance for gaseous exchange. Such patients may develop a low oxygen partial pressure (hypoxaemia) coupled with a low carbon dioxide partial pressure (hypocapnia) in their arterial blood. This may develop into type I respiratory failure. Which is the single best explanation for the low carbon dioxide concentration in arterial blood in these patients?

A Alveolar carbon dioxide partial pressure is lower than that of oxygen.

B Carbon dioxide has a lower alveolar air to capillary blood concentration gradient than oxygen

C Carbon dioxide is more soluble in water than oxygen

D Pulmonary fibrosis reduces total lung capacity

E The diffusion coefficient for carbon dioxide is lower than that for oxygen

12. Measurements on a 66-year-old man with long-standing mild COPD and eating a mixed diet might give the following values:

Respiratory quotient (respiratory exchange ratio) = 0.8

P_ACO_2 (alveolar partial pressure of carbon dioxide) = 8kPa

Assuming a partial pressure of oxygen in inspired air of 21kPa, what will be the predicted alveolar partial pressure for oxygen (P_AO_2)?

A 5kPa

B 6kPa

C 9kPa

D 11kPa

E 13kPa

13. Gas exchange in the lung depends on the alveolar ventilation (Va) and the blood flow, or perfusion, (Q) in pulmonary capillaries. In the upright lung the ventilation-to-perfusion ratio (Va/Q) at the apex (top) is higher than at the base (bottom). What is the single best explanation for the greater ventilation to perfusion ratio (Va/Q) at the apex of the lungs? ★ ★

A The apex has greater perfusion than the base

B The apex has greater ventilation than the base

C The apex has less ventilation and less perfusion than the base

D The apex is relatively over-perfused

E The apex is relatively over-ventilated

14. The alveoli are the site in the lungs specialized for gas exchange between the blood and the air. The alveoli and capillary blood are separated by the blood–air barrier. There are also cells of the immune system that act to prevent infections entering the lungs. Which of the following is the single best description for the type I pneumocytes of alveoli? ★

A They are squamous epithelial cells and comprise 95% of the cells in the alveoli

B They are also known as Clara cells

C They make and secrete the surfactant

D They have an important phagocytic role in the alveoli

E They also fulfil the stem-cell role in the event that the epithelium is damaged

15. Which single property of haemoglobin best accounts for its ability to transport oxygen efficiently in the blood from the lungs to the peripheral tissues? ★

A It has 4 subunits, each with one haem group

B It is a globular protein present at high concentration

C Interactions between its subunits ensure positive cooperative binding of oxygen

D Its presence within the red blood cell protects it from glomerular filtration

E It exists in variant forms with subtly different characteristics

16. In Fig. 8.3 curve A represents the oxygen dissociation curve for normal adult haemoglobin (HbA). Which of the following oxygen binding proteins would have an oxygen dissociation curve represented by curve B?

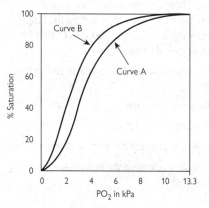

Fig. 8.3

A Carboxyhaemoglobin (HbCO)

B Fetal haemoglobin (HbF)

C Methaemoglobin (HbM)

D Myoglobin (MB)

E Sickle haemoglobin (HbS)

17. A 19-year-old male student is admitted to hospital with moderate carbon monoxide poisoning from a faulty gas central heating boiler in his student flat. He is conscious and when you see him he is breathing normal room air. A sample of blood is taken for blood gas analysis and the air in his lungs is analysed. Which is the single most likely finding from these tests? ★ ★

A Arterial PO_2 would be decreased

B Alveolar PO_2 would be decreased

C Arterial PCO_2 would be increased

D Venous PO_2 would be increased

E Arterial O_2 content would be decreased

18. Carbon dioxide exists in three forms in the blood: dissolved CO_2, HCO_3^-, and complexed to the terminal amine groups of blood proteins as carbamino CO_2. Which of the following is the single most likely amount of carbamino CO_2 in the venous blood? ★

Options

A 5%

B 10%

C 30%

D 60%

E 90%

19. In aerobic muscular exercise the increase in oxygen demand by the muscles is matched by an increase in pulmonary ventilation that increases oxygen uptake in the lungs. As the work level increases it will eventually cross a threshold from aerobic to anaerobic exercise. At this point there is a further increase in ventilation, but this is no longer able to meet fully the oxygen requirement of the exercising muscles. What is the single most likely cause of the increase in ventilation that occurs when exercise moves from the aerobic to anerobic state? ★ ★

A A fall in oxygen concentration detected at peripheral chemoreceptors

B An increase in carbon dioxide concentration detected at central chemoreceptors

C An increase in carbon dioxide concentration detected at peripheral chemoreceptors

D An increase in proton concentration detected at central chemoreceptors

E An increase in proton concentration detected at peripheral chemoreceptors

20. A 64-year-old man who was recently discharged from hospital following a total hip replacement is brought into A&E by ambulance. He has pleuritic chest pain and is hypoxic, hypotensive, and tachycardic. A diagnosis of PE is suspected. Which single investigation is most likely to confirm a diagnosis of pulmonary embolism? ★ ★

A Arterial blood gases

B Chest X-ray

C CT pulmonary angiogram

D D-dimer concentration

E ECG

21. A group of individuals are on a 7-day trekking trip to the summit of Kilimanjaro; the summit is over 5,500 metres above sea level. They are all fit and healthy and they have local guides and porters to assist them on the trek. As they ascend above 2,000m the trekkers notice that they start to experience problems which their guides do not. What is the initial compensation made by the body to the reduction in oxygen as people ascend to high altitudes? ★

A Angiogenesis in the muscles

B Hypoxic pulmonary vasodilation

C Hyperventilation

D Increased kidney excretion of HCO_3^-

E Increased kidney production of erythropoietin (EPO)

22. A blood sample is taken from a patient for analysis of both the plasma and serum constituents. What constituents are absent from serum that are present in the plasma? ★

A Albumin

B Clotting factors

C Glucose

D Insulin

E Urea

23. A 75-year-old woman presented to her general practitioner with a 4-month history of tingling in her feet, fatigue, and increasing breathlessness on exertion. On examination, she was pale and mildly jaundiced and had signs suggestive of a peripheral neuropathy. Her blood count results were as follows:

Hb 4.4g/dL (Normal 11.5–15.5)

MCV 119fL (Normal 80–96)

Reticulocytes 3.0% (Normal 0.5–2.5)

WBC 2.9 × 10^9/L (Normal 4.0–11.0)

Plats 59 × 10^9/L (Normal 150–400)

Examination of the blood film revealed the presence of hypersegmented neutrophils. What is the single most likely reason for the patient's anaemia?

A Chronic liver disease

B Erythropoietin deficiency

C Folate deficiency

D Iron deficiency

E Vitamin B_{12} deficiency

24. A 25-year-old woman who is O RhD⁻ is having her second baby. Her partner is blood group A RhD⁺. Their first child was born and identified as blood group O RhD⁺ in utero, but the mother was not immunized with anti-D within 36 hours of delivery. The blood group of the present fetus is analysed. Which blood group in the fetus is the single most likely one to result in the development of Rhesus disease? ★ ★

A A RhD⁻

B AB RhD⁺

C B RhD⁻

D O RhD⁻

E O RhD⁺

25. A 65-year-old man develops a left-sided chest pain radiating to the left arm and jaw. An ECG on admission shows ST elevation in leads V_2–V_4. He deteriorates and dies. At post-mortem an extensive myocardial infarct is found in the anterior left ventricular wall and the apex of the heart. Which coronary artery is the single one most likely to be occluded? ★

A Circumflex artery

B Left anterior descending artery

C Left coronary artery

D Left marginal artery

E Posterior interventricular artery

26. A 68-year-old woman with a history of ischaemic heart disease presents with nausea, abdominal pain, and anxiety. An ECG shows that the P wave is normal, with the PR interval getting progressively longer with each beat until the QRS complex is dropped, suggesting second degree heart block Mobitz Type I caused by an infarct on the inferior wall of the heart. Which coronary artery is the single most likely one to be occluded in this patient?

A Circumflex artery

B Left anterior descending artery

C Marginal branch of right coronary artery

D Right coronary artery

E Sino-atrial nodal branch

27. When auscultating the heart, two heart sounds are heard. What is the single best description of the valvular actions that account for the second heart sound? ★ ★

A Closure of the aortic and mitral valves

B Closure of the aortic and tricuspid valves

C Closure of the mitral and tricuspid valves

D Closure of the tricuspid and pulmonary valves

E Closure of the aortic and pulmonary valves

28. Which heart valves are closed during systole? ★

A Aortic and pulmonary

B Aortic and mitral

C Aortic and tricuspid

D Mitral and pulmonary

E Mitral and tricuspid

29. A 65-year-old woman complains of shortness of breath over 4 years and needs to sleep with her head elevated on pillows. A chest radiograph shows convexity in the area of the left atrium indicating left atrial enlargement. The profile and size of the left ventricle appear normal. What is the single most likely diagnosis? ★ ★

A Aortic stenosis

B Mitral regurgitation

C Mitral stenosis

D Systemic hypertension

E Ventricular septal defect

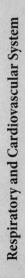

30. The force generated by contraction of cardiac myocytes is dependent on their length, which is in turn related to end-diastolic volume (EDV). Which single law best describes this relationship between ventricular EDV and force of cardiac contraction? ★

A Bernoulli's Law

B Fick–Laplace Law

C Frank–Starling Law

D Henry's Law

E Poiseuille's law

31. Blood pressure is determined by a number of factors including blood volume, cardiac output, and vascular resistance. With regard to vascular resistance, which are the single most important blood vessels for determining blood pressure? ★

A Arteries

B Arterioles

C Capillaries

D Veins

E Venules

32. A 22-year-old man is brought into the A&E department after being knocked off his motorbike. He looks pale and his skin feels cool and clammy. There are diminished peripheral pulses, his heart rate is 115 beats per minute, and he has a blood pressure of 106/94mmHg. What is the single most important factor that causes the diminished peripheral pulses and increased heart rate in this patient? ★ ★

A Acetylcholine

B Nitric oxide

C Noradrenaline

D Prostacyclin

E Renin

33. What is the single most likely mechanism by which beta blockers are thought to exert their primary anti-hypertensive effect? ★ ★ ★

A Inhibition of arterial α-1 receptors

B Inhibition of arterial β-2 receptors

C Inhibition of renal juxtaglomerular cell β-1 receptors

D Inhibition of cardiac β-1 receptors

E Inhibition of CNS sympathetic outflow

34. The response-to-injury hypothesis is the presently accepted model describing the pathogenesis of atherosclerosis, a major cause of morbidity and mortality worldwide. What role does hyperlipidaemia play in the development of atheromatous plaques? ★ ★

A Oxidized LDL constricts vasa vasorum thus reducing oxygen delivery

B Oxidized LDL is cytotoxic to endothelial cells and smooth muscle cells

C Oxidized LDL is ingested by smooth muscle cells to form foam cells

D Oxidized LDL stimulates B lymphocytes to release inflammatory cytokines

E Oxidized LDL stimulates nitric oxide (NO) synthetase thus increasing NO levels

35. Aspirin has important antipyretic, anti-inflammatory and analgesic effects which it exerts via irreversible inhibition of cyclo-oxygenase. Low-dose aspirin is also a cheap and effective means of reducing the risk of thrombotic events, e.g. in patients with coronary artery disease. At which point in the platelet activation pathway does aspirin exert its effect on haemostasis? ★ ★

A ADP receptor-mediated increase in intracellular calcium

B Glycoprotein IIb/IIIa receptor-mediated binding of fibrinogen

C Nitric oxide (NO)-mediated decrease in intracellular calcium

D Phosphodiesterase-mediated lowering of cAMP levels

E Thromboxane A_2 (TXA_2)-mediated platelet degranulation

EXTENDED MATCHING QUESTIONS

Presentation of disease and basic pathophysiology of chronic cough

For each of the following patients, choose the option which best describes the aetiology of chronic cough. Each option may be used once, more than once, or not at all.

A Allergic rhinitis

B Asthma

C Bronchial carcinoma

D Chronic obstructive pulmonary disease

E Congestive cardiac failure

F Cryptogenic fibrosing alveolitis

G Cystic fibrosis

H Foreign body

I Gastro-oesophageal reflux

J Sarcoidosis

K Tuberculosis

L Zenker diverticulum

1. A 25-year-old man complains of night time cough and a periodic sensation of tight chest related to exercise and exposure to cold air. He also gives a history of sensitivity to aspirin. ★ ★

2. A 54-year-old woman with BMI of 30 kg/m² who smokes heavily and drinks 20 units of alcohol per week complains of chronic cough, hoarse voice and sensation of a lump in the throat. ★ ★

3. A 28-year-old black man complains of chronic cough, shortness of breath, fever, and red, painful eyes. A chest radiograph reveals bilateral hilar lymphadenopathy and reticular shadows in the lung fields. ★ ★

4. A 26-year-old man who smokes complains of chronic cough and throat clearing, and has cobblestoning of the oropharyngeal mucosa. Naso-endoscopy reveals bilateral sinonasal polyps. ★ ★

5. A 32-year-old man complains of chronic cough and sinonasal congestion. Further questioning reveals weight loss associated with abnormal, greasy, foul-smelling stools. He also wishes to be investigated for primary infertility. ★ ★

Cardiovascular pharmacology

For each of the following cases, please select the most appropriate drug. Each of the options may be used once, more than once, or not at all.

A Adenosine

B Amiodarone

C Amlodipine

D Atropine

E Bendroflumethazide

F Digoxin

G Doxazosin

H Flecainide

I Isosorbide mononitrate

J Lidocaine

K Lisinopril

L Losartan

M Procainamide

N Propranolol

O Verapamil

6. A 77-year-old man is brought into his local A&E department having collapsed at home. He is attached to a cardiac monitor and found to have a sinus bradycardia rate of 35 beats per minute and to be hypotensive. Which of the drugs opposite is the most appropriate to stabilize him initially? ★ ★

7. This drug can be used to treat atrial fibrillation with rapid ventricular response and also has a positive inotropic effect (increases cardiac contractility). ★ ★

8. This drug is predominantly used for its effects on the cardiovascular system but it also mediates the bradykinin system. ★ ★

9. This drug has been shown to reduce mortality in heart failure and works predominantly by reducing preload. ★ ★

10. This drug is an anti-arrhythmic that acts by reducing action-potential duration, increasing the refractory period and reducing the rate of depolarization. ★ ★

Single Best Answers

1. D ★   OHMS 2nd edn → pp354–60

The correct answer is 5th intercostal space, mid-axillary line (on the left side, in this patient). Chest drains are used to drain air, blood, or fluid from the pleural space. To minimize the risk of complications, they are inserted into the 'safe triangle' on the upper, lateral aspect of the chest. The triangle has an anterior border at the lateral edge pectoralis major, a posterior border at the lateral edge of latissimus dorsi, a superior border at the base of the axilla, and inferior border at the line of the 5th intercostal space. Inserting a needle into the 'safe triangle' avoids the internal thoracic artery and the long thoracic nerve and avoids damage to muscle and breast tissue. This is the most common site for the insertion of chest drains for the drainage of pleural effusions. It is also the location for a large-bore chest drain for a tension pneumothorax. The needle is inserted just above the rib into the lower part of the intercostal space to avoid damage to the intercostal neurovascular bundle which travels superiorly in the intercostal space in the costal groove.

One rib space below the level of dullness on percussion in the mid-axillary line (A) or posteriorly on the chest (B) are areas which can be used during a needle thoracentisis to sample the effusion fluid (i.e. aspirating fluid for analysis). This is a diagnostic pleural tap and is usually performed using ultrasonography. The 2nd intercostal space in the mid-clavicular line (C) is the point of insertion of the needle for thoracocentesis in the immediate management of a tension pneumothorax. This position may also be used for the aspiration of a superior pneumothorax. However, it is not usually recommended as it may leave an unsightly scar and can be more uncomfortable for the patient. The 9th intercostal space in the mid-axillary line (E) is also sometimes recommended as the insertion site for diagnostic taps.

BTS Pleural Disease Guideline 2010. A Quick Reference Guide. *British Thoracic Society Reports* **2** (3) 2010, and http://www.brit-thoracic.org.uk/guidelines/pleural-disease-guidelines-2010.aspx.

2. D ★★   OHMS 2nd edn → pp360–1 OHCM → p824

A spontaneous pneumothorax occurs when air enters the pleural space through damaged visceral pleura. The negative intrapleural pressure draws air into the pleural space and the lung collapses due to its recoil. The air in the pleural space causes hyper-resonance on the affected side and reduces TVF and VR. Pleural effusion, haemothorax, and empyema would all be dull on percussion and increase TVF and VR. Tension pneumothorax, which is a life-threatening condition, would cause more severe symptoms associated with decreased cardiac output and a mediastinal/tracheal shift away from the midline.

3. C ★   OHMS 2nd edn → pp366–70

The recurrent laryngeal nerve is a branch of the vagus nerve which is motor to the intrinsic muscles of the larynx. It courses under the arch of the aorta on the left side and ascends to the larynx in the tracheo-oesophageal groove. Most pulmonary and mediastinal lymph nodes are located close to the lung hilum which is in close proximity to the aortic arch, and therefore a nodular involvement around the lung hilum can impinge on the left recurrent laryngeal nerve.

4. C ★   OHMS 2nd edn → pp372–3

Inhaled material tends to pass through the right main bronchus because it is wider and shorter than the left main bronchus. The course of the right main bronchus into the inferior lobar bronchus is wider and vertical and so the material would lodge here.

5. B ★   OHMS 2nd edn → p376

The functional residual capacity (FRC) is defined as the volume of air remaining in the lungs at the end of a quiet expiration. This occurs when the chest musculature is completely relaxed and airflow has ceased. This natural resting position of the chest arises when the inward elastic recoil of the lungs is just balanced by the outward elastic recoil of the chest wall. This should not be confused with the residual volume (RV), the volume in the chest at the end of a forced expiration (with expiratory muscles contracted). The FRC is equal to the RV plus the expiratory reserve volume.

6. C ★★   OHMS 2nd edn → pp401–2; OHCM → p176

The scenario suggests a history of chronic obstructive pulmonary disease (COPD), a diagnosis which embodies the consequences of both chronic bronchitis and emphysema. The presence of bullae (large air spaces resulting from alveolar destruction) and the reduced plasma α_1-antitrypsin are consistent with emphysema which will have been greatly exacerbated by cigarette smoking. Severe emphysema can produce enlargement of the chest, in part due to air trapping (because of airway obstruction) and in part due to destruction of the lung stroma (and a consequent reduction in lung recoil). The reduced lung recoil leads to the chest becoming larger due to the unopposed chest wall recoil. In these cases the functional residual capacity (FRC) will increase above normal values. Note that air trapping, while a good answer here, is not given in the option list.

Kumar, P, & Clark, M (2007). *Clinical Medicine* 5th edn. pp863–4. London: Saunders Ltd.

7. E ★   OHMS 2nd edn → pp378–9

Compliance is a measure of the distensibility of the lungs, or, more formally, the increase in volume per unit increase in distension pressure. Compliance is therefore the gradient of the static pressure–volume curve. Lung compliance is increased when the lungs are filled with saline because this abolishes the surface tension effects at the air–water interface normally present in the alveoli. These surface tension effects are a major component of lung recoil and therefore of lung compliance. Pulmonary surfactant reduces the surface tension effects in the living lung and lack of surfactant can lead to alveolar collapse due to surface tension effects, especially in the premature newborn.

8. B ★   OHMS 2nd edn → pp380–1

In the Poiseuille equation, resistance to flow of a fluid is equal to 8 times the viscosity times the length of the tube all divided by π times the radius of the tube raised to the fourth power. Although this equation only really applies to rigid tubes (unlike the airways which are flexible), the radius of the tube still exerts the greatest effect on resistance (and therefore on airflow) simply because its value is radius[4]. Thus small changes in airway radius produce significant changes in resistance, as in asthma when there is bronchiolar (small airway) constriction. The question is limited here to breathing room air at sea level. In deep sea diving, the divers breathe a mixture of helium and oxygen. In addition to preventing nitrogen narcosis, the low density of helium greatly reduces the viscosity of the gas mixture, reducing the work of breathing. This work against viscosity would be a significant element of the total work of breathing when a diver is breathing highly compressed oxygen and nitrogen.

9. B ★   OHMS 2nd edn → p400; OHCM → pp172–3

Asthma is defined as a reversible obstruction of the airways. This is caused by broncho-constriction in the smaller airways of the lung which can be reversed by drugs that directly relax the smooth muscle of the airway or reduce inflammation or secretion. If the airway is narrowed, then the effect is to increase airway resistance and to decrease flow. Small changes in airway diameter exert strong effects on airflow (cf the Poiseuille equation). The most sensitive measure of the calibre of the airways is the maximum airflow velocity produced with a forced expiration—the peak expiratory flow rate (PEFR). A reduction of the PEFR to below 70% of normal is strongly indicative of airway obstruction. Air trapping, which increases residual volume and reduces vital capacity, may occur in asthma but residual volume is not measured by simple lung-function tests. Decreased vital capacity is not only seen in obstructive disorders, but also in restrictive disorders (where residual volume is also reduced), so FVC measurement does not readily differentiate between the two sorts of lung condition. Only reduced PEFR is pathognomonic of obstructive disease.

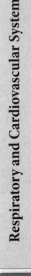

10. B ★★ OHMS 2nd edn → pp378–9

In the dynamic curves of inspiration and expiration, pressure is applied to the lungs and airflows, but airway resistance and inertia mean that volume in the lung takes time to develop. Thus volume lags behind the applied pressure throughout inspiratory and expiratory curves of the respiratory cycle. If the pressure is held constant, and dynamic volume is at point A, then airflow would continue until the maximum volume at that pressure is achieved at point B. This will be at the no-airflow condition, which defines static compliance measurement. Note that the differences between inspiratory and expiratory curves are a form of hysteresis, due in the case of dynamic pressure–volume measurement to the effects of airway resistance and inertia on airflow into and out of the lung. A similar and smaller hysteresis will be seen when the *static* curve is measured during incremental inflation and deflation of the lung. This smaller hysteresis is thought to be due to different surfactant effects in the expanding and contracting lung and to the changes in lung compliance which develop when lung volume is held constant.

Sircar, S (2008). *Principles of Medical Physiology*, p322. Stuttgart & New York: Thieme Medical Publishers.

11. C ★★ OHMS 2nd edn → pp46, 382–5

The rate at which gas moves from a region of high partial pressure to a region of low partial pressure is proportional to the partial pressure difference, the surface are of the intervening barrier, and the diffusion coefficient of the gas. It is also inversely proportional to the thickness of the barrier (Fick's law). The diffusion coefficient of a gas is proportional to the solubility of the gas and inversely proportional to the square root of its molecular weight. Carbon dioxide is 20 times more soluble in water than oxygen and its diffusion coefficient is therefore much larger and the concentration gradient for carbon dioxide exchange is correspondingly lower than that for oxygen. Thickening of the alveolar septum in pulmonary fibrosis increases the diffusion distance for both oxygen and carbon dioxide. Normally the driving force for carbon dioxide, at 0.8kPa between blood and lung, is only one tenth of the 8kPa difference required to move oxygen from alveoli to capillary blood. This is a direct consequence of the higher diffusion coefficient for carbon dioxide. As oxygen uptake is reduced, then the arterial blood becomes hypoxic and eventually ventilation is stimulated by the peripheral chemoreceptors. While increased ventilation will increase the concentration gradients for transfer of both gases, the relative effect on the smaller carbon dioxide gradient will tend to remove more of that gas from the blood than oxygen uptake is increased. Thus the picture of hypoxaemia and hypocapnia will develop. Note that another major cause of the Type I failure picture in the blood gases of these patients is ventilation perfusion (Va/Q) mismatch in the lung. This is not included in the option list.

Naish, J, Revest, P, & Syndercombe-Court, D (2009). *Medical Sciences*, pp710–11. London: Elsevier.

12. D ★   OHMS 2nd edn → pp384–5

You could probably guess an approximate answer from the scenario, since such a patient is likely to have hypoxia, with some carbon dioxide retention due to the COPD. However, the more rigorous way to find the correct answer, 11kPa, is to apply the Alveolar Gas Equation:

$$P_{Alveolar}O_2 = P_{Inspired}O_2 - (P_{Alveolar}CO_2/RQ)$$

where RQ is the respiratory quotient. This is the version given in OHMS 2nd edn, but it is a simplification. This equation is included in the 'four most important equations in clinical practice' because of its role in understanding disturbances in gas exchange and the use of oxygen therapy. Alveolar oxygen partial pressure (P_AO_2) is normally a good estimate of the oxygen partial pressure in systemic arterial blood (P_aO_2). Differences in the P_AO_2 calculated from the equation and the P_aO_2 as measured in the patient can be clinically important. For example, in patients with right to left shunts producing venous admixture, the calculated alveolar oxygen partial pressure (P_AO_2) is higher than the actual measured arterial oxygen partial pressure (P_aO_2). The P_aO_2 is lowered because oxygenated ('arterialized') blood coming from the lungs mixes with deoxygenated blood that has bypassed the lungs, or has passed through the lungs without proper oxygenation. The resulting arterial blood has lower oxygen than the alveolar air.

13. E ★ ★   OHMS 2nd edn → pp386–9

This can be a bit of a brain teaser, but is easy to understand by remembering Fig. 8.4.

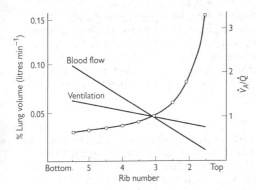

Fig. 8.4

The apex (top) of the lung receives less blood flow *and* less ventilation than the base, but while C is a true statement, it does not explain why the ratio of Va to Q is higher in the apex of the lung than at the base. The high Va/Q at the top is because local ventilation (in L.min⁻¹) is greater than local blood flow; alveoli are therefore relatively over-ventilated compared with those at the lung base. A high Va/Q equates to hyperventilation of the pulmonary capillary blood and low Va/Q to hypoventilation.

14. A ★   OHMS 2nd edn → p374

The type I pneumocytes are squamous cells that make up the majority of the cells in the alveoli, and are responsible for the absorption of surfactant and thus promote its turnover. Their squamous nature makes them ideal for the diffusion of oxygen and carbon dioxide across the alveoli. The type II cells secrete surfactant and are also the stem cell population of the alveoli able to differentiate into type I cells. There are macrophages in the alveoli and Clara cells line the bronchiolar airways.

15. C ★   OHMS 2nd edn → pp10, 390–1

All of the answers are true, but only C explains the ability of haemoglobin to transport oxygen efficiently over the physiological range of PO_2, as illustrated by the sigmoidal oxygen dissociation curve. This cooperative binding ensures rapid uptake of oxygen by the blood perfusing the lungs (high PO_2) and efficient delivery of oxygen to the peripheral tissues (low PO_2).

16. B ★ ★   OHMS 2nd edn → pp390–2, Fig. 6.17

Curve B shows oxygen binding cooperatively (sigmoidal curve) with a higher affinity than that of normal adult haemoglobin (curve shifted to the left, hence less oxygen required to achieve 50% saturation). This property of fetal haemoglobin ensures efficient transfer of oxygen from the maternal blood to the fetus. Myoglobin has a higher oxygen affinity than does Hb, but its oxygen dissociation curve is hyperbolic. The other forms of Hb have an oxygen affinity that is roughly the same as (HbS) or lower than (HbCO, HbM) that of HbA.

17. E ★★   OHMS 2nd edn → pp390–1

The haemoglobin binds CO with high affinity (220 times more than O_2), and thus there will be less O_2 bound to haemoglobin in the arterial blood. Binding of CO to haemoglobin causes an increased binding of oxygen molecules at the other 3 oxygen binding sites that are available on haemoglobin. This then results in a shift to the left of the oxyhaemoglobin dissociation curve, which decreases the availability of oxygen to the already hypoxic tissues. The PO_2 levels should remain normal. Oxygen saturation is accurate only if directly measured, and not if calculated from the PO_2, which is the case for many blood gas anlaysers. The PCO_2 levels are estimated by subtracting the carboxyhaemoglobin (HbCO) level from the calculated saturation. PCO_2 level may be normal or slightly decreased. Metabolic acidosis is secondary to lactic acidosis from ischaemia. If the patient is now breathing room air then the alveolar levels would also now be normal. However, because of the binding of CO irreversibly, the amount of arterial CO_2 would be increased.

18. C ★   OHMS 2nd edn → pp394–5

In arterial blood CO_2 bound to Hb (which is the most significant protein for carrying CO_2) is 5% as it is carrying O_2. However, the deoxygenated Hb of venous blood binds CO_2 more readily than oxygenated Hb of arterial blood, so in venous blood 30% of total CO_2 carriage is by carbamino compounds. Dissolved CO_2 obeys Henry's law and it is 20 times more soluble in blood than O_2, so in arterial blood there is very little (5%), but it increases in venous blood (10%). It is dissolved in both the intra- and extracellular compartments. CO_2 diffuses across the cell membrane into the cytosol where the hydration reaction forms carbonic acid. Carbonic acid that is formed dissociates into protons (H+) and bicarbonate ions (HCO_3^-). The bicarbonate ions are exchanged for chloride ions across the red cell membrane, and this enhances the transport of CO_2 in the blood plasma. 90% of CO_2 in arterial blood is transported as bicarbonate, falling to 60% in venous blood.

19. E ★★   OHMS 2nd edn → pp396–8

During aerobic exercise oxygen demand is matched to oxygen uptake in the lungs by mechanisms which are probably complex and do not simply involve the measurement of arterial blood gas concentrations by central and peripheral chemoreceptors. The resulting increase in ventilation to meet an increased metabolic demand for oxygen is known as the hyperpnoea of muscular exercise. Once anaerobic exercise commences, an oxygen debt is built up with a switch to lactic acid production in the exercising muscles. This lactic acid raises plasma, and therefore, arterial proton concentration. This is detected at peripheral chemoreceptors and stimulates a further increase in ventilation of the lungs. The result is that hyperventilation develops. Hyperventilation is defined as 'ventilation in excess of metabolic requirement', so although it may seem paradoxical, in severe anaerobic exercise arterial carbon dioxide partial pressure may actually decrease below the level seen in steady-state and maximal aerobic exercise. Peak exercise level is in fact limited by the rate at which oxygen can be delivered to the tissues by the blood and not by the ability of the respiratory system to oxygenate the blood.

20. C ★ ★   OHMS 2nd edn → p406

Of all the investigations listed, CT pulmonary angiogram (CTPA) is the only one that will confirm the presence of a pulmonary embolism. The other tests may have results suggestive of pulmonary embolism but are not specific.

21. C ★   OHMS 2nd edn → p407

As air pressure falls, there are fewer oxygen molecules present in a given volume (the percentage of oxygen is the same, 21%) due to Boyle's law. The initial response is to breathe faster and deeper (hyperventilate) at high altitude. CO_2 is constantly being produced and diffuses into the fresh air breathed into the lungs while O_2 goes into the blood. By hyperventilating, the rate at which CO_2 is lost increases and therefore CO_2 is lost from the blood. This makes the blood relatively alkaline; the kidneys correct this over a few days by increasing the excretion of bicarbonate (HCO_3^-) from the blood. The kidneys, in response to hypoxia, also secrete EPO, which stimulates the production of red blood cells, which helps increase the haemoglobin levels and the O_2 carrying capacity. However, this is a slower adaptive process, as red blood cells have to be made. EPO, also along with hypoxia, stimulates the production of new blood vessels in the muscles, which helps with delivering O_2 to the muscles; again, this is a slower adaptive change.

When the blood passing through an area of lung is not picking up enough oxygen, the blood vessels carrying that blood tighten, so that less deoxygenated blood can get through the lungs. This is called hypoxic pulmonary vasoconstriction (not dilation). Normally the mechanism shunts blood from poorly to well-oxygenated alveoli, but at high altitude hypoxia can produce widespread pulmonary constriction and pulmonary hypertension.

22. B ★   OHMS 2nd edn → p408

Blood plasma is isolated from the cellular fractions of the blood sample by centrifugation in the presence of an anticoagulant, which prevents the blood from clotting. Serum, on the other hand, is obtained when no anticoagulant has been added to the blood sample and the blood forms a clot; as a result, serum (the fluid produced by centrifugation in this case) does not contain clotting proteins such as fibrinogen. Therefore plasma and serum are essentially the same except that the clotting factor proteins are absent from serum.

23. E ★★   OHMS 2nd edn → p409; OHCM → pp326–7

Vitamin B_{12} deficiency occurs as a result of inadequate dietary intake (e.g. a vegan diet) or from malabsorption (e.g. pernicious anaemia). The megaloblastic anaemia can be characterized by the presence of hyper-segmented neutrophils. B_{12} deficiency can lead to demyelination of nerves, hence the symptoms of peripheral neuropathy.

24. E ★★   OHMS 2nd edn → p410

The ABO blood groups are inherited via a Mendelian pattern with A and B being co-dominant and O recessive. There are, however, other antigens expressed by red blood cells. Rhesus system antigens are a group of glycoproteins that are expressed in most people (85% of Caucasians and 99% of Orientals are Rhesus positive). The Rhesus system becomes a major issue during pregnancy. When a RhD− mother gives birth to a RhD+ child with the same ABO group as her and there is mixing of the fetal blood with the mother's (usually during childbirth), the mother's immune system will not destroy the red blood cells, as they are the same ABO group. However, they do induce the production of antibodies against the RhD antigens. The first child is unaffected but should the mother have another RhD+ baby, her immune system will destroy the red blood cells of the fetus leading to haemolytic Rhesus disease no matter what the ABO group. The issue is prevented normally by routine screening of pregnant women for RhD and giving an injection of anti-D antibodies within 36 hours of childbirth. This has reduced the incidence of Rhesus disease by 90% but the injection in some countries is not routine. There is no way the fetus can be AB RhD+ as the mother is blood group O, nor can it be BRLD+ given the parents' blood groups.

25. B ★   OHMS 2nd edn → pp418, 424

The correct answer is the left anterior descending coronary artery (LAD), because the ECG changes and post-mortem findings indicate that it was occlusion of an artery supplying the anterior wall of the left ventricle and the apex that caused myocardial infarction. The

LAD lies in the anterior interventricular groove and is the only artery in the option list which supplies that area. An occluded left coronary artery would cause an anterolateral infarct, affecting both the anterior wall supplied by the LAD and the inferior wall supplied by the circumflex artery. ST elevation would be seen in V_2–V_4, I, AVL, and V_5 and/or V_6.

26. D ★ ★ ★   OHMS 2nd edn → pp418–19, 422–8

The right coronary artery descends in the coronary groove on the anterior surface of the heart and then continues on the diaphragmatic surface. It gives off a small atrioventricular (AV) nodal branch before finally branching into the posterior interventricular artery. Ischaemia of the AV node (and in some cases the bundles of His) results in a conduction delay. The arrhythmia is characterized by a delay at the AV node and hence a progressively longer PR interval until the conduction is completely blocked, because the impulse arrives during the refractory period and is not conducted, resulting in a missed ventricular contraction. Nausea and abdominal pain are often symptoms of an inferior infarct and should not be confused with indigestion.

27. E ★ ★   OHMS 2nd edn → pp432–3; OHCM → p42

Heart sounds are the noise made by the heart valves closing. The atrio-ventricular valves (those that lie between atria and ventricles) are the mitral valve on the left and tricuspid on the right. Closure of these two valves is audible as the first heart sound. The pulmonary and aortic valves are at the exit of the right and left ventricles, respectively, and prevent the backflow of blood from the pulmonary trunk or aorta into the ventricles. Closure of these valves can be heard as the second heart sound.

28. E ★   OHMS 2nd edn → pp432–3

During ventricular systole, the ventricles contract, forcing the atrioventricular valves to close. The papillary muscles which are attached to the valve cusps through the chordae tendinae also contract, preventing prolapse of the valves.

29. C ★ ★   OHMS 2nd edn → pp436–7

Almost all cases of mitral stenosis occur with rheumatic heart disease. Because the orifice of the mitral valve between the left atrium and the left ventricle is narrowed, the flow of blood through the valve is restricted. The resulting increase in left atrial pressure leads to atrial dilation. Consequently, pulmonary oedema develops. The left ventricle is usually small.

All the other conditions listed lead to ventricular hypertrophy.

30. C ★ OHMS 2nd edn → pp434–5

The Frank–Starling Law establishes that the force of cardiac contraction is related to end-diastolic volume, and this represents one of a range of adaptive mechanisms employed by the circulatory system in dealing with conditions resulting in cardiac overload (others include myocardial hypertrophy and activation of neurohumoral systems). The Frank–Starling Law is clinically important to understand, because, while arterial tone is regarded as the primary determinant of blood pressure, venous tone, has an impact on cardiac work and thus cardiac output. Pharmacological modulation of venous tone and thus venous return (e.g. by using nitrates) has an important role to play in reducing the amount of work done by the heart in conditions such as acute myocardial infarction and cardiac failure.

Kumar, V, Abbas, A, Fausto, N, & Aster, J (2010). *Robbins and Cotran Pathologic Basis of Disease*, 8th edn., pp533–4. London: Elsevier Saunders.

31. B ★ OHMS 2nd edn → pp442–3, 448–50

The vascular resistance is crucial for determining blood pressure. The resistance determines how hard the heart has to work to pump the blood around the body (afterload). The most important vessels for determining the blood pressure are the arterioles. This is because they are the smallest vessels in the arterial tree and are hence responsible for the resistance to flow. The reason that they have such an impact on peripheral vascular resistance can be explained by Poiseulle's law and the powerful effects of radius on flow together with the fact that they have a thick tunica media relative to luminal diameter and smooth muscle which regulates vessel diameter.

32. C ★ ★ OHMS 2nd edn → pp448–53

This is a case of class II haemorrhage where there is a loss of 15–30% of the blood volume. Clinical symptoms include tachycardia (rate >100 beats per minute). The decrease in pulses is a result of noradrenaline levels being increased, which causes an increased peripheral vascular resistance and a subsequent increase in the diastolic BP. The reduced circulating blood volume also leads to reduced cardiac stroke volume, lowering pulse pressure. The human body responds to acute haemorrhage by activating the following major physiological systems: the haematological, cardiovascular, renal, and neuroendocrine systems. The cardiovascular system initially responds to hypovolaemic shock by increasing the heart rate, increasing myocardial contractility, and constricting peripheral blood vessels. This response is secondary to an increased release of noradrenaline and decreased baseline vagal tone (regulated by the baroreceptors in the carotid arch, aortic arch, left atrium, and pulmonary vessels). The cardiovascular system also responds by redistributing blood to the brain, heart, and kidneys and away from skin, muscle, and GI tract.

The renal system responds to haemorrhagic shock by stimulating an increase in renin secretion from the juxtaglomerular apparatus. Renin converts angiotensinogen to angiotensin I, which subsequently is converted to angiotensin II by the lungs and liver. Angiotensin II has two main effects, both of which help to reverse haemorrhagic shock, vasoconstriction of arteriolar smooth muscle, and stimulation of aldosterone secretion by the adrenal cortex. Aldosterone is responsible for active sodium reabsorption and subsequent water conservation.

The neuroendocrine system responds to haemorrhagic shock by causing an increase in circulating antidiuretic hormone (ADH). ADH is released from the posterior pituitary gland in response to a decrease in BP (as detected by baroreceptors) and a decrease in the sodium concentration (as detected by osmoreceptors). ADH indirectly leads to an increased reabsorption of water and salt (NaCl) by the distal tubule, the collecting ducts, and the loop of Henle.

Nitric oxide (NO) and prostacyclin cause vasodilation in arteries and thus lower peripheral resistance.

33. C ★ ★ ★   OHMS 2nd edn → pp456–9;
OHCM → pp108, 130, 132–4

One of the main mechanisms by which beta blockers lower blood pressure is thought to be through inhibition of beta receptors on juxtaglomerular cells in the kidney which normally activate renin synthesis and thus the conversion of angiotensin I to angiotensin II (causes vasoconstriction and Na+ and water retention). Beta blockers have little effect on the heart at rest (but may be useful in certain clinical conditions where there is increased sympathetic drive e.g. myocardial infarction and CCF), and non-selective beta blockers may increase peripheral vascular resistance through inhibition of β-2 receptors on arteries (results in unopposed α receptor-mediated vasoconstriction). Conversely, certain newer beta blockers (e.g. carvedilol) have additional vasodilatory effects due to blockade of α-2 receptors.

Qi Che *et al.* (2009). Beta-blockers for hypertension: Are they going out of style? *Cleveland Clinical Journal Medicine*, **76**(9): 533–42.

34. B ★ ★   OHMS 2nd edn → pp460–3

Chronic hyperlipidaemia contributes to the production of oxygen-free radical species which have the effect of deactivating NO (an important endothelial relaxing factor), and are directly toxic to endothelial cells and smooth muscle cells. Lipid is ingested by macrophages which acquire a foamy appearance and release growth factors and cytokines, which amongst other effects increase leukocyte adhesion. Ultimately, the foamy macrophages die, releasing free lipid into the centre of the plaque, which contributes to plaque instability. T lymphocytes are central to the inflammatory response (not the B lymphocyte), releasing inflammatory cytokines such as interferon-γ, which further stimulate macrophages, endothelial cells, and smooth muscle cells.

Kumar, V, Abbas, A, Fausto, N, & Aster, J (2010). *Robbins and Cotran Pathologic Basis of Disease*, 8th edn., pp500–2. London: Elsevier Saunders.

35. E ★★   OHMS 2nd edn → pp464–71

Platelet degranulation is an important step in haemostasis, leading to release of vasoconstrictor agents and the recruitment of more platelets. Degranulation is brought about by TXA_2 and substances that increase intracellular calcium, which in turn leads to a change in platelet shape, exposure of glycoprotein IIB/IIIa, and further degranulation. ADP receptor blockers, e.g. clopidogrel, block the recruitment phase of thrombosis that is, in part, mediated by ADP secreted from activated platelets. GPIIb/IIIa inhibitors (e.g. abciximab) are particularly powerful anti-thrombotic agents with a significant risk of haemorrhage. NO donor drugs could potentially block the increase in intracellular calcium mediated by cGMP. Dipyridamole has the same effect on intracellular calcium through inhibition of phosphodiesterase and thus increased cAMP levels and lowered intracellular calcium. Aspirin inhibits cyclo-oxygenase, which controls the conversion of arachidonic acid to TXA_2; this, in turn, stimulates platelets to degranulate. This inhibition is irreversible and will persist for the lifetime of the platelet (8–10 days).

Kumar, V, Abbas, A, Fausto, N, & Aster, J (2010). *Robbins and Cotran Pathologic Basis of Disease*, 8th edn., pp117–21. London: Elsevier Saunders.

Extended Matching Questions

1. B ★★

Bronchospasm in patients with asthma is often triggered by exercise or cold air. Nocturnal symptoms suggest chronicity and a possible need for inhaled steroid therapy.

2. I ★★

This patient has significant risk factors for gastro-oesophageal reflux disease and although she may not be experiencing heartburn, it is likely that her symptoms are related to this.

3. J ★★

This young black male with constitutional symptoms, cough, dyspnoea, and suggestive chest radiograph changes, is likely to have sarcoidosis. He probably also has uveitis which further supports the diagnosis. Multiple other systems may also be involved.

4. A ★★

Allergic rhinitis with chronic postnasal discharge is an important (if underestimated) cause of chronic cough, and the presence of mucosal changes and polyps are suggestive of this. Allergen testing may be helpful in further management.

5. G ★★

The clinical presentation, age at diagnosis, and severity of symptoms can vary widely in cystic fibrosis. The combination of respiratory symptoms, malabsorption, and infertility are highly suggestive of cystic fibrosis, which is caused by defects in the gene for cystic fibrosis transmembrane conductance regulator (CFTR), a chloride channel.

General feedback on 1–5: OHMS 2nd edn → pp25, 400, 404; OHCM (8) p48

Kumar, V, Abbas, A, Fausto, N, & Aster, J (2010). *Robbins and Cotran Pathologic Basis of Disease*, 8th edn. pp465, 701. London: Elsevier Saunders.

6. D ★★

Atropine is an acetylcholine muscarinic receptor antagonist which prevents the slowing effect of parasympathetic (vagal) stimulation of the heart and can therefore be used in cases of bradycardia to help raise the heart rate in the short term to give enough time for definitive treatment such as surgical implementation of a cardiac pacemaker if this is not a reversible problem.

7. F ★★

Digoxin is a cardiac glycoside. It works by inhibiting the Na^+/K^+ -ATPase of cardiac myocytes leading to an increase in intracellular sodium ions. These are then exchanged for calcium ions leading to an increase in sarcoplasmic reticulum calcium stores, which therefore release more calcium ions when stimulated, leading to an increase in cardiac contractility. Digoxin also increases vagal activity via action on the central nervous system, thereby reducing heart rate. It is a very useful drug used to control heart rate in AF, especially if associated with heart failure.

8. K ★★

ACE inhibitors, such as lisinopril, exert their cardiovascular effects via the renin–angiotensin aldosterone system. They inhibit the enzyme that converts angiotensin I to angiotensin II, thus lowering salt retention and reducing vasoconstriction. In addition they mediate the metabolism of bradykinin, which is important when considering the side-effect profile. Increase of bradykinin in the bronchial mucosa is responsible for stimulation of the cough reflex and this is why persistant dry cough is a common side-effect in patients taking ACE inhibitors.

9. I ★★

Isosorbide mononitrate is a veno-selective nitric oxide donor. Nitric oxide is normally synthesized by vascular endothelium and causes local vasodilation. Therefore isosorbide mononitrate is a vasodilator, increasing the venous capacity, decreasing central venous pressure and thus reducing preload and cardiac workload.

10. J ★★

Lidocaine is a class Ib anti-arrhythmic that can be used to treat ventricular tachycardia.

General feedback on 6–10: OHMS 2nd edn → pp420–31, 434, 440, 457–8

CHAPTER 9
URINARY SYSTEM

The kidneys are responsible for maintaining the constant chemical composition of body fluids. This process begins with high-pressure filtration in specialized glomerular capillaries located in the renal cortex. The pressure filtration produces an ultrafiltrate of plasma made up of the water and smaller molecules. As the fluid passes along the renal tubules, water, electrolytes, and non-electrolytes are reabsorbed in the required amounts by a process of selective reabsorption. Some active secretion of unwanted substances also occurs. Following this reabsorption the remaining tubule fluid is passed to the renal pelvis and then down the ureters to the bladder for storage until voided.

The effort involved in all this is quite staggering. One-fifth of the daily cardiac output, about 1400 litres of whole blood, including 840 litres of plasma, passes through the kidneys. Of the 540 litres of plasma (the effective renal plasma flow) passing each day through the glomerular capillaries, one-fifth of the plasma water and small molecules are freely filtered at the glomeruli to produce about 170–180 litres per day of glomerular filtrate for the renal tubules. Since typically only 1–2 litres of urine are passed each day (that is about 1 ml per minute) 99% of the initial filtrate is reabsorbed as the fluid passes along the renal tubules. In oliguria, urine production can fall below 300ml per day, as in severe dehydration. In situations causing polyuria, urine output can rise to several litres per day, or more, as in excessive water intake or untreated diabetes mellitus or diabetes insipidus.

The kidney's main functions are osmoregulation, acid–base balance, and the excretion of waste products of metabolism, notably urea. Osmoregulation is mostly under endocrine control by antidiuretic hormone and the renin–angiotensin–aldosterone system. Acid–base balance is driven mainly by the carbon dioxide partial pressure in renal tubule cells, although kidneys work together with lungs and the control of breathing in overall acid–base balance. The kidney has important endocrine functions. It is the source of erythropoietin, the hormone that stimulates red blood cell production in hypoxia. The kidney is also important in calcium metabolism, producing the activated form of vitamin D that promotes calcium uptake from the gut.

If the renal filter becomes leaky, then plasma proteins may be lost from the body leading to hypoproteinaemia and oedema. If osmoregulation fails, then plasma volume will alter, usually rising, to produce increased venous volume, oedema, and raised arterial blood pressure. If glomerular filtration rate falls, the patient will develop acute or chronic renal failure with retention of sodium, potassium, water, acid, urea, and other substances. Clinically, the ureters and bladder have their own pathologies, including obstruction of urine flow, retention of urine, infections, and tumours. The causes and clinical importance of urinary system symptoms and signs, such as oliguria, polyuria, glycosuria, proteinuria, and haematuria, should be fully understood. ■

SINGLE BEST ANSWERS

1. In Fig. 9.1, which single anatomical term describes A on the CT taken through L1 of the vertebral column? ★

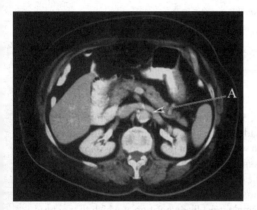

Fig. 9.1

A Hepatic portal vein

B Left renal artery

C Left renal vein

D Splenic vein

E Superior mesenteric artery

2. A 21-year-old man was kicked in the loins during a rugby game. He presents to A&E complaining of left loin tenderness. On examination he has a rigid anterior abdominal wall and a palpable loin mass. He develops ureteric colic, and urinalysis reveals haematuria with blood clots. CT shows that the left kidney is ruptured and that retroperitoneal blood is causing kidney tamponade. Which single structure prevents haemorrhage into the surrounding area, and extravasation to the opposite side? ★ ★

A Perirenal fascia

B Peritoneum

C Renal capsule

D Transversalis fascia

E Thoracolumbar fascia

3. A 52-year-old man with a 6-year history of gout has sudden onset of severe left flank pain that comes and goes in waves all night long. Urinalysis shows haematuria. He is sent for radiological investigation, which confirms a ureteric calculus ('kidney stone') that is seen at the tip of the transverse process of the 2nd lumbar vertebra. Which is the single most likely position at which the ureteric calculus has lodged? ★

A Major calyx

B Minor calyx

C Pelvic brim

D Pelvi-ureteric junction

E Vesico-ureteric junction

4. A 52-year-old previously healthy man presents to A&E pale, sweating, and vomiting. He complains of a sudden, severe colicky pain over his left flank that radiates over his left groin and testicle. Urinalysis reveals no glucose, nitrite, or protein, although blood is present. Urine microscopic analysis shows RBCs, but very few WBCs. What is the single most likely diagnosis? ★ ★

A Benign prostatic hypertrophy

B Prostatic carcinoma

C Pyelonephritis

D Transitional cell carcinoma of the bladder

E Ureteric calculus

5. A schematic of the normal glomerular filtration barrier (similar to that seen with the transmission electron microscope) is depicted in Fig. 9.2. Which single component of the glomerular filtration barrier is involved in minimal change disease (the commonest cause of nephrotic syndrome in children)? ★ ★ ★

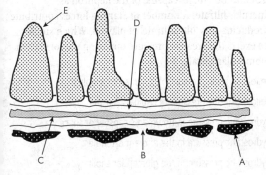

Fig. 9.2

A Endothelial cell

B Endothelial fenestration

C Glomerular basement membrane (lamina densa)

D Glomerular basement membrane (lamina rara externa)

E Podocyte foot process

6. A 73-year-old man complains of blood in his urine and intermittent sharp suprapubic pain on voiding which sometimes passes to the tip of his penis. He reports blood-stained urine and that pain occurs towards the end of micturition. When he passes urine the urine is initially clear and the blood and pain only appear towards the end of micturition. He obtains relief by lying down, but finds that after 10 minutes he feels the urge to urinate again. Which single condition is the most likely cause of these symptoms? ★ ★

A Benign prostatic hypertrophy

B Bladder calculus

C Transitional cell carcinoma of the bladder

D Stricture of the urethra

E Urinary tract infection

7. About 20% of the water and small molecules of plasma flowing though renal glomerular capillaries passes into Bowman's capsule of the nephron as glomerular filtrate. A number of Starling forces contribute to producing this 'ultrafiltrate' of plasma. Which single force exerts the greatest pressure opposing the formation of glomerular filtrate? ★

A Colloid osmotic pressure of Bowman's capsule fluid

B Colloid osmotic pressure of capillary plasma

C Hydrostatic pressure in Bowman's capsule or space

D Hydrostatic pressure in the efferent arteriole

E Hydrostatic pressure in the glomerular capillary

8. Substances such as inulin (or for routine, and less accurate, clinical measurement, endogenous creatinine) have special properties that make them suitable for the measurement of glomerular filtration rate (GFR). Their molecular size means that they are freely filtered at the glomerulus and once in the tubular fluid they remain there until passed out of the body in the final urine. This allows measurement of the volume of plasma from which inulin is removed (or cleared) in one minute and this is the GFR. The 'clearance value' for inulin is therefore the GFR (125ml/min). The normal (non-diabetic) value for glucose clearance is 0ml/min. Which is the single most likely explanation for this observation? ★

A Filtered glucose is metabolized by the tubule cells

B Filtered glucose is reabsorbed from the tubule fluid

C Glucose is actively secreted into the tubule fluid

D Glucose is not normally filtered at the glomerulus

E Glucose is synthesized by the tubule cells

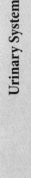

9. Fig. 9.3 shows a renal nephron with five regions labelled I to V. Which single region of those labelled is essential for the production of urine that is both more dilute and more concentrated than plasma? ★ ★

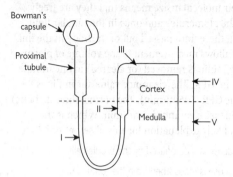

Fig. 9.3

A I

B II

C III

D IV

E V

10. A 35-year-old woman, who is keen on dieting, has become slightly confused in recent days. She collapses at home and falls down the stairs. She bumps her head on the wall and is briefly unconscious. When she recovers consciousness she appears uninjured but is more confused and her partner takes her to A&E where she is kept in overnight. The admitting staff note that she is producing high volumes of very dilute urine on admission, but both urine volume and osmolarity are close to normal the following morning when she appears well and is discharged. Which is the single most likely cause of the large volume of dilute urine produced by the patient? ★ ★

A Diabetes insipidus due to lack of antidiuretic hormone (ADH) secretion

B Diabetes insipidus due to lack of antidiuretic hormone (ADH) synthesis

C Increased cortisol secretion

D Renal insensitivity of ADH (nephrogenic diabetes insipidus)

E Water intoxication

11. One of the main functions of the kidney is to regulate the volume and osmolarity of extracellular fluid. The kidney achieves this by varying the volume of water excreted in the urine and varying the reabsorption of sodium in the distal tubules, allowing excess sodium to be excreted. These processes regulating volume and osmolarity show some overlap. Reduction in circulating blood volume stimulates cardiovascular stretch receptors in the great veins and right atrium, and any fall in arterial pressure will stimulate the arterial baroreceptors. Decreased plasma volume results in increased sympathetic output from the medulla of the brain. In the kidney this causes constriction of renal efferent arterioles and causes renin release by the juxtaglomerular apparatus (JGA). Renin activates the renin-angiotensin-aldosterone system. Which single most important effect does aldosterone have on the kidney? ★

A Activates Na^+-K^+ ATPase in the collecting duct

B Decreases secretion of K^+ into the urine

C Down-regulates epithelial sodium channel (ENaC)

D Inserts aquaporin II channels into distal tubule and collecting duct epithelial cells

E Stimulates Na^+–H^+ exchange in the proximal tubule

12. If a patient suffering from respiratory acidosis (due to hypoventilation and carbon dioxide retention) lasting several days has his/her acid–base balance corrected too quickly (perhaps by inappropriate mechanical ventilation) s/he may develop a 'rebound' metabolic alkalosis, which, untreated, can persist for 1–3 days. Which single renal mechanism is most likely to be responsible for the metabolic alkalosis in the patient described above?

A Readjustment of the tubular fluid HPO_4^{2-} / $H_2PO_4^-$ buffer system

B Reduction in free protons in tubular fluid

C Reduction in partial pressure of CO_2 in tubule cells

D Reduction in reabsorption of filtered bicarbonate

E Reduction in the production of NH_4^+ in the tubular fluid

13. A 71-year-old man complains of dysuria and incontinence of urine. He also notes a 1-month history of severe lower back pain and pain in his right thigh. He was diagnosed 8 years previously with prostate cancer, for which he was treated with surgery alone. He was subsequently lost to clinical follow-up. The attending doctor wisely performs a digital rectal examination (DRE) and tests perineal sensation, revealing loss of perianal sensation and poor anal tone. Which is the single most likely underlying cause of his symptoms? ★ ★

A Faecal impaction secondary to opioid analgesic use and severe constipation

B Prostatic adenocarcinoma involving the bladder neck causing obstruction and overflow incontinence

C Prostatic adenocarcinoma metastasis to the lumbar spine causing damage to L2–4 nerve roots

D Prostatic adenocarcinoma metastasis to the lumbar spine causing damage to S2–4 nerve roots

E Prostatic adenocarcinoma metastasis to pelvic lymph nodes causing damage to the hypogastric sympathetic plexus

14. A 65-year-old man undergoes an elective right hemicolectomy for a caecal adenocarcinoma, for which he receives antibiotic prophylaxis. While under anaesthetic he experiences a significant hypotensive episode. On the second post-operative day he develops oliguria and a rising serum creatinine. Which is the single most likely cause of the acute renal failure in this scenario? ★ ★

A Acute glomerulonephritis

B Acute interstitial nephritis

C Acute obstructive uropathy

D Acute renal vein thrombosis

E Acute tubular necrosis

15. A 49-year-old woman with insulin-dependent diabetes mellitus (IDDM) presents with recurrent fever, right-sided flank pain, and malaise. Investigations reveal proteinuria, haematuria and pyuria, normal serum creatinine and right-sided hydronephrosis (obstructing lesion at right ureteropelvic junction). She also reports having a long history of lower back pain, for which she regularly uses high doses of analgesics. Which is the single most likely cause of her clinical presentation? ★ ★ ★ ★

A Congenital pelvi-ureteric junction obstruction

B Renal calculus

C Renal papillary necrosis

D Retroperitoneal fibrosis

E Urothelial carcinoma of ureter

EXTENDED MATCHING QUESTIONS

Urology

From the option list choose the single most appropriate substance for each of the following statements. Each option may be used once, more than once, or not at all.

A Acetazolamide

B Amiloride

C Amlodipine

D Bendroflumethiazide

E Furosemide

F Hydralazine

G Mannitol

H Ramipril

I Spironolactone

J Verapamil

1. The diuresis produced by this substance, which acts in the thick-walled ascending limb of the loop of Henle, may cause a patient to develop a metabolic alkalosis. ★

2. This substance produces a modest diuresis by antagonising aldosterone receptors in the distal tubule and collecting duct of the renal nephron. ★ ★

3. This substance is no longer used clinically as a diuretic but is still used to manage the effects of high altitude. ★ ★

4. This substance is sometimes used in renal transplant surgery to check if the donor kidney is responding to the recipient's blood supply. ★ ★

5. This substance produces diuresis by inhibiting sodium chloride co-transport on tubule cell apical membrane in the distal tubule. It is commonly used in the management of hypertension. ★ ★

Single Best Answers

1. C ★   OHMS 2nd edn → pp474–6

This is the left renal vein, which is longer than the right renal vein. The kidneys are found between T12 and L3 and so a CT through L1 bisects both kidneys. Note how the vessel passes from the kidney anterior to the circular aorta and drains to the inferior vena cava, which is on the right side of the aorta. The renal veins are normally anterior to the renal arteries and the ureters are positioned more posteriorly within the hilum of the kidney. The splenic vein is found more anteriorly, grooving the posterosuperior pancreas.

Remember that CT scans are orientated as if viewed from the feet, so that left is on the right side of the image.

2. A ★★   OHMS 2nd edn → p474

The perirenal fascia (Gerota's fascia) is a membranous layer that surrounds the kidney, the adrenal glands, and the perirenal fat. It is continuous with the transversalis fascia laterally; superiorly it blends with the fascia of the diaphragm, and it fuses over the renal vessels medially. Only inferiorly does it remain relatively open as it surrounds the ureters.

Gerota's fascia is also important when staging renal carcinoma, where extension of the tumour beyond the fascia indicates Stage 4 disease.

3. D ★   OHMS 2nd edn → p478

Fig. 9.4 of an intravenous pyelogram (IVP) shows normal urinary tract structures: A, major calyx; B, minor calyx; C, pelvic brim; D pelvi-ureteric junction; E vesico-ureteric junction. Renal stones can form and can become located in the renal calyces (A and B). However, the scenario describes ureteric colic, the pain felt by excessive distension and peristalsis of the ureter. There are three constrictions along the ureters, which are potential sites of obstruction. The pelvi-ureteric junction is where the renal pelvis narrows to form the ureteric tube, and is anterior to the transverse process of L2. The pelvic brim (C) is where the ureter descends over the bifurcation of the common iliac arteries, anterior to the sacroiliac joint. The vesico-ureteric junction (E) is the one-way flap valve located where the ureter enters the bladder, medial to the iliac spine. These three areas need to be examined carefully when locating a calculus.

When the stone is high in the ureter the pain signals will run along the ilioinguinal and the iliohypogastric nerves, which enter the cord at T12 and L1. The ureteric pain is therefore referred to the skin dermatome associated with the relevant parts of T12 and L1 sensory inflow. In this case these will be the loin region. As the stone descends the ureter the patient may start to feel the pain descend over the groin and into scrotum or labia majora ('from loin to groin') areas. This is because the pain is now reaching the cord via the genitofemoral nerve, which innervates the lower ureter and enters the cord at L1 and L2. The pain is therefore referred to a different sensory dermatome region.

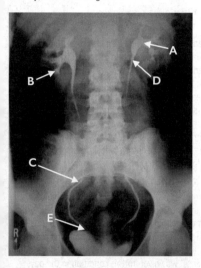

Fig. 9.4

4. E ★ ★   OHMS 2nd edn → p478

An ureteric calculus, which is gradually forced down, or is stuck in the ureter, can cause agonizing pain which is intermittent and which is referred from the spinal segments that supply the ureter (T11–L2). The pain is carried by iliohypogastric, ilioinguinal and genitofemoral nerves, down over the flank towards the genitals. It may sometimes also project over the anteromedial thigh (femoral branch of genitofemoral nerve).

The presence of a ureteric calculus can be confirmed by an abdominal X-ray and IV-pyelogram. Ureteric calculi will normally be seen in one of the three classical anatomical locations: at the renal pelvis; at the pelvic brim; or at the vesico-ureteric junction (see feedback to SBA 3). A CT scan of kidneys, ureter, and bladder (CT KUB) would usually be performed on such patients to confirm the presence and location of a calculus.

All of the other conditions listed can cause haematuria, but the symptoms will usually evolve gradually instead of showing the sudden onset described in the scenario. Pyelonephritis can occasionally present with pain over the loin, although it is usually referred to the back and urinalysis would show increased nitrite and leukocytes.

5. E ★★★ OHMS 2nd edn → pp482–3; OHCM(8) → pp296–7

Minimal change disease is the commonest cause of nephrotic syndrome (NS) in children (but also seen in 20% of adults with NS), who only undergo renal biopsy if there is no response to empirical steroid therapy. Light microscopy is essentially normal, but electron microscopy (EM) reveals diffuse effacement (or fusion) of the podocyte foot processes. Interestingly, a hereditary form of congenital NS (Finnish type) has been found to be associated with a mutation in the nephrin gene (nephrin is a component of the slit diaphragm which lies between podocyte foot processes) and results in minimal change glomerular morphology.

Nephrotic syndrome is characterized by the presence of all of the following: oedema, marked proteinuria, and hypoalbuminaemia. Heavy proteinuria is the cause of the reduced plasma albumin. This loss, in turn, reduces the colloid osmotic pressure of plasma, which impedes the normal reabsorption of tissue fluid formed by pressure filtration in tissue capillaries, leading to tissue oedema. The term 'minimal change disease' was given to this condition in the days when light microscopy alone could not distinguish the tissue abnormalities. These abnormalities became evident with the introduction of the higher resolutions available with electron microscopy.

Kumar, V, Abbas, A, Fausto, N, & Aster, J (2010). *Robbins and Cotran Pathologic Basis of Disease*, 8th edn, pp923–6. London: Elsevier Saunders.

Typical symptoms of a bladder stone include intermittent pain and terminal haematuria (haematuria towards the end of micturition). The bleeding is caused at the end of micturition as the urine empties from around the calculus. Lying down will move the stone from the internal urethral orifice. The pain is typically felt suprapubically and is referred down to the tip of the penis because the calculus is lodged in the inferior portion of the bladder. This is inferior to the 'pelvic pain line' and so pain will be referred to S2–4. The roof of the bladder and the ureters lie superiorly and will refer pain to T11–L2. Fig. 9.5 of an abdominal X-ray shows a radio-opaque filling defect in the left side of the bladder (the stone).

Urinary System

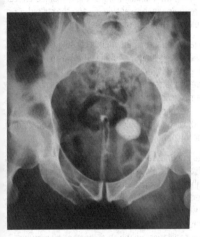

Fig. 9.5

The physical examination of this patient should include a rectal examination to rule out benign prostatic hypertrophy (A). A transitional cell carcinoma of the bladder (C) would also produce haematuria, but the tumour would be less likely to shift with body posture, and diagnosis would be by biopsy obtained during cystoscopy. Blood at the beginning of urine flow is characteristic of a urethral source, such as urethral stricture (D). An enlarged prostate can obstruct the urethra, preventing the bladder from completely emptying and leading to stone formation. Bleeding anywhere in the urinary tract, for example as a consequence of a urinary tract infection (E), especially in the mid- or upper urinary tract, can cause total haematuria. In total haematuria, mixing of blood and urine causes uniform red coloration of urine throughout urine flow.

The pelvic pain line divides pelvic structures on the basis of whether their visceral afferent fibres pass back to the CNS via the thoracolumbar route taken by the sympathetic outflow (above the line) or the sacral route taken by the parasympathetic outflow (below the line). Pain sensation is less well perceived from structures below the pelvic pain line.

7. B ★   OHMS 2nd edn → p486

The net filtration pressure for the formation of glomerular filtrate is the hydrostatic pressure in the capillary (E), less the combined effects of hydrostatic pressure in Bowman's capsule (C) and the colloid osmotic pressure of plasma (B), both of which oppose filtration.

Normally, the hydrostatic pressure in Bowman's capsule is kept low, since filtrate fluid flows away along the tubule. The plasma colloid osmotic pressure (B) exerted by the plasma proteins is the larger of these two forces opposing filtration. The large size of plasma proteins prevents their passage out of the plasma compartment during filtration, and the colloid osmotic pressure of the fluid in Bowman's capsule (A) will be negligible and its effects are omitted from the equation for the net filtration pressure.

Glomerular capillaries are unusual in having both afferent and efferent arterioles. Hydrostatic pressure in the afferent arteriole of the glomerulus is higher than for a normal arteriole, but hydrostatic pressure in the efferent arteriole (D) is not. An important aspect of renal function is the way that afferent and efferent arterioles vary their vascular resistance to autoregulate the high and constant pressure in glomerular capillaries, on which a constant glomerular filtration rate depends.

8. B ★   OHMS 2nd edn → p490

Glucose is freely filtered at the glomerulus, so 125ml of plasma water containing glucose at the plasma concentration pass into the nephrons each minute. Thus 125ml/min of plasma are 'cleared' of glucose, but normally all of that glucose is reabsorbed back into plasma, most of it in the proximal tubule, and none appears in the final urine.

The renal clearance of a substance, $C = (U \times V)/P$

Where:

    C = is the plasma volume cleared (in ml/min),

    U = urine concentration of the substance,

V = urine production (ml/min), and

P = plasma concentration of the substance.

For glucose, final urine concentration is normally at zero, so C, the clearance, must also be equal to zero. In diabetes mellitus, the plasma concentration of glucose rises above normal values. When it reaches about 10mmolesL⁻¹ the transport maximum for the active reabsorption process in the renal tubule is exceeded. Unabsorbed glucose now remains in the tubule, increasing the solute concentration and attracting water. The excess glucose causes the osmotic diuresis and glycosuria from which diabetes mellitus takes its name.

Inulin, used historically as a marker to measure GFR, is a polysaccharide originally derived from *dahlia* tubers. It is freely filtered at the glomerulus, neither reabsorbed nor secreted into the tubule, and neither synthesized nor metabolized along the tubule. These five special properties mean that all the inulin that is filtered ('cleared') from the plasma will appear in the final urine, and the option list is derived from these properties. Newer, more sensitive, methods for GFR measurement now exist, among them the use of chromium[51] ethylenediamine tetraacetic acid.

9. B ★ ★   OHMS 2nd edn → pp492–5

The area labelled II is the thick-walled segment of the ascending limb of the loop of Henle, sometimes called the 'diluting segment' of the nephron. It pumps sodium chloride into the surrounding medullary interstitium, but water is effectively unable to follow as the water permeability of the thick ascending limb is low. Consequently, the tubular fluid entering the distal tubule is more dilute than the cortical interstitium, which has the same osmolarity as plasma. In the absence of antidiuretic hormone (ADH), this, the default state of the kidney, produces final urine which removes excess water from the body.

In conditions of body water conservation, ADH secretion will rise and water will now be reabsorbed from distal tubule (III) and from cortical (IV) as well as medullary (V) regions of the collecting duct. To produce urine more concentrated than plasma, water is reabsorbed as the collecting duct passes through the gradient of osmolarity established across the medulla. The source of the additional interstitial sodium chloride required to establish this gradient is the thick-walled, ascending limb of the loop of Henle About 65%–70% of all the filtered salt and water are reabsorbed in the proximal tubule (I) without any alteration to osmolarity of tubular fluid.

10. E ★ ★   OHMS 2nd edn → p494

Classic diabetes insipidus (DI) results from the loss of the ability to produce concentrated urine. The result is production of up to 18 litres per day of very dilute urine. There are two main forms of DI: cranial DI, in which either the hypothalamus fails to synthesize ADH, or the posterior pituitary fails to release the ADH into the blood, and nephrogenic DI, in which the V2 cells of the collecting duct become insensitive to ADH action. Another possible cause of high levels of urine production (not perhaps as high as 18 litres per day) is excessive water consumption leading to water intoxication (E). This can be the result of intentional or emotional water drinking leading to hyponatraemia. The low plasma sodium can lead to mental confusion, coma and even death. Some dieting regimens which involve drinking large amounts of water can cause water intoxication if electrolyte balance is not properly maintained.

In the above scenario, both cranial (A and B) and nephrogenic (D) DI are ruled out because following admission with a high urine output, the patient's urine output falls because of her reduced opportunity to continue to consume large volumes of water unobserved by hospital staff. A patient with true DI would maintain high levels of urine output even if water intake is restricted and may in consequence become acutely unwell. Head trauma can cause DI by severing the infundibular stalk, cutting off ADH secretion by the posterior pituitary. The increased urine flow would develop rather slowly, producing high urine output by the time of discharge from hospital. Low (not high as in option C) levels of cortisol, as in Addison's disease, can also cause hyponataemia.

11. A ★   OHMS 2nd edn → pp500–1

The enzyme renin converts inactive circulating angiotensinogen into active angiotensin I. Angiotensin converting enzyme (ACE) converts angiotensin I to angiotensin II. Angiotensin II triggers aldosterone release from the adrenal cortex (zona glomerulosa cells).

Aldosterone promotes Na^+ reabsorption in the distal tubule and collecting duct of the kidney nephrons. It does this by activating and increasing transcription of the Na^+-K^+ ATPase of the basolateral membrane and up-regulating the ENaC (epithelial sodium channel) of the apical membrane of tubule cells. The net effect of this is to also increase urinary K^+ loss. The Na^+ reabsorption leads to salt and then water retention, restoring plasma volume.

Note that K^+ secretion into the urine K is increased (not decreased as in B) and that ENaC is up-regulated, not down-regulated as in (C). Antidiuretic hormone (ADH) is responsible for increasing water reabsorption by insertion of vesicles containing aquaporin II (D) into the apical membrane of distal tubular and collecting duct epithelial cells. Na^+–H^+ exchange in the proximal tubule (E) is regulated primarily by the prevailing partial pressure of carbon dioxide (PCO_2) within tubule cells, proton excretion increasing as PCO_2 rises.

Angiotensin II is a potent vasoconstrictor responsible for efferent arteriole vasoconstriction in response to renin release (via ACE-mediated conversion of angiotensin I to II) as well as stimulating Na^+–H^+ exchange in the proximal tubule. A low perfusion pressure in the renal glomerulus is also detected by the JGA and this will also increase renin release.

12. E ★ ★   OHMS 2nd edn → pp502–3

Hypoventilation results in arterial hypoxaemia and hypercapnia. The retention of CO_2 causes a respiratory acidosis and, if this persists for several days, full renal compensation for this acidosis will develop. In this compensation the rise in tubule cell PCO_2 leads to the increased secretion of protons into the tubular fluid with an accompanying diffusion of HCO_3^- back into plasma. The concentration of free protons in tubular fluid rises, the phosphate buffer system moves to the more acid state, and deamination of glutamine produces ammonia which reacts with protons to form ammonium ion which effectively traps protons in the tubular fluid. When the respiratory acidosis is corrected, all of these mechanisms reverse (as described in options A to E) and all except ammonium ion production (E) will correct very promptly. Ammonia production, which can increase renal acid excretion from 60 to 600 mmoles per day, requires the induction of enzymes. These enzymes can take 1–3 days to build up the maximum level of renal compensation and they can take many hours to reverse. Therefore, slowness of the reduction in the production of ammonium ion is the cause of the rebound metabolic alkalosis, since more protons are now excreted (and more HCO_3^- restored to the plasma) than normal acid–base balance demands. Remember that filtered HCO_3^- is not reabsorbed in the proper sense. Tubular HCO_3^- is broken down by protons secreted by tubule cells, and newly produced HCO_3^- moves back into plasma. Remember, too, that both proton secretion and effective HCO_3^- reabsorption are proportional to tissue PCO_2.

13. D ★ ★   OHMS 2nd edn → pp504–5; OHCM(8) → pp470, 650–1

The clinical scenario describes the symptoms of cauda equina syndrome, a medical emergency. A digital rectal examination (DRE) and assessment of lower limb motor and sensory function (including perineal sensation) is mandatory in any patient presenting with back pain and bowel or bladder symptoms. His serum PSA (prostate-specific antigen) is also likely to be elevated, given the history of prostatic cancer. In this patient, the most likely scenario is that of metastatic disease in the lumbar spine, resulting in damage to the S2–4 nerve roots which supply the pudendal nerve. The pudendal nerve is important for voluntary contraction of the external urethral sphincter and for sensing bladder filling, pain, and urinary flow. The pudendal nerve also provides sensory information from anal and perineal muscles and skin as well as erectile tissues of the perineum, including the penis or clitoris.

While constipation and faecal impaction (A) may present with urinary incontinence, there should not be any symptoms referable to the limbs or loss of perineal sensation or anal tone. Similarly for bladder outlet obstruction (B), which is more likely to present simply with acute or chronic urinary retention. The L2–4 nerve roots (C) do not mediate any components of the micturition reflex. Damage to the hypogastric plexus (E) could conceivably cause detrusor muscle contraction and relaxation of the internal urethral sphincter (via loss of sympathetic outflow) and urinary incontinence, but this would not adequately explain the pain in the lower back and thigh, nor loss of perineal sensation etc.

14. E ★ ★ OHMS 2nd edn → p506; OHCM(8) → pp298, 306–7

Acute tubular necrosis (ATN) is the commonest cause of acute renal failure (ARF), accounting for 50% of cases of ARF in hospitalized patients, and is often related to ischaemia (as in this case), but can also be caused by nephrotoxins (such as antibiotics, radiographic contrast agents, NSAIDs, etc.).

The history makes acute glomerulonephritis (A) unlikely, but the administration of an antibiotic pre-operatively makes acute interstitial nephritis (B) a possibility, although this usually presents a few days to 2 weeks after drug exposure and is characterized by fever, eosinophilia, skin rash, and oliguria. With any surgical intervention in the abdomen or pelvis, the possibility of iatrogenic damage to the ureters causing acute urinary obstruction (C) should be borne in mind, but this would have to be bilateral (or unilateral in the case of a single functioning kidney) to cause ARF. Acute renal vein thrombosis (D) is usually seen in the setting of nephrotic syndrome, but may occur in patients with altered renal blood flow (e.g. severe gastrointestinal fluid loss in neonates), after trauma, or in other conditions causing a hypercoagulable state. It may result in ARF if both renal veins are affected.

15. C ★ ★ ★ ★ OHMS 2nd edn → pp508–9; OHCM(8) → pp640–3, 646

Renal papillary necrosis is considered to be a consequence of ischaemia within the renal medulla and pyramids and has several well-documented associations, the commonest of which are infection, obstruction, diabetes mellitus, analgesic abuse, and sickle-cell disease. Over 50% of patients have two or more of these associated conditions.

Congenital ureteropelvic obstruction (A) is the commonest cause of unilateral hydronephrosis in the paediatric age group, where boys are affected twice as often as girls. Renal calculi (B) can present similarly, but affect men more often than women, and with a peak age of 20 to 40 years. The radiographic appearance of nephrolithiasis (renal calculi or kidney stones) is often quite distinctive, and one could expect to find a metabolic condition predisposing to stone formation (e.g. gout, cystinuria). Retroperitoneal fibrosis (D) typically causes bilateral hydronephrosis (unilateral in about 20%) and pathological associations include HLA-B27 haplotype, elevated serum IgG4, malignancy, and methysergide or ergot-derivative use. Urothelial (or transitional cell) carcinoma (E) of the ureter would also be a consideration and should be excluded by performing urine cytology and ureteroscopic biopsy.

Extended Matching Questions

1. E ★

Furosemide is a loop diuretic and acts primarily by blocking Na^+ - K^+ -$2Cl^-$ pumping at the luminal border of tubule cells of the thick-walled ascending limb of the loop of Henle. Na^+ (and K^+) remain within the tubule and these ions attract water osmotically to produce an increased urine flow. Na^+ reabsorption in the distal tubule has a different mechanism from that in the thick-walled ascending limb. The increased Na^+ concentration of fluid delivered to the distal tubule stimulates increased Na^+ reabsorption there, in this case in exchange for K^+ or H^+— a mechanism mediated by aldosterone action. This causes further K^+ loss. The K^+ losses can lead to hypokalaemia. The amounts of K^+ or H^+ secreted during Na^+ reabsorption in the distal tubule depend on the relative abundance of the two ion species. When plasma and interstitial K^+ are low then more H^+ than normal is secreted in exchange for Na^+ by this mechanism. The loss of H^+ from the body in the urine results in metabolic alkalosis. Since about 30% of the filtered load of sodium is reabsorbed in the thick-walled ascending limb, loop diuretics exert a more powerful effect.

2. I ★★

Spironolactone is a potassium-sparing diuretic and acts by blocking aldosterone receptors in the distal tubule and collecting duct. Aldosterone promotes Na^+ reabsorption, so when its action is prevented Na^+ remains in the tubule, attracts water, and produces a diuresis. However, only about 2–3% of the filtered load of Na^+ is reabsorbed in the distal tubule, and so any diuretic effect is modest. Potassium-sparing diuretics can be combined with loop or thiazide diuretics. The combined effect is to produce a good diuresis and to minimize the loss of K$^+$ and consequent alkalosis produced by distal tubule actions (see Question 1). Amiloride is another example of another potassium-sparing diuretic, in this case acting by blocking the luminal sodium channels activated by aldosterone binding to its receptors.

3. A ★★

Acetazolamide is a carbonic anhydrase (CA) inhibitor. This enzyme catalyses the formation of carbonic acid from carbon dioxide and water. The carbonic acid partially dissociates to form protons and bicarbonate, which together form an important buffer system. Large amounts of bicarbonate are filtered into the renal tubules and rather than being simply reabsorbed, the bicarbonate is annihilated (broken down into water and carbon dioxide) by protons secreted into the tubule lumen and fresh bicarbonate is synthesized within tubule cells and passed into the plasma. Blocking CA prevents this effective reabsorption. Bicarbonate remains in the tubule and attracts water to produce a modest diuresis. Loss of bicarbonate (a base) can produce a metabolic acidosis. This effect helps counterbalance the respiratory alkalosis which develops at high altitude. The respiratory alkalosis occurs because low inspired oxygen partial pressure leads to hypoxia, causing increased ventilation so that carbon dioxide is lost from the body and plasma bicarbonate falls.

4. G ★★

Ultimately, all diuretics produce an increase in solute concentration in renal tubular fluid. These solutes attract water osmotically and cause an increased urine flow. Osmotic diuretics exert this solute effect directly, without interfering with renal metabolism. Mannitol is one such substance. It is freely filtered and then remains in the tubular fluid producing an osmotic diuresis. When connecting a donated kidney to a recipient's blood vessels and before joining the ureter to the transplanted kidney, mannitol can be injected into the recipient's arterial system supplying the kidney. The mannitol produces a prompt flow of urine, which demonstrates that the renal function is likely to be normal. Mannitol-induced diuresis can also be used in an attempt to reduce raised intracranial pressure.

5. D ★★

Bendroflumethiazide, as the name indicates, is a thiazide diuretic. This class of diuretic acts by inhibiting Na$^+$-Cl$^-$ co-transport in the early distal tubule of the nephron. Like loop diuretics, thiazides also cause potassium loss, but their diuretic action, while greater than that of potassium sparing diuretics, is weaker than that of loop diuretics.

General feedback on 1–5: OHMS 2nd edn → p498

CHAPTER 10

DIGESTIVE SYSTEM

In essence, the digestive system is a four-layered tube that extends from mouth to anus. Its main purpose is the enzymatic digestion of food to produce smaller molecules that can then be absorbed into the body as nutrients. To achieve this the gut is regionally specialized to enable the serial processing of food and the absorption of food, water, and electrolytes as materials pass along the bowel.

The four layers of the bowel are:

1) A mucosa surrounding the lumen, made up of a specialized epithelium, a lamina propria of connective tissue, and a layer of smooth muscle—the muscularis mucosae.

2) A submucosa, a layer of connective tissue often containing glands.

3) A muscularis externa with, usually, an inner layer of circular smooth muscle and an outer layer of longitudinal smooth muscle, responsible for peristalsis.

4) An outermost layer of epithelia and connective tissue called the adventitia, or serosa if the bowel is enfolded by peritoneum or mesentery.

Despite this common arrangement along the whole bowel, the four layers show characteristic differences in each region, reflecting the specialization of function found in the oesophagus, stomach, small intestine, and large intestine. Indeed, differences can also be seen between the subdivisions of these regions.

Associated with the gut are two major organs, the liver and the pancreas. The liver processes the newly absorbed nutrients passed to it from the bowel by the hepatic portal vein. It also produces bile, which is eventually secreted into the bowel. Bile, stored and modified between meals in the gallbladder, is a vehicle for the removal from the body of conjugated bile pigments from the breakdown of haemoglobin. Bile also delivers to the small intestine the bile salts essential for the proper digestion of fats. The pancreas is divided into an exocrine pancreas, whose secretions of pro-enzymes, bicarbonate, and water pass to the small intestine to neutralize gastric acid and support digestion, and islets of endocrine tissue that produce insulin, glucagon and somatostatin—hormones concerned, in part, with glucose regulation.

Control of bowel function is complex. There are two nerve plexuses within the gut's four-layered structure, and digestion—both in terms of the bowel and of liver and pancreatic function—is controlled by local and remote autonomic neural signals and by endocrine (and, in some cases, paracrine) mechanisms. In such a complex system there is much that can go wrong. The bowel is a portal for the entry of pathogens of all sorts, and the barrier functions of gastric acid and the gut's own immune system may be overcome by infection with micro-organisms or infestation with parasites. Gut epithelia contain rapidly dividing cells, making many regions of the bowel prone to malignancy. Obstruction of the common bile duct or excessive gastric acid secretion can both cause major problems. It is important know the causes and clinical significance of the many symptoms and signs of gastrointestinal disturbance such as haematemasis and melaena, diarrhoea and malabsorption, constipation, jaundice, discoloration of urine, and anaemia, as well as the possible causes of abdominal pain. ■

SINGLE BEST ANSWERS

1. Which single structure is usually located most posteriorly in the free border of the lesser omentum, anterior to the epiploic foramen? ★ ★

A Bile duct

B Common hepatic artery

C Hepatic artery proper

D Hepatic vein

E Portal vein

2. A 36-year-old man is found to have a mass approximately 3cm in diameter in the right scrotum. The hernia sac lies superior and medial to the pubic tubercle and lateral to the inferior epigastric vessels. The patient had not undergone any previous surgery. Which is the single most likely diagnosis? ★ ★

A Acquired hernia

B Direct hernia

C Femoral hernia

D Indirect hernia

E Umbilical hernia

3. At surgery, the presence of taeniae coli helps to distinguish the large bowel from the small bowel. Which single histological layer of the bowel forms the taeniae coli of the large intestine? ★ ★

A Circular layer of muscularis propria

B Longitudinal layer of muscularis propria

C Mucosa

D Muscularis mucosae

E Submucosa

4. A 30-year-old man complains of diarrhoea, fatigue, and abdominal pain. Coeliac disease is suspected and at endoscopy duodenal biopsies are taken to confirm the diagnosis. Which single group of structures is found uniquely in the duodenum? ★

A Brunner's glands

B Goblet cells

C Paneth's cells

D Peyer's patches

E Villi

5. A 51-year-old woman with a 20-year history of heavy drinking suffers from violent vomiting followed by haematemesis. Her abdomen is swollen, and examination confirms that she has hepatosplenomegaly. Examination of her stools shows no evidence of melaena. Which is the single most likely cause of the haematemesis? ★

A Barrett's oesophagus

B Hiatus hernia

C Oesophageal stricture

D Oesophageal squamous cell carcinoma

E Oesophageal variceal rupture

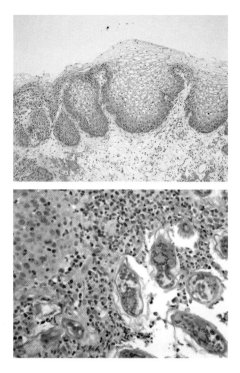

Plate 1 (Fig. 1.2 a and b)

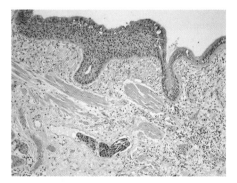

Plate 2 (Fig. 5.1)

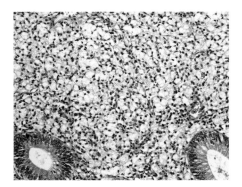

Plate 3 (Fig. 5.2)

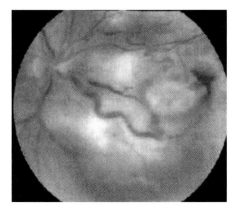

Plate 4 (Fig. 5.3)

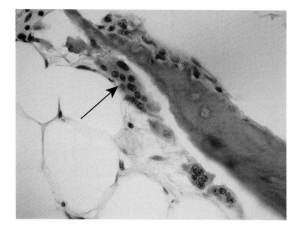

Plate 5 (Fig. 7.1)

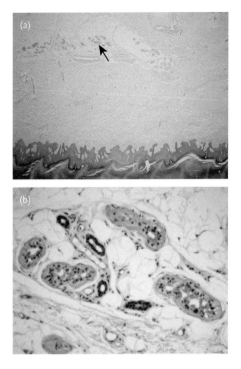

Plate 6 (Fig. 7.2 a and b)

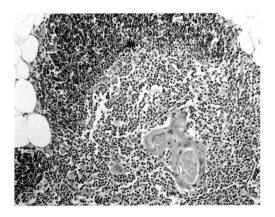

Plate 7 (Fig. 14.1)

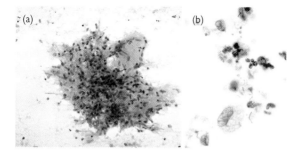

Plate 8 (Fig. 14.2 a and b)

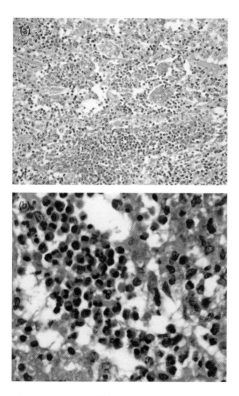

Plate 9 (Fig. 14.3 a and b)

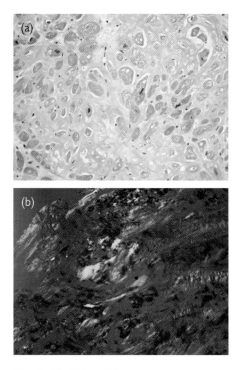

Plate 10 (Fig. 15.1 a and b)

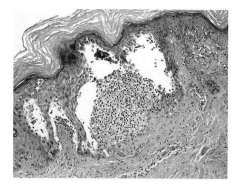

Plate 11 (Fig. 15.4)

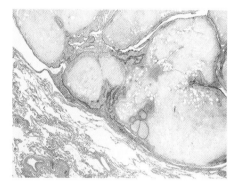

Plate 12 (Fig. 15.5b)

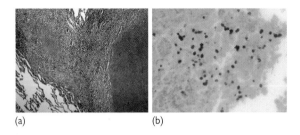

(a) (b)

Plate 13 (Fig. 15.6 a and b)

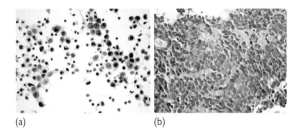

(a) (b)

Plate 14 (Fig. 15.7 a and b)

6. A gastric ulcer on the lesser curvature of the pyloric antrum of the stomach perforates. There is gastrointestinal bleeding when the ulcer erodes one of the underlying blood vessels. Which single artery is most likely to be eroded in this case? ★

A Gastroduodenal artery

B Left gastric artery

C Left gastroepiploic artery

D Right gastric artery

E Right gastroepiploic artery

7. In Fig. 10.1 which single structure does the label 'A' identify on this CT taken at the transpyloric plane? ★ ★

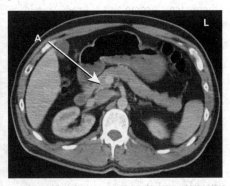

Fig. 10.1

A Duodenum

B Head of the pancreas

C Hepatic flexure of colon

D Jejunum

E Stomach

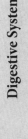

8. A 25-year-old man complains of abdominal pain that initially started around the umbilicus but then shifted towards the right. Examination reveals tenderness in the right lower quadrant which is aggravated by flexion and extension of the thigh. Which is the single most common location to which pain from the affected organ is localized? ★ ★

A Left iliac fossa

B Paracaecal

C Pelvic

D Retrocaecal

E Retro-ileal

9. A 72-year-old heavy smoker who suffers from severe atherosclerosis complains of severe pain in the lower abdomen. Occlusion of which single artery would cause ischaemia of the descending colon? ★ ★

A Iliocolic artery

B Left colic artery

C Right colic artery

D Sigmoidal artery

E Superior rectal artery

10. In achalasia, swallowed food accumulates in the oesophagus. This can cause dysphagia, regurgitation, substernal cramps and weight loss. Which single mechanism of swallowing is most likely to have failed in patients with achalasia? ★

A Constriction of the pyloric sphincter

B Contraction of pharyngeal muscles

C Oral phase of swallowing

D Receptive relaxation of the lower oesophageal sphincter

E Relaxation of the upper oesophageal sphincter

11. Acinar cells of the exocrine pancreas secrete a fluid containing inactive digestive enzyme precursors (to prevent autolysis of the pancreas). The fluid then passes to pancreatic tubules where tubule cells add isotonic sodium bicarbonate to the fluid. The bicarbonate will neutralize gastric acid and provide an optimal pH for pancreatic enzymes when the pancreatic secretion enters the duodenum via the common bile duct and enzyme precursors become activated by duodenal enterokinase. Pancreatic exocrine secretion is controlled by three groups of neural and endocrine mechanisms during digestion, the so-called cephalic, gastric, and duodenal phases. Which single substance produces the greatest increase in pancreatic acinar cell secretion during the cephalic phase? ★ ★

A Acetylcholine

B CCK (Cholecystokinin)

C Gastrin

D Histamine

E Secretin

12. A 58-year-old woman with a body mass index (BMI) of 34 presents with nausea and sudden, severe pain in the right epigastrium which sometimes radiates to the right shoulder. Her temperature is 38.5°C, and she is mildly jaundiced and tachycardic. Raised serum lipase levels confirm a diagnosis of acute pancreatitis. Endoscopic retrograde cholangiopancreatography (ERCP) identifies a gallstone in the biliary tree. Which is the single most likely location of the gallstone in this case? ★ ★

A Common bile duct

B Cystic duct

C Gallbladder

D Hepatic duct

E Sphincter of Oddi

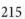

13. Patients with excessive breakdown of their red blood cells will usually develop a mild form of jaundice, known as haemolytic jaundice. In these patients the urine is colourless when voided whereas patients with obstructive jaundice or cholestatic jaundice void urine that is dark on production. However, the colourless urine of patients with haemolytic jaundice darkens on exposure to air. In those patients with haemolytic jaundice, which single substance is the most likely cause of the dark coloration of their urine that develops on exposure to air? ★ ★

A Biliverdin

B Conjugated bilirubin

C Unconjugated bilirubin

D Urobilin

E Urobilinogen

14. Two families of membrane proteins facilitate movement of monosaccharides such as glucose, fructose, and galactose into and out of cells in the body. One group comprises the glucose transporter proteins (GLUT1–GLUT11) and the other comprises the sodium-glucose linked transporters (SGLT1–SGLT2). Such proteins are important for glucose absorption in many body tissues, especially small intestine and kidney where large loads of glucose, fructose, and galactose absorption or reabsorption are handled. Which single membrane transport protein, located at the apical (luminal) border of the cell, is responsible for the absorption of fructose by epithelial cells of the small intestine? ★ ★

A GLUT1

B GLUT2

C GLUT3

D GLUT5

E SGLT1

15. Surgical resection of more than 50% of the ileum can result in the patient developing anaemia, diarrhoea, steatorrhoea, or renal stones. Which single alteration in gastrointestinal function is most likely to cause steatorrhoea in a patient with small bowel resection? ★ ★

A Increased bile salt synthesis by the liver

B Increased bile salts in the colon

C Lack of bile salt reabsorption in the ileum

D Lack of vitamin B_{12} absorption in the ileum

E Reduced absorption of water and electrolytes in the ileum

16. A 40-year-old woman with Peutz–Jeghers syndrome presents with abdominal pain, nausea, and vomiting. Double contrast barium study shows a protruding terminal ileal loop with coiled spring appearance. Colonoscopy reveals multiple polyps in the colon and terminal ileum. Which is the single most likely cause of intestinal obstruction in this patient? ★ ★

A Congenital abnormality

B Diffusely infiltrating tumour

C Hernia

D Intussusception

E Volvulus

17. A 19-year-old previously healthy medical student suffers from watery diarrhoea, bloating, and flatulence following return from an elective abroad. Biopsies show, on light microscopy, sickle-shaped organisms adjacent to the duodenal surface epithelium. Infection with which single organism is the most likely cause of his symptoms? ★ ★

A *Amoeba*

B *Giardia*

C *Salmonella*

D *Shigella*

E *Vibrio cholerae*

18. Blood clotting factors are synthesized in the liver. Severe liver disease results in lower blood levels of clotting factors and increased bleeding tendency. Which single clotting factor is most likely to remain normal in liver disease? ★ ★

A II

B VII

C VIII

D IX

E X

19. Synthesis of the intracellular storage protein ferritin, and of the transferrin receptor (TfR), are reciprocally linked to cellular iron content. In patients affected by hereditary haemochromatosis (HH) there is excessive storage of iron in tissues, leading to tissue damage. Which single statement best describes the expression of ferritin and TfR when the levels of iron are high? ★ ★

A Decreased ferritin mRNA synthesis and decreased TfR mRNA synthesis

B Decreased ferritin mRNA synthesis and increased TfR mRNA synthesis

C Increased ferritin mRNA synthesis and decreased TfR mRNA synthesis

D Increased ferritin mRNA synthesis and increased TfR mRNA synthesis

E Unchanged ferritin mRNA synthesis and increased TfR mRNA synthesis

20. A 30-year-old man diagnosed with tuberculosis (TB) is started on isoniazid. This is one of the drugs used in a 'triple therapy' for TB. Three weeks into his therapy he develops liver toxicity secondary to this drug. Which single form of conjugation reaction is isoniazid subjected to in the liver? ★ ★

A Acetylation

B Conjugation with glutathione

C Glucuronidation

D Methylation

E Sulphation

21. A 65-year-old known alcoholic is brought unconscious into the A&E department. On examination he is jaundiced, confused, and has multiple bruises and gynaecomastia. Ascites and bilateral peripheral leg oedema are also found. Failure of which single liver function is most likely to be responsible for this man's ascites? ★

A Detoxification of ammonia

B Detoxification of endogenous oestrogens

C Excretion of bile pigments

D Synthesis of albumin

E Synthesis of clotting factors

EXTENDED MATCHING QUESTIONS

Hormones and the digestive system

For each of the following statements, choose the single most appropriate hormone from the option list. Each option may be used once, more than once, or not at all.

A Bradykinin

B CCK (Cholecystokinin)

C Gastrin

D GIP (Gastric inhibitory polypeptide)

E Glucagon

F Histamine

G Insulin

H Motilin

I Neurotensin

J Secretin

K Somatomedin

L Somatostatin

N VIP (Vasoactive intestinal peptide)

1. Gastric infection with *Helicobacter pylori* inhibits the release of this substance from endocrine D-cells of the gastric epithelium, leading to higher levels of gastric acid secretion. ★ ★

2. The actions of this substance on gastric glands include a decrease in acid production by parietal cells and an increase in pepsin secretion by peptic (chief) cells as well as the production of bicarbonate-rich pancreatic secretion. ★

3. The receptors to this substance are blocked by drugs such as cimetidine, leading to reduced gastric acid secretion. ★

4. Originally named pancreozymin, this substance causes relaxation of the sphincter of Oddi. ★

5. This substance stimulates the production of migrating motor complexes (MMCs) in the stomach and duodenum, which occur in the so-called 'interdigestive period'. ★ ★

ANSWERS

Single Best Answers

1. E ★★   OHMS 2nd edn → p515, Fig. 8.2

There are three structures found running in the free border of the lesser omentum. Normally, the most posterior structure is the portal vein (E). Anteriorly, on the right is the bile duct (A) and on the left is the hepatic artery proper (C).

The short common hepatic artery (B) arises from the coeliac artery and supplies blood to the liver, pylorus of the stomach, duodenum, and pancreas. The hepatic artery proper (C), which supplies the liver, is a branch of the common hepatic artery that joins the triad of vessels found within the fold of the lesser omentum. The hepatic veins (D) form two groups of vessels that drain venous blood from the liver to the inferior vena cava. The (usually) three veins in the upper group arise posteriorly and drain the left and quadrate lobes of the liver. The variable number of smaller veins that form the lower group arise from the right and caudate lobes of the liver.

2. D ★★   OHMS 2nd edn → pp517–18

An indirect or congenital hernia is due to a patency of the processus vaginalis, meaning that the deep inguinal ring failed to close in the weeks surrounding the time of birth. The herniation passes through the deep inguinal ring (lateral to inferior epigastric vessels) and travels through the inguinal canal to the superficial inguinal ring.

An acquired inguinal hernia (A), or direct hernia (B) is due to a weakness in the inguinal triangle area medial to the inferior epigastric vessels (Hesselbach's triangle) and lateral to the spermatic cord. Acquired hernias rarely descend into the scrotum. A femoral hernia (C) occurs via the femoral canal, inferior to the inguinal ligament. An obturator hernia is difficult to diagnose in many cases, although it can cause irritation of the obturator nerve leading to shooting pains in the groin and medial thigh. An umbilical hernia (E) is located at the site of the umbilicus.

Note that femoral hernias are usually below and lateral to the pubic tubercle while inguinal hernias are normally above and medial.

3. B ★★   OHMS 2nd edn → pp520–3

It is the outer longitudinal layer of the muscularis propria of the large intestine that forms three longitudinal bands of muscle seen macroscopically as taeniae coli.

Because the longitudinal muscle of the large intestine is divided into three strips, a characteristic bulging or pouching of the colon occurs when the taenia contract. These bulges in the gut wall (indicating pouches within the gut lumen) are called haustra. When the circular layer of muscularis propria (A) contracts, segmentation movements occur, moving large intestine contents back and forth between haustral compartments. The mucosa (C), comprising epithelium, lamina propria, and muscularis mucosae (D), surrounds the lumen of the large intestine. The submucosa (E) surrounds the mucosa and separates it from the muscularis propria (muscularis externa) containing circular and longitudinal muscle layers. The outermost layer of the bowel is the serous membrane or serosa.

4. A ★   OHMS 2nd edn → pp520–3

The duodenum can be distinguished from the jejunum and ileum by the presence of mucus-secreting glands, called Brunner's glands, in the submucosa and muscularis mucosae. These glands secrete alkaline mucus.

All of the structures in options B to D are found throughout the duodenum, jejunum, and ileum. Goblet (B) cells have a characteristic goblet shape and secrete mucus. Paneth's cells (C) contain eosinophilic granules, secrete lysosomes and are antimicrobial. Peyer's patches (D) are areas of lymphoid tissue with antigen-presenting cells and are located in the lamina propria and submucosa. Villi (E) are the finger-like extensions of the mucosa that greatly increase the area of epithelial surface available for the absorption of the products of digestion.

Coeliac disease results from sensitivity to gliadin found in the gluten protein of wheat-based food products. The reaction to gliadin damages villi of the small intestine, flattening them (sub-total villous atrophy) and producing the typical histological features of coeliac disease as seen in biopsies of the small intestine. The reduction in area for intestinal reabsoption so produced causes many chronic problems including weight loss, fat malabsorption, steatorrhoea, diarrhoea, and various deficiency anaemias.

OHMS 2nd edn → p524

The answer is oesophageal variceal rupture. The most likely diagnosis in this patient, with a history of excessive alcohol intake, is liver cirrhosis. Cirrhosis increases the vascular resistance in the liver leading to back pressure in the hepatic portal vein, producing portal hypertension. This back pressure opposes reabsorption of circulating tissue fluid in bowel tissue, and the excess accumulates in the abdominal cavity as oedema, a condition known as ascites. With blood flow through the liver reduced, blood bypasses the liver, flowing instead through porto-systemic anastomoses, in order to return to the systemic system. One such anastomosis is located around the oesophagus. The raised pressure causes dilation of these veins, eventually producing oesophageal varices. These frequently rupture causing serious blood loss and haematemesis.

Barrett's oesophagus (A), a premalignant metaplasia of the epithelium of the lower oesophagus, usually results from the chronic regurgitation of gastric acid seen in GORD (gastro-oesophageal reflux disease). Hiatus hernia (B) can cause GORD, and chronic acid erosion of the oesophageal mucosa can lead to scarring and narrowing of the oesophagus, producing oesophageal stricture (C). Dysphagia is the most common symptom of oesophageal stricture and is also associated with squamous cell carcinoma of the oesophagus (D). Oesophageal carcinoma can result in bleeding and haematemesis, but the clinical presentation is likely to be different from that given in the scenario.

The black, tarry stools described by the term 'melaena' arise from the action of gastric acid on the iron of the haemoglobin. Melaena is associated with bleeding into the upper GI tract (stomach and duodenum), typically in peptic ulcer. Bleeding of the oesophageal mucosa can lead to to melaena if the blood is swallowed, but melaena is less likely if blood is vomited, as in haematemesis.

6. D ★ OHMS 2nd edn → pp527–8

The right gastric artery supplies the antral part of the lesser curvature of the stomach and is likely to be the vessel that is eroded in this case.

The gastroduodenal artery (A) supplies the pylorus and the duodenum. The left gastric artery (B) supplies the fundal part of the stomach. The left gastroepiploic (C) and right gastroepiploic (E) arteries supply areas of the greater curvature of the stomach (Fig. 10.2).

Before the advent of drugs such as histamine H_2 receptor antagonists and proton pump inhibitors, able to reduce excessive gastric acid secretion, erosion of the mucosa by gastric or duodenal ulcers, and subsequent gastrointestinal haemorrhage were common emergencies.

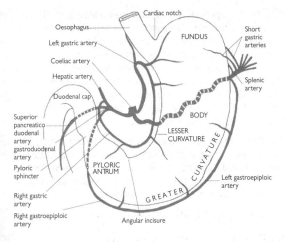

Fig. 10.2

7. B ★★   OHMS 2nd edn → p530

The answer is head of the pancreas. L1–L2 is the level known as the transpyloric plane. The surface anatomy description of this horizontal plane is that it lies midway between the jugular notch of the sternum and the pubic symphysis. The plane passes through the second part of the duodenum and the head of the pancreas.

The duodenum (A) is on the right side of the pancreas and is not clearly shown in this image. The head of the pancreas (B) can be seen lying behind the stomach. The body and tail of the pancreas can be seen to traverse the abdomen towards the spleen on the left. The kidneys and the renal vasculature can be clearly seen on this CT. The hepatic flexure (C) and splenic flexures of the colon are positioned more inferiorly and are not visible at this level on a CT scan. The duodenojejunal junction lies on the transpyloric plane, but the jejunum itself begins at the level of L2. The stomach (E) is positioned anteriorly in the abdomen and its contents and air can clearly be delineated in this CT.

Of interest, posterior to the pancreas, this image shows the superior mesenteric artery as it branches from the abdominal aorta, and the left renal vein joining the inferior vena cava.

8. D ★★   OHMS 2nd edn → pp533–4

The answer is retrocaecal. The patient has signs and symptoms consistent with acute appendicitis. The point at which the appendix arises from the caecum is fairly constant, and the surface landmark is McBurney's point—a position one-third of the distance from the

ASIS (anterior superior iliac spine) on a line towards the umbilicus on the right side of the lower abdomen. While the base of the appendix may have a constant location, the organ itself varies in length (2 to 20 cm or more) and position in the abdomen of different individuals. In about 75% of cases the appendix lies behind the caecum (retrocaecal) but it may be paracaecal (B), pelvic (C), or retro-ileal (E) in location. The appendix is usually located in the region of the right iliac fossa, but in rare cases of situs inversus it may be located in the left iliac fossa (A).

Pain from appendicitis is frequently referred to the umbilical area, and movement of the adjacent iliopsoas muscles can exacerbate the pain. Because the appendix may lie in different positions in different individuals, pain can be referred to a variety of locations and this can make the diagnosis of appendicitis difficult.

http://en.wikipedia.org/wiki/Vermiform_appendix

9. B ★★   OHMS 2nd edn → p535

The left colic artery supplies the descending colon. It is the first branch of the inferior mesenteric artery (IMA) and divides into an ascending and a descending branch.

The sigmoidal arteries (D) are typically smaller branches of the left colic artery, which supply the sigmoid colon. The superior rectal

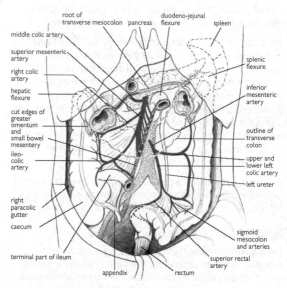

Fig. 10.3

artery (E) is the terminal branch of the IMA. The iliocolic artery (A) and the right colic artery (C) are branches of the superior mesenteric artery and supply the area of the caecum and the ascending colon (Fig. 10.3).

10. D ★ OHMS 2nd edn → p548; OHCM → p240

The answer is receptive relaxation of the lower oesophageal sphincter. The upper third of the oesophagus propels each food bolus towards the stomach by means of skeletal muscle under voluntary control. The middle third uses a mixture of skeletal muscle and smooth muscle. In the lower third of the oesophagus, food is propelled by smooth muscle contractions, controlled by autonomic efferents. These efferents modulate ongoing activity in the submucosal (Meissner's) plexus and the myenteric (Auerbach's) plexus of the gut wall. Together these form the enteric nervous system of the gut. In achalasia, normal function of the enteric system is disturbed, and peristalsis in the lower third of the oesophagus and reflex, receptive relaxation of the lower oesophageal sphincter produced by the passage of the food bolus both fail (D). The lower oesophageal sphincter remains closed and food accumulates in the oesophagus, producing the symptoms of achalasia.

The pyloric sphincter (A) is, of course, located between stomach and duodenum. Note that options B, C, and E are all aspects of swallowing controlled by voluntary, skeletal muscle and not controlled by the enteric system or autonomic nervous system. Finally, while oesophageal peristalsis also fails in achalasia, it is not included in the option list.

11. A ★ ★ OHMS 2nd edn → p553

The answer is acetylcholine. 'Cephalic phase' implies control from higher centres in the central nervous system. In this case this will be by vagal efferents of the autonomic nervous system that are activated by the sight and smell of food and by food entering the mouth. Since it is the parasympathetic (the vagus nerve) which increases motility and secretion generally in the GI tract and also relaxes GI sphincter tone, it will be the acetylcholine released from the parasympathetic postganglionic efferents that activates the acinar cells. Some gastrin (C) may also be released from gastric G-cells during the cephalic phase, but acetylcholine is thought to have a greater effect on pancreatic acinar cells in this phase.

In the gastric phase, vagovagal loops stimulate pancreatic secretion. These loops are activated by stomach distension and the presence of digested protein in the stomach. This, in turn, causes gastrin release, which maintains pancreatic acinar cell secretion.

In the intestinal phase CCK (B) is released by duodenal I-cells in response to monoglycerides and free fatty acids in the duodenum. It acts on acinar cells to produce enzyme-rich secretion, although whether by direct or indirect (vagovagal) action remains unclear. Secretin (E), synthesized by duodenal S-cells, is released mainly by the presence of hydrochloric acid in the chyme entering the duodenum. Secretin acts mainly on pancreatic duct cells to produce an alkaline, bicarbonate-rich pancreatic fluid. Although histamine (D) is better known for its role in stimulating gastric acid secretion, there is also evidence that it increases pancreatic acinar secretion in animals.

Naish, J, Revest, P, & Syndercombe-Court, D (2009). *Medical Sciences*, p805. London: Saunders Elsevier.

12. E ★ ★   OHMS 2nd edn → pp544–6

The answer is sphincter of Oddi. Gallstones lodged in the upper parts of the biliary tree can cause painful biliary colic. If the gallstone lodges at the lower part of the tree in the sphincter of Oddi, and causes stenosis (narrowing) rather than complete obstruction of the entrance of the common bile duct to the duodenum, then reflux of duodenual contents into the pancreatic ducts can occur (see Fig. 10.4). The digestive enzymes in the duodenal contents will both damage the pancreas and activate pancreatic enzyme precursors, leading to tissue damage and acute, painful pancreatitis.

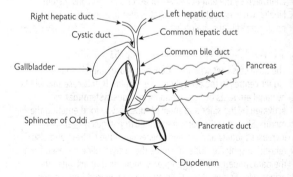

Right hepatic duct — Left hepatic duct
Cystic duct — Common hepatic duct
Common bile duct
Gallbladder — Pancreas
Sphincter of Oddi — Pancreatic duct
Duodenum

Fig. 10.4

Biliary colic, due to gallstones, and cholecystitis (inflammation of the gallbladder) are painful conditions, and the pain commonly radiates to the right shoulder. An altered sensitivity to touch below the right scapula (Boas's sign) can be indicative of cholecystitis.

13. D ★★   OHMS 2nd edn → pp544, 583

The answer is urobilin. In haemolytic jaundice, there is increased breakdown of the haem moieties from haemoglobin giving increased biliverdin (A) production and an increase in plasma levels of unconjugated bilirubin (C). This unconjugated bilirubin causes jaundice. Liver function is usually unimpaired in these patients so the liver will excrete maximal amounts of conjugated bilirubin (B) into the bowel. Bacterial action in the large intestine converts this to urobilinogen (E), some of which is reabsorbed into the blood and then excreted in the urine. Higher than normal urinary urobilinogen concentration is a feature of haemolytic jaundice. If left to stand in room air, the clear urobilinogen in the urine of these patients is oxidized to urobilin (D), which gives the urine a dark brown coloration.

In obstructive jaundice, where the bile ducts are obstructed either by gallstones or by a tumour of the head of the pancreas, entry of conjugated bilirubin into the bowel is reduced or prevented, and plasma-conjugated bilirubin concentration rises. This conjugated bilirubin gives the urine a dark colour without being left to stand. Obstructive jaundice is characterized by low urine urobilinogen, with higher than normal urine conjugated bilirubin. Haemolytic jaundice is characterized by high urine urobilinogen.

14. D ★★   OHMS 2nd edn → p560

GLUT5 (glucose transporter-5) is a fructose-selective protein transporter which facilitates the diffusion of fructose into the cell along its concentration gradient. Intestinal epithelial cells also contain GLUT2 transporter (B) on the basal membrane to facilitate transport of glucose, galactose, and fructose out of the cell into interstitial fluid. Other members of the GLUT family given as options are GLUT1 (A), found mostly in erythrocytes and the blood–brain barrier, and GLUT3 (C), which is mostly expressed in neurones. SGLT1 (sodium-glucose linked transporter-1) (E) is perhaps the most famous of the glucose transporters and differs from the GLUT family in that it uses co-transport of the monosaccharide neurones with sodium ions entering the cells. As sodium ions move into the cell down their concentration and electrochemical gradients, glucose can be transported into the cell against the glucose concentration gradient, a process not possible with the simple facilitated diffusion of GLUT family transporters.

15. C ★★   OHMS 2nd edn → pp566, 588; OHCM → p281

The answer is lack of bile salt reabsorption in the ileum. Bile salts assist the formation of the microscopic fat micelles required for hydrophilic pancreatic lipase to digest hydrophobic fat (triglyceride) molecules into fatty acids and glycerol. Bile salts, produced in the liver, are normally reabsorbed in the terminal ileum and recycled, often more than once after each meal. This recycling is known as the enterohepatic circulation of bile salts. When there is large-scale resection of the ileum, this recycling cannot occur and bile salts enter the colon and are lost from the body. There will be insufficient bile salts in the small intestine for proper fat digestion, and steatorrhoea will develop.

The liver can increase the synthesis of bile salts (A), but with a reduced enterohepatic circulation, production may not be sufficient to replace the lost bile salts and prevent steatorrhoea. Increased bile salts passing into the colon (B) will attract water, producing an osmotic diarrhoea, and this will be worsened by the reduced absorption of water and electrolytes in the shortened ileum (E). Since the absorption of the complex of intrinsic factor and Vitamin B_{12} (D) occurs in the terminal ileum, then small bowel resection will reduce B_{12} absorption, leading in time to a macrocytic, megaloblastic B_{12} deficiency anaemia.

Kumar, P, & Clark, M (2009). *Clinical Medicine* 7th edn, p295. London: Saunders Ltd.

16. D ★ ★   OHMS 2nd edn → p567

Intussusception occurs when one segment of the bowel, constricted by a wave of peristalsis, herniates or telescopes into the immediately distal segment of bowel. It is the commonest cause of intestinal obstruction in children but can occur in adults when a precipitating factor is present, e.g. polyps or an intraluminal tumour. Peutz–Jeghers syndrome is an autosomal dominant disease in which hamartomatous polyps develop in the bowel. While Peutz–Jeghers syndrome is rare it is an important risk factor for intussusception in adults.

Various congenital abnormalities (A) can cause atresia (complete obstruction or partial obstruction) of the bowel in newborn infants. A diffusely infiltrating tumour (B) can obstruct the bowel, but is likely to have a different presentation and radiography from the case described here. Sometimes, abdominal and inguinal hernias (C) can trap a loop of bowel causing obstruction and this can progress to strangulation with ischaemia, necrosis and gangrene of the trapped bowel. In volvulus (E) a section of bowel becomes twisted upon itself, leading to obstruction and bowel ischaemia and necrosis. It is commonest among men in middle to late life.

17. B ★ ★   OHMS 2nd edn → p568

The characteristic sickle-shaped organisms indicate that this is protozoal infection by *Giardia lamblia*, a common cause of watery diarrhoea and malabsorption. *Giardia* characteristically causes excessive gas production, such as flatulence or foul belching.

Although *Giardia* does secrete enterotoxins, it also has a cysteine-rich surface protein that resembles diarrhoea-causing toxins. *Giardia* also possesses cell-surface glycoproteins that cause fluid to accumulate in the intestine. The physical presence of rapidly proliferating trophozoites (which are sickle-shaped) and their toxic proteins mask and damage the intestinal epithelium in several ways, shortening microvilli and damaging the epithelial cell brush border. These effects produce malabsorption. Giardiasis is treated with oral antibiotics, such as metronidazole.

The other organisms listed all cause diarrhoea, either by the action of a bacterial toxin as in the cholera bacterium, *Vibrio cholerae* (E), which promotes secretion of fluid into the bowel, or by direct damage to the epithelium leading to fluid leakage into the bowel. Protozoan (options A and B) and bacterial organisms (C, D, and E) causing diarrhoea are usually identified by microscopy or culture of stool samples.

18. C ★ ★   OHMS 2nd edn → pp578–9

The answer is factor VIII. The vitamin K-dependent factors II, VII, IX, and X are usually first affected in liver disease. Factor VII (B) decreases first due to short half-life (6h), followed by reductions in factor II (A) and X (E) levels. Factor IX (D) levels are usually only modestly reduced until advanced stages of liver disease.

In contrast, factor VIII levels (C) may be normal, or even elevated, in advanced liver disease and may be associated with elevated levels of von Willibrand's factor, although whether the raised plasma factor VIII is due to increased biosynthesis in the liver, or another mechanism, is unclear.

19. C ★ ★   OHMS 2nd edn → pp580–1

When iron levels are high, cells use stored ferritin mRNA to synthesize ferritin to promote iron storage in cells and the TfR mRNA is degraded. In contrast, when iron levels are low, TfR mRNA levels rise and increased synthesis of receptors occurs, while ferritin mRNA is stored in an inactive form. This is an important example of control of expression of proteins at the translational level. Patients with HH have increased serum iron and ferritin, and the saturation of transferrin with iron is much greater than normal.

20. A ★ ★   OHMS 2nd edn → pp582–3

The answer is acetylation. Xenobiotics are substances foreign to the body, such as drugs. Prior to their elimination from the body they usually undergo two phases of metabolic alteration in the liver: Phase 1 involves a hydroxylation reaction; Phase 2 involves a conjugation. This second phase assists the eventual excretion of the products in bile or urine. Five types of conjugation reactions are carried out, as listed in the option list. Isoniazid undergoes acetylation in the liver to a variety of metabolites that are eventually excreted in the urine.

One such metabolite is acetylhydrazine, a potent hepatotoxin. Individuals can be classified as slow or fast acetylators, which influences the rate of clearance of isoniazid metabolites from blood. Slow acetylators are more subject to toxic effects of the metabolites because they persist longer in these patients. With long-term administration at therapeutic doses, isoniazid can cause clinically significant liver injury in 1% of patients and elevated liver enzyme levels in 10–20% of patients.

21. D ★   OHMS 2nd edn → pp576–7, 585

This man has liver failure secondary to alcohol abuse. Failure of synthesis of albumin results in reduced plasma oncotic pressure. Clinically, low serum albumin causes the accumulation of fluid in the peritoneal cavity (ascites). Low serum albumin is also responsible for the peripheral oedema of the legs.

All of the options are a consequence of reduced liver function. A decreased level of consciousness due to hepatic encephalopathy results from failure of detoxification of ammonia (A). Gynaecomastia results from failure to detoxify endogenous oestrogens (B). Jaundice is the consequence of raised plasma levels of bilirubin. This occurs in alcoholic liver disease because insufficient bilirubin is being conjugated with glucuronic acid in the liver and excreted as bile pigments (C) in the bile. Bleeding abnormalities may occur if the liver's ability to synthesize clotting factors (E) is impaired.

Extended Matching Questions

1. L ★★

Antral somatostatin concentration has been found to be significantly decreased in patients infected with *H. pylori*. One of the actions of somatostatin is to inhibit the secretion of gastrin by G-cells in the gastric antrum. Lowering somatostatin will remove inhibition of G-cells leading to enhanced gastrin secretion. As a consequence gastric acid secretion by parietal (oxyntic) cells is increased above normal levels.

2. J ★

Secretin secretion is stimulated by low duodenal pH. Secretin has many actions, but lowering acid production in the stomach and stimulating the production of a bicarbonate-rich secretion by pancreatic duct cells are obvious actions in response to acidity in the small intestine.

3. F ★

The gastric paracrine hormone histamine, acting on H_2 receptors of parietal (oxyntic) cells, promotes hydrochloric acid secretion. This interaction is the common pathway for the acid-promoting actions of gastrin and acetylcholine, which bind to gastrin receptors and M_1 receptors on enterochromaffin-like cells that then release histamine. In blocking gastric H_2 receptors by competitive inhibition, drugs such as cimetidine and ranitidine prevent histamine-activated acid secretion. Other routes to stimulate parietal cells exist (M_3 and CCK_8/gastrin receptors on parietal cells) but cimetidine and ranitidine have been found to be valuable for reducing gastric acid secretion in patients with indigestion and peptic ulcers.

4. B ★

The hormone originally named pancreozymin by its discoverers is now called cholecystokinin (CCK). It is released in response to fat- or protein-rich chyme in the duodenum. The hormone has many actions including, as its full name suggests, contraction of the gallbladder as well as the production of a pancreatic secretion rich in digestive enzymes. CCK also relaxes the smooth muscle of the sphincter of Oddi to allow secretions to enter the small intestine. CCK slows gastric emptying to allow emulsification and digestion of fats when fats are abundant in the duodenum.

5. H ★ ★

The hormone motilin, released from endocrine cells of the duodenum, initiates migrating motor complexes (MMCs) in the stomach in periods between episodes of digestion. The MMCs generate contractions, which spread from stomach to small intestine, sweeping stomach contents, including acid, into and through the small intestine. This is thought to be an important housekeeping function for the GI system. MMCs cease with the onset of feeding, possibly through the action of neurotensin.

General feedback on 1–5: OHMS 2nd edn → pp549, 553, 554, 559

Naish, J, Revest, P, & Syndercombe-Court, D (2009). *Medical Sciences*, pp795, 797. London: Saunders Elsevier.

Digestive System

CHAPTER 11

ENDOCRINE SYSTEM

omplex animals have evolved two separate systems for the control of body tissues. One is the nervous system, which makes direct connections with specific muscles and glands and regulates their activity by the focal release of neurotransmitters. The other system is the endocrine system, where hormones, secreted into the circulation, can exert effects on remote tissues in many different locations simultaneously. The classical distinction between the two systems is, however, blurred. Some hormones, such as antidiuretic hormone and oxytocin, are released into the bloodstream by neurones, rather than by typical endocrine cells. In other situations, hormones are released only to act locally, not all over the body, as with paracrine cells. Occasionally, the hormone feeds back on to the cell that secreted it, as in autocrine regulation.

The interface between neural and endocrine control lies in the hypothalamus and related areas of the brain. This region also helps integrate the output of the autonomic nervous system, which controls visceral function. Hypothalamic areas also regulate appetite behaviours for food, water, sex, etc. Autonomic nervous system, appetites, and hormones all contribute to homeostasis—the regulation of the internal environment of the body. The hypothalamus and the pituitary gland form the 'hypothalamic–pituitary endocrine axis'. This axis regulates much of the body's endocrine activity through a system of hypothalamic factors. These factors, which are hormones in their own right, regulate the release of individual pituitary hormones. Each pituitary 'trophic' hormone then controls a part of the overall endocrine system. Thus, pituitary hormones control hormone production by thyroid, adrenal cortex, liver, and gonads. This complex cascade of hormonal control is regulated by various types of negative feedback based on plasma hormone concentrations. The hypothalamus and pituitary are also controlled by higher centres in the brain.

Other endocrine tissues also use negative feedback control, but rather than the level of the hormone itself, it is the level of stimulus that regulates hormone secretion. Thus, rising plasma osmolarity (or decreasing blood volume) stimulates antidiuretic hormone secretion, and rising plasma glucose stimulates insulin secretion. Combinations of hormones are sometimes used to regulate an aspect of the internal environment. The control of plasma calcium by calcitonin, parathormone, and calcitriol (1,25-dihydroxycholecalciferol), and of plasma glucose by insulin and glucagon, are examples.

Disorders of endocrine function often produce an excess or deficit of individual hormones. The change in circulating hormone level leads to characteristic alterations to normal physiology and metabolism. To interpret correctly endocrine disturbance in a clinical setting requires a good understanding of normal hormonal actions and the likely consequences of abnormal variation in levels of individual hormones or groups of hormones. Because hormones affect many body systems, endocrine disorders can produce very diverse symptoms and signs. ■

1. A 58-year-old male visits his GP because he has noticed a slow and progressive increase in the size of his tongue, hands and feet (with an increase in shoe and collar size) over the past 4 years. Recently, he has been 'bumping into things'. In taking a history, his GP finds that the patient's libido is reduced and examination shows bitemporal hemianopia ('tunnel vision'). The GP notices the patient's coarse facial features and large, spade-like hands. Investigations show glycosuria. Which single underlying pathology explains all of the features mentioned in the above scenario? ★ ★

A A growth-hormone-secreting pituitary adenoma

B Compression of the optic chiasma

C Enlargement of the pituitary gland

D Lowered plasma cortisol levels

E Lowered plasma gonadotrophin levels

2. A 28-year-old woman visits her GP with a 3-month history of weight loss, mild anxiety, and restlessness. She often feels hot and has 'clammy hands'. On examination, the doctor finds a bounding pulse with a rate of 120 beats per minute and hand tremor. The patient's thyroid gland is bilaterally swollen and palpation reveals a smooth surface to the gland, with no evident nodules. A blood sample is sent for analysis and the results show lower than normal levels of thyroid-stimulating hormone (TSH) and high levels of the thyroid hormones tri-iodothyronine (T_3) and thyroxine (T_4). Which is the single most likely diagnosis? ★

A de Quervain's thyroiditis

B Graves' disease

C Hashimoto's disease

D Sheehan's syndrome

E Thyroid adenoma

3. A 67-year-old woman is brought comatose to the A&E by ambulance. Her husband says that for some weeks she has complained of abdominal pain and muscular weakness. She has vomited on several occasions. Two days ago she became feverish and developed a cough and today she collapsed suddenly. On examination she is found to be very thin, with tanned skin and deep pigmentation of the skin creases of her palms. She is hypotensive with blood pressure at 70/55mmHg and her pulse rate is 110 beats per minute. She has some difficulty breathing. Which is the single most likely underlying cause of the patient's comatose state? ★ ★

A ACTH-secreting pituitary adenoma

B Diabetic ketoacidosis

C Non-secreting pituitary adenoma

D Pneumonia infection

E Primary adrenal insufficiency

4. Excess circulating aldosterone results in an increased plasma volume and hypertension. In primary hyperaldosteronism, the cause is excess secretion of ACTH or of aldosterone itself. In secondary hyperaldosteronism, the cause of the raised aldosterone is secondary to some other problem, such as renal artery stenosis. Which single investigation of plasma biochemistry will differentiate between primary and secondary hyperaldosteronism? ★

A Plasma cortisol concentration

B Plasma osmolarity

C Plasma pH

D Plasma potassium concentration

E Plasma renin concentration

5. A 63-year-old man who is known to have type II diabetes mellitus is started on a new medication by his GP. He returns to his GP complaining that he is experiencing 'hypos', or low blood sugar levels (hypoglycaemia), so the GP changes his medication. Which single treatment is the GP most likely to choose to reduce the risk of hypos? ★ ★

A Acarbose

B Gliclazide

C Metformin

D Repaglinide

E Subcutaneous long-acting low-dose insulin

6. A 48-year-old obese woman is experiencing heartburn and reflux which her GP explains are due to the reflux up into the oesophagus of the acid produced in her stomach. Increased secretions from which single cell type found in the stomach are most likely to reduce gastric acid production? ★ ★

A Chief cells

B D-cells

C Enterochromaffin-like (EC-like) cells

D G-cells

E Parietal cells

7. A 62-year-old man with end-stage renal disease is prescribed a vitamin D analogue. Which is the single best description of the important role the kidney has in vitamin D synthesis? ★

A Converts dietary vitamin D to plasma D_3

B Converts 7-dehydrocholesterol to vitamin D_3

C Converts D_3 to 1-hydroxy D_3

D Converts D_3 to 25-hydroxy D_3

E Converts 25-hydroxy D_3 to 1,25-dihydroxy D_3

8. The control of feeding behaviour involves a complex interplay of hormonal and neuronal factors. Defects in certain hormones (such as leptin) or their receptors can lead to obesity. Which single tissue or organ secretes the hormone leptin as part of the control of feeding behaviour? ★

A Adipose

B Adrenal

C Hypothalamus

D Pituitary

E Thyroid

9. A 27-year-old man is involved in a road traffic accident (RTA) and is admitted into the intensive therapy unit (ITU). The nurse looking after him becomes worried that the adrenaline infusion he is being given is causing problems. Which single problem is most likely to be caused by excess adrenaline? ★ ★ ★

A Ankle oedema

B Breathlessness

C Poor sleep pattern

D Pupil constriction

E Toe necrosis

10. A 68-year-old man with chronic obstructive pulmonary disease (COPD) sees his GP as he is increasingly short of breath, and is started on 40mg prednisolone OD (once daily, from the Latin: *omne in die*) for an exacerbation. Which single side-effect is most likely to occur with this medication? ★ ★ ★

A Alopecia

B Hyperkalaemia

C Hypoglycaemia

D Psychosis

E Skin thickening and bruising

EXTENDED MATCHING QUESTIONS

Hypothalamic and pituitary hormones

From the option list choose the single most appropriate hormone described in each of the following statements. Each option may be used once, more than once, or not at all.

A Adrenocorticotrophic hormone (ACTH)

B Corticotrophin-releasing hormone (CRH)

C Dopamine

D Follicle-stimulating hormone (FSH)

E Gonadotrophin-releasing hormone (GnRH)

F Growth hormone (GH)

G Growth hormone-releasing hormone (GRH)

H Luteinizing hormone (LH)

I Oxytocin

J Prolactin (PL)

K Somatostatin

L Thyroid-stimulating hormone (TSH)

M Thyrotrophin-releasing hormone (TRH)

N Vasopressin (antidiuretic hormone, ADH)

1. Cold and stress increase secretion of this hypothalamic hormone and ultimately its actions will result in increased basal metabolic heat production. ★

2. Secretion of this pituitary hormone shows a marked diurnal rhythm, peaking in the early morning. Its hypothalamic-releasing factor is inhibited by raised plasma glucocorticoid. ★

3. This pituitary hormone is responsible for the normal amenorrhoea in women following childbirth. ★ ★

4. This hypothalamic hormone controls the release of two pituitary hormones, both of which peak in concentration around day 14 of the ovarian cycle. ★

5. Synthetic analogues of this pituitary hormone, which acts on smooth muscle, can be used to induce labour in childbirth. ★ ★

Physiology and pathology of hormones

From the option list choose the single most appropriate hormone described in each of the following statements. Each option may be used once, more than once, or not at all.

A Adrenaline

B Adrenocorticotrophic hormone

C Aldosterone

D Cholecystokinin

E Cortisol

F Glucagon

G Growth hormone

H Insulin

I Oestrogen

J Parathyroid hormone

K Prolactin

L Somatostatin

M Testosterone

N Thyroid hormone

6. A pituitary adenoma of cells producing this hormone may lead to truncal obesity, hirsutism, proximal muscle weakness, and decreased immunity. ★

7. Deficient synthesis of this hormone, largely eliminated in the UK by dietary supplementation, can cause goitre and myxoedema in adults. ★

8. This hormone can be used instead of intravenous glucose administration in patients with hypoglycaemic coma. ★ ★

9. Sulphonylurea drugs, by inhibiting ATP-dependent K^+ channels, promote release of this hormone. ★

10. This hormone stimulates secretion of pancreatic enzymes and contraction of the gallbladder. ★ ★

ANSWERS

Single Best Answers

1. A ★★   OHMS 2nd edn → p592; OHCM → p230

The most likely diagnosis is acromegaly. A pituitary adenoma secreting growth hormone (GH) elevates plasma GH and causes growth of hands, feet, and facial bones (something that does not normally occur after puberty). Soft-tissue changes to tongue and skin are also associated with excess GH. Circulating GH inhibits glucose uptake into muscle and fat, promotes gluconeogenesis, and inhibits insulin's action at insulin receptors to produce insulin resistance. With excess GH these effects lead to high plasma glucose and eventually to glucosuria. Most of the other changes described in the scenario result from enlargement of the pituitary gland (C) within the confined space of the sella turcica, causing pressure to rise. Pressure on the roof of the sella turcica initially affects the medial part of the optic chiasma (B). The fibres here are those that cross from one side of the brain to the other and come from the nasal retina of each eye. The image formed on the nasal retina of each eye comes from the lateral (temporal) part of the visual field, so loss of fibres from the nasal retinae produces loss of both lateral visual fields, causing 'tunnel vision'. Fibres in the lateral (temporal) part of the retina do not cross over at the optic chiasma; they provide the nasal fields of vision and are initially spared damage. Increased pressure on the pituitary itself can cause loss of secretion of some or all of the pituitary hormones. ACTH suppression would lead to lower plasma cortisol levels (D), and loss of gonadotrophin secretion by the pituitary (E) will lead to sexual dysfunction. Note that option A is ultimately the cause of options B to E. You may find it helpful to look at Fig. 13.8 in Chapter 13 which shows the visual pathway and a diagram of bitemporal hemianopsia (tunnel vision).

2. B ★   OHMS 2nd edn → pp594–5; OHCM → p210

The scenario points to hyperthyroidism, and the most likely cause is Graves' disease. This is an autoimmune condition in which circulating antibodies bind to thyroid TSH receptors, causing secretion of high levels of T_3 and T_4. The increased activity leads to smooth enlargement of the thyroid. The high plasma levels of thyroid hormones suppress the production of thyrotrophin-releasing hormone (TRH) in the hypothalamus and this inhibits pituitary TSH secretion. The resulting picture is of high plasma T_3 and T_4 and low plasma TSH. A similar picture for plasma hormone levels would result from a secreting thyroid adenoma (E), but this is likely to be palpable as a single nodule on examination of the thyroid.

de Quervain's thyroiditis (A) results from viral infection of the thyroid and is associated with transient hyperthyroidism followed by transient hypothyroidism and then return to normal. Hashimoto's disease (C) and Sheehan's syndrome (D) both cause hypothyroidism. Hashimoto's is another autoimmune disorder where antibodies acting on the thyroid reduce T_3 and T_4 production. The low plasma T_3 and T_4 produce high plasma TSH due to hypothalamic feedback. Sheehan's syndrome (post-partum hypopituitarism) describes the consequences of an avascular necrosis of the pituitary following severe blood loss during or after childbirth. Pituitary function is lost and one consequence can be low circulating levels of T_3 and T_4 (hypothyroidism) due to the lack of TSH secretion.

3. E ★★   OHMS 2nd edn → p598; OHCM → pp218–19, 846

This is a classical Addisonian crisis resulting from loss of cortisol and aldosterone secretion due to destruction of the adrenal cortex (primary adrenal insufficiency). Adrenal androgens are also depleted. Cortisol has many functions and is important in the response to stress and infection. Aldosterone plays a key role in regulating body sodium content, plasma volume, and blood pressure. In Addison's disease an autoimmune process destroys the adrenal cortex in about 80% of cases in the UK. Worldwide, tuberculosis infection is the commonest cause of this rare and difficult-to-diagnose disorder. The low levels of circulating cortisol and aldosterone can mean that any cause of stress, such as a chest infection, can provoke an Addisonian crisis and life-threatening collapse. Blood tests on the patient will reveal low plasma cortisol and high levels of adrenocorticotrophic hormone (ACTH). The low circulating cortisol can stimulate very high levels of ACTH-secretion by the pituitary leading to an increase in skin pigmentation, especially in the creases of the palms. An ACTH-secreting pituitary adenoma (A) would give high plasma ACTH and high cortisol; a non-secreting pituitary adenoma (C) might compress pituitary ACTH cells reducing their secretion, but this would lead only to decreased plasma cortisol since the intact adrenal cortex will still produce aldosterone in response to angiotensin action. Diabetic ketoacidosis (B) is a distractor for the comatose state of the patient. Pneumonia (D), while it could trigger the crisis, is not the underlying cause.

4. E ★
OHMS 2nd edn → pp598–9, 602; OHCM → p220

In secondary hyperaldosteronism, high renin levels drive the elevated plasma aldosterone. This will occur, for example, in renal artery stenosis, which reduces glomerular perfusion pressure and causes renin to be released from the juxtaglomerular apparatus. Activation of the renin–angiotensin–aldosterone system raises aldosterone levels. In secondary hyperaldosteronism, renin levels are therefore high, whereas in primary disease, due to adrenal cortical hyperplasia or an aldosterone-secreting tumour (Conn's syndrome) renin levels will be low.

None of the other options differentiate between primary and secondary disorders. In excess, the glucocorticoid cortisol (A) can have mineralcorticoid effects, but does not directly affect aldosterone levels. Aldosterone leads to sodium and water retention, but sodium and plasma osmolarity (B) remain normal or only slightly raised in hyperaldosteronism. Aldosterone also causes potassium (D) to be lost from the body and this can lead to metabolic alkalosis, altering plasma pH (C).

5. C ★★
OHMS 2nd edn → p608; OHCM → p200

Metformin is a drug that increases the body's sensitivity to insulin—it does not increase the amount of insulin released. It therefore is not known to cause hypoglycaemic episodes alone—only in combination with other medication. Acarbose (A) inhibits gut enzymes that digest complex carbohydrates, so reducing the uptake of glucose into the blood. This does not generally lead to hypoglycaemia, but the drug is not very effective and has significant side-effects including diarrhoea and anaemia. Gliclazide (B) is a sulphonylurea drug which stimulates insulin release from pancreatic B-cells. Repaglinide (D) binds sulphonylurea receptors and has the same effect. Both of these medications can result in a patient experiencing hypoglycaemia. Any form of insulin (as in E) can cause hypoglycaemic episodes.

6. B ★★
OHMS 2nd edn → pp610–11

D-cells are sensitive to acid levels in the stomach and when pH is low they increase release of the hormone somatostatin. This inhibits factors that promote acid secretion. Chief cells (A) secrete pepsinogen and renin; the pepsinogen becoming the active proteolytic enzyme pepsin in the presence of gastric acid.

Fig. 11.1 summarizes the major factors controlling gastric acid secretion.

Parietal cells (E) in the epithelium of the body of the stomach secrete gastric acid.

G-cells (D) found in the antral part of the stomach secrete gastrin which acts on gastrin cholecystokinin (CCK_8)

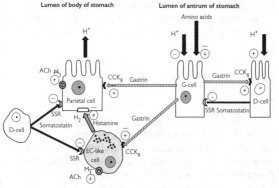

Fig. 11.1

receptors. Gastrin stimulates acid secretion by parietal cells and also stimulates EC-like cell and D-cell secretion.

EC-like cells (C) are enterochromaffin-like cells. These secrete histamine which acts via histamine H_2 receptors on parietal cells to promote acid secretion.

D-cells (B) secrete somatostatin which binds to somatostatin receptors and has inhibitory actions on the secretions of parietal cells, G-cells, and EC-like cells.

The neurotransmitter acetylcholine **(ACh)** is released by post-ganglionic parasympathetic neurones (not shown in the diagram) and acts at muscarinic receptors on parietal cells, EC-like cells, and D-cells.

During feeding, the sight, smell, and taste of food produce a 'cephalic phase' of acid secretion mediated by the vagus nerve. In the stomach, postganglionic parasympathetic fibres release ACh to act on parietal cells (at M_3 muscarinic receptors), promoting acid secretion, and on EC-like cells (at M_1 receptors), causing the release of histamine which acts locally on parietal cells, producing further acid secretion into the body of the stomach. When the products of gastric digestion reach the antral region of the stomach, amino acids stimulate G-cells to release gastrin into the bloodstream. The gastrin passes to parietal cells in the body of the stomach helping to maintain the acid secretion. In this way G-cells support the 'gastric phase' of acid secretion activated when food is present in the stomach. If proton secretion is in excess of requirement, as may occur at the end of gastric digestion, proton concentration in the antral region rises. The falling pH here inhibits gastrin release by G-cells and stimulates D-cells to release somatostatin. Somatostatin acts to reduce acid secretion by inhibiting the secretions of G-cells, EC-like cells and parietal cells.

Although this may look complex, it is in fact a simplification and some interactions have been omitted.

7. E ★   OHMS 2nd edn → p613

The conversion of 25-hydroxy D_3 to 1,25-dihydroxy D_3 (the active form of vitamin D) is an important role of the kidney. This function is impaired in chronic renal failure, accounting for some of the blood abnormalities, for example secondary hyperparathyroidism, found in those patients with the condition. Vitamin D analogues are often given to these patients to compensate for the impaired vitamin D metabolism. Untreated, this impaired metabolism can lead to bone reabsorption and renal osteodystrophy ('renal rickets').

Dietary vitamin D (A), derived from fish oils and eggs yolks, is already in the D_3 form (cholecalciferol) when ingested and absorbed. Some dietary intake may be in the D_2 (ergocalciferol) form produced by some fungi and invertebrate species. Although sometimes used as a food supplement, D_2 is not an effective replacement for D_3. Sunlight aids conversion of 7-dehydrocholesterol to vitamin D_3 (B) in the skin, and the liver converts D_3 to 25-hydroxy D_3 (D). 1-hydroxy D_3 (C), also known as alfacalcidol, is a synthetic vitamin D analogue.

8. A ★   OHMS 2nd edn → p614

Adipose tissue is often considered to be merely a fat depot, but it is, in fact, metabolically highly active. Apart from responding to metabolic signals leading to mobilization or deposition of triglyceride, it also secretes the hormone leptin. This polypeptide acts on receptors in the hypothalamus to inhibit the action of neuropeptide Y (a neurotransmitter which increases food intake and inhibits physical activity) and to influence the activity of several other neurotransmitters contributing to the control of feeding behaviour. Leptin does so by decreasing appetite through signalling satiety (the sense of feeling full).

9. E ★ ★ ★   OHMS 2nd edn → pp615–16

The answer is toe necrosis. Adrenaline is a stress hormone often used in ITU to help support very sick patients. It is predominantly used for its cardiovascular effects, which lead to increased cardiac output. To do this, adrenaline produces peripheral vasoconstriction as well as increasing rate and strength of cardiac contractions. This peripheral vasoconstriction can cause peripheral tissue necrosis in those patients with an already compromised circulation. Adrenaline also slows gastric motility and can cause poor absorption of parenterally administered nutrients which ITU patients may require.

Since it produces arteriolar constriction, adrenaline will lower capillary pressure and may reduce the likelihood of peripheral oedema (A). Breathlessness (B) is not a common side-effect of adrenaline infusion and, in fact, the drug is used to treat the causes of breathlessness in asthma and anaphylactic shock. Although adrenaline may cause anxiety and restlessness, any consequent poor sleep pattern (C) would not be an immediate cause for concern in an ITU patient. Adrenaline causes pupil dilation not constriction (D).

10. D ★ ★ ★ OHMS 2nd edn → p618

The answer is psychosis. Prednisolone is a corticosteroid drug with mainly glucocorticoid actions, mimicking endogenous cortisol. Glucocorticoids are released into the blood in response to ongoing stress such as infection and this property is often used in clinical treatment, as in this example. The anti-inflammatory actions of corticosteroids can be helpful, particularly in acute exacerbations, in those COPD patients who show a good response to a trial of the drug. However, as well as having beneficial effects, the corticosteriods have significant side-effects, especially with prolonged use. One such side-effect is psychosis.

Alopecia (hair loss), or baldness, as in option A, comes in a variety of forms. Alopecia areata or spot baldness can improve during corticosteroid treatment. Hyperkalaemia (B) is unlikely in prednisolone treatment. High doses of glucocorticoids can have mineralocorticoid effects (mimicking aldosterone). This can sometimes lead to excessive sodium retention and consequent potassium loss by the kidney, leading to hypokalaemia in patients taking glucocorticoids. Hypoglycaemia (C) is unlikely in those patients taking glucocorticoids, since the drug elevates circulating glucose levels and extended use can lead to 'steroid-induced diabetes'. Long-term corticosteroid use can lead to thinning of the skin, collagen loss, and purpura rather than skin thickening (E).

Extended Matching Questions

1. M ★

Thyrotrophin-releasing hormone is produced by neurones acting on secretory cells in the hypothalamus. The blood transports the hormone in the hypophyseal–pituitary portal system to act on the cells in the anterior pituitary that secrete thyroid-stimulating hormone (TSH). The TSH then passes in the blood to the thyroid gland where it causes secretion of thyroxine (T_4) and the more active tri-iodothyronine (T_3). T_4 is converted to T_3 in the liver. These thyroid hormones increase basal metabolic rate, increasing heat production, and also have many other actions in various body tissues.

2. A ★

Adrenocorticotrophic hormone (ACTH) is notable for showing a diurnal rhythm in plasma concentration. ACTH acts on zona facsiculata cells of the adrenal cortex to stimulate the production of glucocorticoid hormones: ACTH and cortisol peak at around 7 a.m. and are at their lowest levels around midnight. The diameter of those small airways in the lung, which become constricted in asthma, shows a similar diurnal pattern, with airways narrowest (and asthma often more severe) in the early morning hours after midnight. Although corticosteroids such as prednisolone and related compounds can be used to treat asthma, the relationships, if any, between diurnal cycles of ACTH, cortisol, and airway diameter remain unclear.

3. J ★ ★

Prolactin (PL) is responsible for the maintenance of milk production in mothers who breastfeed their infants. Suckling by the infant stimulates receptors in the nipple and areola of the breast, and the neural signals pass to the hypothalamus. Hypothalamic factors, which pass to the anterior pituitary to regulate PL release, include dopamine, vasoactive intestinal peptide (VIP) and thyrotrophin-releasing hormone (TRH). Dopamine probably has the greatest effect and it acts to inhibit PL release. Suckling inhibits dopamine release in the hypothalamus, increasing PL secretion. PL activates the transcription of the genes that produce milk proteins and enzymes that produce lactose in mammary gland tissue. With regular breastfeeding of an infant, lactational amenorrhoea will usually occur with a loss of the normal, monthly ovulation. One of the effects of high circulating PL that results from suckling is inhibition of hypothalamic gonadotrophin-releasing hormone (GnRH), with disruption to the normal secretion of luteinizing hormone (LH) and follicle-stimulating hormone (FSH) responsible for the normal ovarian cycle and ovulation. PL also reduces gonad tissue response to these hormones.

4. E ★

As mentioned in the feedback to Question 3, gonadotrophin-releasing hormone (GnRH) is released from cells in the hypothalamus and passes to the anterior pituitary via the hypophyseal–pituitary portal system where it causes secretion into the bloodstream of luteinizing hormone (LH) and follicle-stimulating hormone (FSH).

These are the gonadotrophic hormones. In the male LH controls testosterone production by testicular Leydig cells while FSH stimulates Sertoli cells and sperm production. In females FSH and LH regulate development of ovarian follicles and oestrogen and progesterone production by the ovaries. The plasma concentration of both LH and FSH peak at the time of ovulation and both help maintain progesterone secretion by the corpus luteum after ovulation.

5. I ★★

Syntocinon® is the synthetic version of the naturally occurring posterior pituitary hormone oxytocin, which can be used to induce uterine contractions in childbirth. It is also important in suckling, when stimulation of the nipple by the infant causes oxytocin release; this produces contraction of smooth muscle in the ducts of the glandular tissue of the breast and milk ejection.

General feedback on 1–5: OHMS 2nd edn → pp590–1

6. B ★

Tumours of endocrine glands can cause over-secretion of the relevant hormone in a way that does not respond to the usual feedback control. Overproduction of ACTH will lead to excessive release of glucocorticoids by the adrenal glands, and the excess hormones will cause the characteristic features of Cushing's syndrome.

7. N ★

The thyroid hormones thyroxine and tri-iodothyronine are iodinated versions of the amino acid tyrosine. Addition of sodium iodide to table salt in the UK has largely eliminated the deficient synthesis of thyroid hormones caused by a dietary lack of iodine. In some parts of the world, though, this condition is prevalent, leading to the characteristic features of goitre (thyroid gland hypertrophy) and myxoedema (thyroid hormone deficiency).

8. F ★★

Glucagon, secreted by α-cells of the pancreatic islets of Langerhans, is the hormone that antagonizes the actions of insulin. It mobilizes glucose from glycogen stores in liver and from lipolysis to raise plasma glucose levels. The effect of intramuscular glucagon injection is nearly as quick as that of intravenous glucose, but it does not produce effects in patients who are intoxicated by alcohol. In general, intravenous glucose will be a cheaper and generally easier method for dealing with acute hypoglycaemic comas.

Insulin release by the β-cells of the pancreatic islets of Langerhans is promoted by a raised intracellular concentration of Ca^{2+}. The latter, in turn, is brought about by the depolarization of the cell membrane caused by ATP-activated K^+ channels. The normal stimulus to this overall process is a rise in plasma glucose concentration. In type II diabetes, treatment with sulphonylurea drugs can also be effective by the same mechanism.

Continued digestion in the duodenum must coordinate the post-prandial release of the gastric contents with secretion of bile and of pancreatic enzymes. The key hormone involved is cholecystokinin, whose secretion by the I-cells of the duodenum is stimulated by the presence of fat or protein-rich acidic chyme. It promotes contraction of the gallbladder to release bile and stimulates secretion of digestive enzymes by the exocrine pancreas.

General feedback on 6–10: OHMS 2nd edn → pp590, 594–600, 604–5, 608, 610–11; OHCM p844

CHAPTER 12

REPRODUCTION AND DEVELOPMENT

R eproduction and development are large topics, knowledge of which underpins several medical specialities including sexual health, fertility, gynaecology, urology, reproductive endocrinology, obstetrics, and neonatology. Doctors need to know the structure, function, and endocrine control of both male and female systems in order to diagnose and manage conditions specific to either male or female organs, as well as conditions such as impotence and infertility.

Not surprisingly, the reproductive system is the only body system that shows major differences in both structure and function between males and females. However, sexual differences go beyond the primary sexual characteristics present at birth and the secondary sexual characteristics that emerge under the influence of sex hormones at puberty. Sexual dimorphism in some brain structures commences at an early age, and differences in the endocrine profiles of males and females produce characteristic changes in morphology, physiology, and behaviour that go beyond simple sexual dimorphism to affect many aspects of life, including sexual differences in susceptibility to disease and the longer life expectancy of women as compared to men that is seen around the world. Whether these differences, mainly beneficial to women, are because females are 'biologically superior' or because of a complex mix of genetic, behavioural, and social factors is a matter for discussion and research.

Some knowledge of embryology is important to every medical student. As a minimum it provides explanations for the congenital malformations and their consequences that are encountered in many areas of clinical practice. Deeper knowledge will assist those seeking real insights into the structure of the human body. It is the study of embryological development and the knowledge of how each tissue type arises, how one tissue meets another, and how tissues move and change shape during development that explains the relations between tissues and organs in the adult human form. Achieving a full understanding of the dynamics of the formation of the body's organs and tissues is demanding, but it can replace some of the rote learning of anatomical structures, familiar to many students, with a deeper understanding of form and function. ■

REPRODUCTION AND DEVELOPMENT
SINGLE BEST ANSWERS

1. During a painful childbirth a 25-year-old female is given a regional nerve block to provide analgesia for the relief of perineal pain. With the patient in the lithotomy position, the physician palpates the ischial spine through the wall of the vagina and uses it as a landmark to administer a local anaesthetic. Which single nerve is most likely to be blocked in this procedure? ★

A Anococcygeal nerve

B Anterior labial nerve

C Genital branch of the genitofemoral nerve

D Ilioinguinal nerve

E Pudendal nerve

2. A 17-year-old male presents with a slightly swollen and very painful left testis which has developed over the last 3 hours. He also has pain in the lower abdomen. On examination, his left testis is high within the scrotum, and the ipsilateral cremasteric reflex is absent. A diagnosis of testicular torsion is made and he is immediately sent for detorsion surgery. Which single nerve is involved in the cremasteric reflex? ★

A Genitofemoral nerve

B Iliohypogastric nerve

C Ilioinguinal nerve

D Medial femoral cutaneous nerve

E Pudendal nerve

3. A 17-year-old male presents with a left-sided scrotal swelling. There is a palpable enlarged vein and so he is sent for scrotal ultrasonography. A diagnosis of testicular varicocoele is made. Which is the single blood vessel into which the left testicular vein drains? ★

A External iliac vein

B Inferior epigastric vein

C Inferior vena cava

D Internal iliac vein

E Left renal vein

4. The parents of a 4-week-old boy have brought him to see their GP. They are worried because the child has developed a large scrotal swelling. The GP notes that it is possible to palpate above the swelling, which feels soft and smooth, although the testes and the epididymis cannot be felt. The swelling appears translucent when a pen light is held behind the scrotum. Which is the single most likely diagnosis? ★

A Cryptorchidism

B Epididymal cyst

C Hydrocoele

D Inguinal hernia

E Varicocoele

5. A 41-year-old female suffering from menorrhagia due to multiple fibroids had a complete hysterectomy a week ago. She is readmitted with persistent left-sided loin pain. Which single structure that lies in close proximity to the uterine arteries may have been inadvertently damaged during her surgery? ★ ★

A Internal iliac artery

B Uterine vein

C Ureter

D Urethra

E Urinary bladder

6. In the production of male germ cells, exposure of gametes (which are antigenically different from somatic cells) to the immune system is prevented by a blood–testis barrier. Which single cell type forms the blood–testis barrier? ★ ★

A Leydig cells

B Myofibroblasts

C Peritubular capillary endothelium

D Sertoli cells

E The basement membrane of the seminiferous tubule

7. There are numerous stages in the development of the ovum, which can be seen while examining ovarian tissue under the microscope. Which single type of post-ovulatory follicle is formed in the absence of fertilization? ★

A Antral follicle

B Atretic follicle

C Corpus albicans

D Corpus luteum

E Primordial follicle

8. The placenta is an important endocrine organ, secreting a variety of steroid and peptide hormones. Which single placental hormone softens the connective tissue of the symphysis pubis, facilitating parturition? ★

A Human chorionic gonadotrophin (hCG)

B Human placental lactogen (hPL)

C Oestrogen

D Progesterone

E Relaxin

9. A 25-year-old man is investigated for infertility. On examination, he is tall and has long extremities, enlarged breasts, and atrophied testes. Genetic analysis reveals a 47,XXY karyotype. Which single name describes excessive development of male mammary tissue? ★ ★

A Amastia

B Athelia

C Gynaecomastia

D Polymastia

E Polythelia

10. A 7-year-old boy presented with precocious puberty. On examination, there was bilateral enlargement of the testes. An MRI scan showed an intracranial tumour. Which is the single most likely cause of precocious puberty in this child? ★ ★

A Congenital adrenal hyperplasia

B Exogenous sex steroids

C Primary hypothyroidism

D Raised intracranial pressure

E Testicular tumour

11. A baby is born to a homeless 18-year-old. The baby is small and has several characteristic facial abnormalities. These include a smooth philtrum and thin upper lip, and there are small palpebral fissures. Which is the single most likely cause of the facial abnormalities? ★ ★

A Alcohol exposure

B Gestational diabetes

C Rubella infection

D Thalidomide exposure

E Trisomy 21 (Down's syndrome)

12. A 12 weeks' pregnant 42-year-old woman attends the antenatal department. On examination her uterus is larger than expected for 12 weeks of gestation and she has higher than normal levels of human chorionic gonadotrophin. Transabdominal ultrasound showed there was no intrauterine gestation but revealed many small round anechoic spaces within the uterus, consistent with a molar pregnancy. Which is the single tissue from which a molar pregnancy arises? ★ ★ ★

A Embryoblast

B Epiblast

C Hypoblast

D Smooth muscle

E Trophoblast

13. Which single labelled stage (A to E) in Fig. 12.1 identifies an early morula composed of up to 16 blastomeres? ★

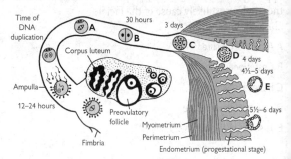

Fig. 12.1

A A

B B

C C

D D

E E

14. A 6-month-old baby boy presents with abdominal distension. On taking a history from the parents it is noted that the baby failed to pass meconium within the first 48 hours after birth and has since suffered with chronic constipation. He also has had repeated bouts of vomiting. The developmental failure of which single germ layer derivative is the cause of the problem described in the scenario? ★ ★

A Intermediate mesoderm

B Lateral plate mesoderm

C Neural crest

D Non-neural ectoderm

E Paraxial mesoderm

15. A baby boy is born at term by normal vaginal delivery. He develops respiratory distress soon after birth and a chest X-ray confirms the presence of a left congenital diaphragmatic hernia. Which single tissue has failed to complete the closure of the diaphragm? ★ ★ ★

A Dorsal mesentery

B Endoderm

C Pleuroperitoneal membrane

D Septum transversum

E Ventral mesentery

16. A baby girl is born with syndactyly (webbing or joining of skin of fingers or toes) of both hands. The failure of which single developmental process has caused this problem? ★ ★ ★

A Cell death

B Cell proliferation

C Patterning of the anteroposterior axis

D Patterning of the dorsal–ventral axis

E Patterning of the proximal–distal axis

17. A 40-year-old woman is referred to the cardiology department for evaluation of a cardiac murmur and dyspnoea on exertion. The electrocardiogram (ECG) shows incomplete right bundle branch block. Echocardiography shows a large atrial septal defect (ASD), with dilated right-sided heart chambers. At cardiac catherization she is found to have a significant left-to-right shunt. During the development of the heart, which single septal tissue is most likely to have led to the ASD in this woman? ★

A Conus swellings

B Endocardial cushions

C Myocardium

D Septum secundum

E Truncal swellings

18. The recurrent laryngeal nerve, a branch of the vagus, is found under the right subclavian artery; on the left side the nerve loops under the ligamentum arteriosum, which is the remnant of the ductus arteriosus that connects pulmonary and aortic trunks in the fetus. Which single fetal artery forms the ductus arteriosus? ★ ★

A 4th aortic arch artery

B 5th aortic arch artery

C 6th aortic arch artery

D Left 7th intersegmental artery

E Right 7th intersegmental artery

19. Fig. 12.2 shows the three main arteries that supply the regions of the developing gut. Which single region, or group of regions, of the gut does the inferior mesenteric artery supply? ★

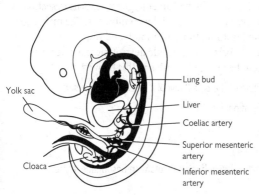

Lung bud

Yolk sac

Liver

Coeliac artery

Superior mesenteric artery

Cloaca

Inferior mesenteric artery

Fig. 12.2

A Anus inferior to the pectinate line

B Caecum, appendix, and ascending colon

C Inferior half of duodenum, jejunum, and ileum

D Left third of the transverse colon, descending colon, sigmoid colon, and rectum

E Right two-thirds of the transverse colon

20. A baby is born with omphalocele, with the majority of his small intestine lying outside the abdomen but covered by an intact layer of amnion. Which single error in a developmental process has caused this condition? ★ ★ ★

A Defect in the abdominal wall musculature

B Failure of the division of the cloaca

C Failure of the formation of the enteric nervous system

D Incorrect return of the physiological herniation of the mid-gut

E Malrotation of the mid-gut

21. A 25-year-old woman developed polyhydramnios at 34 weeks after her last menstrual period and underwent ultrasound assessment to rule out fetal anomalies. Fetal biometry corresponded to 34 weeks and polyhydramnios. There was no demonstrable fluid in the fetal stomach. She had an emergency Caesarian section at 36 weeks after rupture of the membranes. The male baby showed frothing from the mouth and respiratory distress with cyanosis. Which single developmental defect has caused the polyhydramnios in this baby? ★ ★

A Failure of the type II alveolar cells to produce surfactant

B Gestational diabetes

C Placental insufficiency

D Renal agenesis

E Tracheo-oesophageal fistula with oesophageal atresia

22. In Fig. 12.3 which single region (A to E), forms the philtrum of the face? ★ ★ ★

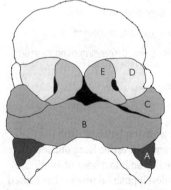

Fig. 12.3

A A

B B

C C

D D

E E

23. A 68-year-old woman dies of bronchopneumonia and donates her body for anatomical dissection. On dissection of the abdomen and pelvis it was noted that she had a horseshoe kidney located in front of the aorta and inferior vena cava at the level of L4. The lower poles of both kidneys are fused to form an isthmus. Which single failure of kidney development has produced a horseshoe kidney? ★

A Ascent of the kidneys

B Failure of the mesonephros to regress

C Metanephric blastema failure

D Renal dysplasia

E Ureteric bud failure to form the collecting ducts

24. Which single structure or structures does the paramesonephric duct become in the female? ★

A Broad ligament

B Epoophoron

C Fallopian tube and uterus

D Ovarian ligament

E Vagina and hymen

EXTENDED MATCHING QUESTIONS

Hormones and steroids involved in reproduction and development

For each of the following, choose the single option which best describes the hormone/steroid described. Each option may be used once, more than once, or not at all.

A Dopamine

B Follicle-stimulating hormone (FSH)

C Gonadotrophin-releasing hormone (GnRH)

D Human chorionic gonadotrophin (hCG)

E Human placental lactogen (hPL)

F Luteinizing hormone (LH)

G Oestrogens

H Oxytocin

I Progesterone

J Prolactin

K Prostaglandin E2

L Relaxin

M Testosterone

1. It stimulates the uterine glands to secrete glycoproteins during the secretory phase of the menstrual cycle. ★

2. It promotes the maintenance of the corpus luteum at the beginning of pregnancy. ★

3. Its synthesis in the testes requires both FSH and LH. ★

4. It is secreted in response to suckling. ★

5. A sharp rise in this hormone precedes ovulation. ★

REPRODUCTION AND DEVELOPMENT
ANSWERS

Single Best Answers

1. E ★   OHMS 2nd edn → p622

The pudendal nerve (S2–4) leaves the pelvis through the greater sciatic foramen and travels around the ischial spine and the sacrospinous ligament to enter the perineum through the lesser sciatic foramen. The pudendal canal (of Alcock) courses anteriorly in the fascia of the obturator internus muscle and divides into the inferior rectal nerve, the perineal nerve, and the dorsal nerve of the clitoris.

The anococcygeal nerve (A) is sensory to the skin in the area of the coccyx. The anterior labial nerves (B) are derived from the ilioinguinal nerve (L1—option D) and the genital branch of the genitofemoral nerve (L1,2—option C) and are sensory to the mons pubis and anterior labium majus. These nerves are also anaesthetized during childbirth.

2. A ★   OHMS 2nd edn → p624

The answer is the genitofemoral nerve. Testicular torsion is the rotation (usually medial rotation) of the testes around the spermatic cord, which results in ischaemic necrosis within 6 hours and is considered to be a surgical emergency.

The cremasteric reflex is considered to be an evaluation of testicular torsion, and is a neurological test both for upper and lower motor neurone lesions and for spinal injury at L1–L2. The reflex is elicited by stroking the upper medial thigh. The afferent fibres of the femoral branch of the genitofemoral nerve are stimulated in this procedure. The reflex activates the motor fibres of the genital branch of the genitofemoral nerve, causing the cremaster muscle to contract, which elevates the testes. This reflex is almost always absent in those patients with testicular torsion. The cremaster muscle is skeletal muscle derived from internal oblique muscle.

The iliohypogastric nerve (B) arises from T12 and L1 and provides sensory information from the skin of the posterior–lateral aspect of the gluteal region and from the skin of the hypogastric region of the lower abdomen. The ilioinguinal nerve (C) arises from L1 and supplies a cutaneous field on the upper anterior thigh lateral to the area supplied by the genitofemoral nerve. The medial femoral nerve (D) is sensory to the anterior and medial aspects of the thigh and knee. The pudendal nerve (E) arises at S2, S3, and S4 and provides cutaneous sensory information from rectal, perineal, and genital areas.

3. E ★   OHMS 2nd edn → p624

The answer is left renal vein. Varicocoele is the dilation of the pampiniform plexus formed from the several small veins which drain the testes. The plexus is located in the spermatic cord. It is not known why the majority of cases are found to be on the left side (>85%). One theory is that the left testicular vein drains to the left renal vein at right angles and so is obstructed by the angulation of the venous junction. The left renal vein crosses anterior to the abdominal aorta under the superior mesenteric artery, and could be compressed between the two arteries (nutcracker syndrome or left renal vein entrapment). Another theory is that the left testicular vein could be compressed by a distended sigmoid colon. Note that on the right side the testicular vein drains directly to the inferior vena cava (C).

The external iliac vein (A) is a large vein connecting the femoral vein to the common iliac vein. The superior epigastric vein drains into the inferior epigastric vein (B), which then joins the external iliac vein close to the femoral ring. The internal iliac vein (D) is a large vein draining many structures within the pelvic region. It joins with the external iliac vein to form the common iliac vein.

Left-sided variocoele can be an important sign in renal cell carcinoma, where spread of the tumour to the left renal vein will block drainage of the pampiniform plexus.

4. C ★   OHMS 2nd edn → p624

A hydrocoele is a collection of fluid in the scrotum. In newborn males it is usually a collection of peritoneal fluid which has drained from the peritoneal cavity through a patent processus vaginalis, which is a diverticulum of peritoneum that has failed to close. This is a common condition although most will close spontaneously within 18 months.

Cryptorchidism (A) is the failure of testicular descent into the scrotum during development. Unilateral cryptorchidism is more common than bilateral, and the testis can often be palpated in the inguinal canal. An epididymal cyst (B) does transilluminate, but the epididymis and the testes can be palpated, and this condition usually occurs between the ages of 20 and 40. Inguinal hernias (D) can accompany hydrocoele because of the patent processus vaginalis, but these do not transilluminate, since the scrotum now contains bowel as well as fluid. A varicocoele (E) feels like a 'bag of worms' and does not transilluminate.

5. C ★★ OHMS 2nd edn → pp626–7

In females, the ureters pass through the broad ligament as they course towards the urinary bladder. Each ureter passes about 12mm from the lateral fornix and the cervix where it is crossed superiorly by the uterine artery. The ureter may be damaged during ligation of the uterine artery, particularly when the pelvic anatomy has been altered by a mass of fibroids.

The uterine artery arises from the internal iliac artery (A). None of options B (uterine vein), D (urethra), or E (urinary bladder), even if damaged, are likely to produce loin pain as the predominant symptom.

 A damaged ureter is a serious complication and may require surgical intervention in an attempt to restore normal function, depending on the nature of ureteral injury. Healing of a crush injury from a clamp or ligature may be helped by placing a stent in the ureter. More extensive and serious damage may require resection or re-routing of the ureter.

http://emedicine.medscape.com/article/454617-overview

6. D ★★ OHMS 2nd edn → pp630–1

Protection from blood-borne products is provided by Sertoli cells, which are bound one to another by junctional complexes containing extensive tight junctions. Sertoli cells are responsible for all metabolic exchange with the systemic circulation compartment.

Leydig cells (A) synthesize and secrete the male sex hormone testosterone. Myofibroblasts (B) adhere to the basal lamina of the seminiferous tubules. Peritubular capillary endothelium (C) is responsible for the production of tissue fluid from blood plasma. Sertoli cells rest on the basement membrane of the seminiferous tubule (E) and their cytoplasm extends to the lumen of the tubule.

7. C ★ OHMS 2nd edn → pp634–7;
OHMS → pp614–17

Following ovulation, in the absence of fertilization, the corpus luteum degenerates into a corpus albicans, which can be recognized under the microscope as a whitish scar within the ovarian tissue.

Options A (antral follicle), B (atretic follicle), and E (primordial follicle) refer to pre-ovulatory follicles. A preantral follicle that does not develop hormone receptors to become a mature antral follicle degenerates and dies, hence its name, atretic follicle. A primordial follicle comprises an oocyte surrounded by mesenchymal cells on a basement membrane. The oocyte arrests in the diplotene of the first meiotic prophase until signalled to resume further development during the reproductive life of a woman. The corpus luteum is the structure that remains following the release of the oocyte and, following successful fertilization, will continue to secrete progesterone under the influence of hCG.

The various stages of follicular development are shown in Fig. 12.4.

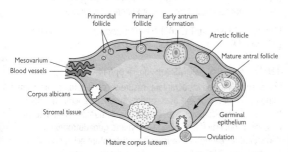

Fig. 12.4

8. E ★   OHMS 2nd edn → p640

During pregnancy relaxin is secreted by the placenta. Its main role is to soften the connective tissue of the symphysis pubis during parturition.

Human chorionic gonadotrophin (A) prevents regression of the corpus luteum to ensure continued progesterone secretion to maintain the uterine endometrium. Human placental lactogen (B) is secreted by the trophoblast cells during pregnancy and produces increased maternal plasma glucose, amino acid, and free fatty acid levels to provide nutrients for the embryo. Oestrogens (C) prepare the body for labour and lactation. Progesterone (D) is produced by the placenta from week 10 to maintain the endometrium and reduce myometrial excitability.

9. C ★★   OHMS 2nd edn → pp642–3

This patient suffers from Klinefelter's syndrome, which is characterized by postpubertal testicular failure. About 80% of males with this syndrome have gynaecomastia. Gynaecomastia also occurs in most newborn males due to stimulation of the glandular tissue by maternal sex hormones, but this effect disappears in a few weeks.

Absence of breasts is referred to as amastia (A). Absence of nipples is called athelia (B). Both are rare congenital anomalies. An extra breast (polymastia, option D) or nipple (polythelia, option E) occurs in about 1% of the female population and is a heritable condition. Hypoplasia of the breast is more often found in Turner's syndrome (commonly a 45,X karyotype).

Klinefelter's syndrome is associated with primary testicular failure. The consequences are small testes and low levels of plasma testosterone. The lack of testosterone feedback inhibition to the pituitary results in high levels of plasma gonadotrophins. The lack of androgens is a cause of the gynaecomastia and hypogonadism, as well as other feminizing features of Klinefelter's syndrome.

Moore, K, & Persaud, T (2003). *The Developing Human: Clinically Orientated Embryology*, 7th edn. New York: Saunders.

10. D ★ ★   OHMS 2nd edn → pp644–5

The answer is raised intracranial pressure secondary to an intracranial tumour. The development of secondary sexual characteristics before 8 years of age in females and 9 years of age in males is defined as precocious puberty (PP). PP is classified into gonadotrophin-dependent (or central) PP, arising from premature activation of the hypothalamic–pituitary–gonadal axis, and gonadotrophin-independent (or peripheral) PP, arising from excess sex steroids. The most likely cause of this child's PP is activation of the gonadotrophin axis by raised intracranial pressure secondary to an intracranial tumour. The raised pressure causes the hypothalamus to secrete larger amounts of gonadotrophin-releasing hormone which activates the hypothalamic–pituitary–gonadal endocrine axis, leading to premature development of secondary sexual characteristics.

Primary hypothyroidism (C) can present with delayed or precocious puberty. High levels of thyrotrophin-releasing hormone can stimulate prolactin and gonadotrophin release. Peripheral causes of PP include: congenital adrenal hyperplasia (A), exogenous sex steroids (B), and testicular tumours (E). However, in adrenal causes of PP, such as congenital adrenal hyperplasia, the testes are small on examination. Gonadal tumours, such as Leydig cell tumour, tend to present with a unilaterally enlarged testis. From the clinical history, there is no evidence of this patient being exposed to exogenous sex steroids.

Lissauer, T, & Clayden, G (2001). *Illustrated Textbook of Paediatrics*, 2nd edn, London: Mosby.

11. A ★ ★   OHMS 2nd edn → p649 OHCM → p282

Fetal alcohol syndrome is thought to be the commonest cause of mental retardation in the Western world. Alcohol is able to cross the placental barrier and causes distinctive facial abnormalities (those mentioned in the scenario) as well as stunting fetal growth. No amount of alcohol is safe and therefore the best recommendation is to not drink at all during pregnancy.

Babies born to mothers who have maternal diabetes (B) are at risk of being large for gestational age or small for gestational age. As neonates they are also more likely to have low blood glucose, jaundice and polycythaemia, and hypocalcaemia and hypomagnesaemia. Congenital rubella syndrome (C) can occur as a result of the mother contracting rubella in her 1st trimester. Neonates present with a classic triad: sensorineural deafness, eye abnormalities (cataracts and microphthalmia) and congenital heart disease—usually patent ductus arteriosus. Thalidomide (D) causes limb defects such as phocomelia (derived from the Greek *phoke*, seal, and *melos*, limb; meaning a shortened limb with long bones reduced or absent). Trisomy 21 (E) may cause a small chin (microgenia), oblique eye fissures with epicanthal folds, a flat nasal bridge and protruding tongue and a single palmar fold.

Environmental factors account for around 7–10% of congenital abnormalities. Genetic causes have been estimated to cause around a third of congenital defects. Most defects have multifactorial causes.

12. E ★ ★ ★   OHMS 2nd edn → pp650–1

The answer is trophoblast. The normal developing embryo consists of two parts: the embryoblast or inner cell mass, which gives rise to the embryo proper, and the trophoblast or outer cell mass, which gives rise to the placenta. In a molar pregnancy, the trophoblast develops into an abnormal mass that often resembles a bunch of grapes. The embryo either does not form or is severely malformed and incompatible with life. Molar pregnancies are caused by an abnormal fertilization of the egg. In a complete mole all the fertilized egg's chromosomes are derived from the father and are therefore YY. Either the sperm fertilized an oocyte containing no female chromosomes or else the female DNA is lost. In a partial mole, the mother's 23 chromosomes remain but there are two sets of chromosomes from the father. This can happen when the egg is fertilized by two sperms, or when the father's chromosomes are duplicated. Normally the placenta is derived from the paternal genetic material while the embryoblast is derived from the maternal.

In normal development the embryoblast (A) gives rise to separate layers, the epiblast (B) and hypoblast (C), which together form the bilaminar germ disc.

Fig. 12.5 shows implantation of a normal embryo into the endometrium at about 14 days after fertilization.

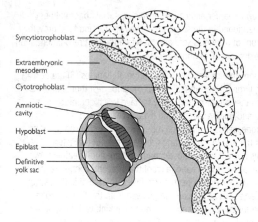

Syncytiotrophoblast

Extraembryonic mesoderm

Cytotrophoblast

Amniotic cavity

Hypoblast

Epiblast

Definitive yolk sac

Fig. 12.5

13. C ★   OHMS 2nd edn → p651

The fertilized ovum is diploid and once the 2nd meiotic division is complete the 1st cleavage into 2 cells can take place. Each cell so produced is called a blastomere. The 1st cleavage takes place around 30 hours after fertilization (B). There are then rapid mitotic divisions over a period of 3 days (C) to produce the 16-cell stage (early morula). By this stage the morula is at the end of the uterine tube and at the opening of the uterus. During cleavage division, while the number of cells doubles, the size of the cells diminishes so that the size of the morula is roughly the same as for the 1-cell and 2-cell stage. The morula (from the Latin for mulberry) is a solid ball of cells and each blastomere is pluripotent (can produce any cell type). The morula continues to divide and by the time it reaches 32 blastomeres it enters the uterus at around day 4 (D). Cavities then start to form by a process of compaction of some of the cells in the morula. There is one main cavity that forms in the morula—the blastocoele—and the embryo becomes the blastocyst (E). This blastocyst will finally start to become embedded into the endometrium on around the 6th day after fertilization.

14. C ★ ★   OHMS 2nd edn → pp652–4

The answer is arrest in the migration of neural crest cells. The child in the scenario has Hirschprung's disease. This results from the absence of enteric neurones within the myenteric and submucosal plexuses of the rectum and/or colon. The ability of the large intestine to propel faecal material is impaired, leading to constipation and distension of the large bowel. The enteric neurones are derived from the neural crest and in development these ganglionic cells migrate caudally along the intestine with the vagal nerve fibres. The cells arrive in the proximal colon by week 8 of gestation and the rectum by week 12. The arrest in the migration of these neural crest cells produces an aganglionic segment of bowel, leading to Hirschprung's disease, which has an occurrence of 1 : 5000 live births, and is more common in males. Nearly all children are diagnosed during the first 2 years of life and half are diagnosed within the first year.

The neural crest cells are found at the lateral borders of the neural plate ectoderm and form a wide variety of cell types including the enteric nervous system, sensory neurones and Schwann cells as well as non-neural derivatives such as melanocytes. The intermediate mesoderm (A) develops into the urogenital system. The lateral plate mesoderm (B) gives rise at limb level to limb connective tissue and at inter-limb level to the gut wall and vascular system. The non-neural ectoderm (D) primarily forms the skin. The paraxial mesoderm (E) forms the somites that give rise to the vertebrae, ribs, and muscles of the trunk and limbs.

15. C ★ ★ ★   OHMS 2nd edn → p656

The answer is failure of a pleuroperitoneal membrane to close a pleuroperitoneal canal. The diaphragm forms between the seventh and tenth week of fetal development. In the scenario, the baby boy has a Bochdalek hernia (a form of congenital diaphragmatic hernia) which occurs on the posterior left side of the diaphragm in approximately 85% of cases. Loops of small and large bowel passing through the diaphragm into the thoracic cavity can cause compression and deformity of the left lung and, in severe cases, the right lung as well.

Four structures fuse during development to form the diaphragm: the dorsal mesentery (A) of the oesophagus, the pleuroperitoneal membranes (C), the septum transversum (D), and the paraxial mesoderm of the body wall. The septum transversum (D) is a sheet of mesoderm that forms rostral to the developing heart. Because of cranial folding, the heart is brought into what will be the thoracic region. The septum transversum, which started more cranially, is now wedged between the heart and the neck of the yolk sac forming an incomplete partition between the thoracic and abdominal cavities. On either side are the pericardioperitoneal canals, which in development are closed off by the pleuroperitoneal membranes. If one of the pleuroperitoneal canals fails to close, a diaphragmatic hernia can arise, usually on the left side as in this case.

16. A ★ ★ ★   OHMS 2nd edn → pp658–60

The answer is failure of normal cell death between the digits. Limbs are patterned along three axes at right angles to each other.

The proximal to distal axis (E) patterns the shoulder to fingertips. Patterning is controlled by the progress zone found underneath the apical ectodermal ridge (AER) of the growing limb. This area secretes growth factors that maintain the cell proliferation in the progress zone. As the cells move out of the progress zone they leave the influence of the growth factors and differentiate. Damage to the AER causes truncation of the limb; the earlier the damage the more severe it is, as more of the limb will be missing.

In the second dimension, the anteroposterior (thumb to little finger) axis (C) is patterned by another signalling centre located on the posterior side of the limb, the zone of polarizing activity (ZPA). If an additional ZPA arises inappropriately on the anterior side of the limb, then mirror image polydactyly arises.

The final axis is the dorsal–ventral (back of hand to palm, extensor to flexor) axis (D). The patterning of this axis is controlled by the factors produced by the ectodermal ridge. This causes the dorsal ectoderm to secrete short-range growth factors. Cell proliferation (B) is important in producing enough tissue for the limb. Cell death (A) is vital to shape the limb appropriately as the early limb is a simple paddle. Cell death shapes the armpit and elbow and separates the digits. Syndactyly is webbing of the digits, which is a failure of normal cell death, or programmed apoptosis, which occurs between the digits.

17. D ★   OHMS 2nd edn → p666

The scenario describes an atrial septal defect (ASD) produced by incomplete closure of the foramen ovale in the septum secundum. An ASD is a deficiency of the septum that separates left and right atria. The atria are separated in development by the growth of two pieces of tissue. The first is the septum primum, which grows down, closing the large ostium primum space between the two forming atria and eventually fusing with the endocardial cushions (B) that form the atrioventricular canals. Before full fusion occurs, programmed cell death creates a hole in the developing septum primum to allow fetal blood to continue to flow from the right to the left side of the heart and, substantially, to bypass the developing lungs, since fetal oxygen is obtained from the placenta and the lungs are collapsed. This hole is called the ostium secundum. A second septum (the septum secundum) now grows downwards and over the septum primum. A hole is formed in this new septum, the foramen ovale, which is covered by a flap valve made from part of the septum primum. This valve only allows blood to flow from right to left atrium. Normally, this flap closes soon after birth, forming the fossa ovale. Closure occurs when right atrial pressure falls below left atrial pressure as the lungs inflate and the pulmonary circulation becomes a low-pressure, low-vascular resistance circuit. Incomplete closure of the foramen ovale will give rise to a patent foramen ovale, an ASD, which can allow blood to pass from left to right sides of the heart. Depending on its size, the defect may not cause significant problems until later in adult life.

The conus (A) and truncal (E) swellings are neural-crest-derived tissue that separate the single outflow tract into the aorta and pulmonary trunk. The myocardium (C) is vital for the separation of the ventricles. Atrial septal defects account for about 10–15% of all congenital cardiac anomalies and are the most common congenital cardiac lesion presenting in adults.

18. C ★ ★   OHMS 2nd edn → pp664-5

As the heart develops, it produces a sequence of paired vessels to take blood away from the heart—the aortic arches (see Fig. 12.6). These are numbered 1 to 6 in order of development in a rostral to caudal direction. They are never all present at the same time and all or part of each pair of arteries may disappear over time. The 1st, 2nd and 3rd arches are symmetrical; the first two disappear while the 3rd becomes the left and right carotid arteries.

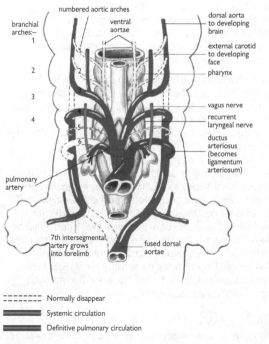

Fig. 12.6

The answer is the distal part of the 6th aortic arch on the left side. From the 4th aortic arch (A) onwards, the fate of the arteries on the left and right sides is different. On the right side the proximal part of the 4th arch artery forms the start of the right subclavian artery. On the left side the 4th aortic arch artery contributes to the arch of the aorta. The 5th pair (B) either disappears soon after appearing or may not develop at all. The most proximal part of the 6th aortic arch arteries on both the left and right will form the pulmonary arteries. The distal part of the 6th aortic arch artery on the right side disappears so the recurrent laryngeal nerve loops higher as the next artery above is the 4th arch, which forms the start of the subclavian artery. On the left side, the distal part of the 6th aortic arch persists and become the ductus arteriosus, an important fetal shunt connecting systemic and pulmonary arterial outputs from the heart. The recurrent laryngeal nerve is therefore lower and loops under the 6th aortic arch on the left side of the embryo. The left subclavian is formed from the left 7th intersegmental artery (D). On the right the distal part of the right subclavian is formed by the right 7th intersegmental artery (E).

19. D ★   OHMS 2nd edn → pp668–9

The gut tube can be divided into three regions, foregut, mid-gut, and hind-gut, each supplied by its own artery and its tributaries. The hind-gut is supplied by the inferior mesenteric artery, and is made up of the left third of the transverse colon, the descending colon, the sigmoid colon, and the rectum.

The embryonic gut tube is blind, ending at both ends. The first region is the foregut. The foregut in the thorax is supplied by the aortic arch arteries. Below the diaphragm the foregut and derivative structures are supplied by the branches of the coeliac trunk. The foregut gives rise to the oesophagus, trachea, lung buds, stomach, and superior half of the duodenum and is associated with the gallbladder, liver, and pancreas as well. The next region is the mid-gut, supplied by the superior mesenteric artery. The mid-gut gives rise to the inferior half of the duodenum, the jejunum, and the ilieum (C) and also the caecum, appendix, and ascending colon (B) as well as the right two-thirds of the transverse colon (E). The blind-ending tube at the end of the hind-gut will form the anus by ectodermal invagination. Where the ectodermal invagination meets the hind-gut is the pectinate line and this marks a change in the blood supply. The anus below the pectinate line (A) is supplied by terminal branches from the internal iliac artery. The fetal blood supply is maintained into the adult.

20. D ★ ★ ★   OHMS 2nd edn → pp669–70

The answer is abnormal physiological herniation of the mid-gut. The mid-gut gives rise to the majority of the gastrointestinal system and so elongates and expands rapidly. This causes a problem as the abdominal cavity is not large enough to contain the large haematopoietic liver as well as all the mid-gut. As a consequence the mid-gut has to herniate out of the abdominal cavity into the umbilical cord around the end of the 6th week and beginning of the 7th week. As it does so it rotates anticlockwise by 90 degrees. Once the abdominal cavity has expanded and grown the mid-gut is able to return and rotates a further 180 degrees anticlockwise, resulting in a total rotation of the mid-gut of 270 degrees. The rotation takes place around the vitello-intestinal duct and superior mesenteric artery axis. Abnormal physiological herniation of the mid-gut, as in option D, is the cause of omphalocoele as the rotation takes place but the loops of intestine do not completely return to the abdomen.

Gastroschisis is similar but the loops of intestine are not covered by the amnion and usually lie to the right of the umbilical cord. Gastroschisis is caused by failure of the abdominal wall to close mainly due to the failure of the abdominal muscle (A) to migrate and close the abdomen. The hind-gut and future urogenital system are connected at the end of the hind-gut in the cloaca (Latin: sewer); the cloaca is separated into the hind-gut and bladder/urethra by the urogenital membrane (septum) as implied in option B. The failure of the development of the enteric nervous system (C) causes Hirschprung's disease, where peristalsis is compromised. Malrotation of the mid-gut (E) predisposes to volvulus and intestinal obstruction.

21. E ★ ★   OHMS 2nd edn → p671

The answer is failure of the tracheo-oesophageal septum to separate the trachea from the oesophagus. The volume of the amniotic fluid increases throughout most of pregnancy, with a volume of about 30ml at 10 weeks of gestation, and reaches a peak of about 1l at 34–36 weeks. Amniotic fluid is constantly circulating, with an estimated exchange rate as high as 3600ml/h. Excretion of fetal urine is the major source of amniotic fluid production in the 2nd half of pregnancy. Fluid is also secreted by the fetal respiratory tract which contributes to the amniotic fluid. The fetus swallows amniotic fluid and it passes through the developing gastrointestinal tract. The respiratory system develops as a budding-off from the foregut and if the tracheo-oesophageal septum fails to separate the trachea from the oesophagus then a tracheo-oesophageal fistula with oesophageal atresia (failure of oesophageal development) can develop, as in option E. The failure of connection of distal and proximal oesophagus means that the fetus is no longer able to swallow and absorb amniotic fluid effectively to circulate it via the placenta; as a result as urine production continues, fluid accumulates within the amniotic sac producing polyhydramnios.

Failure of the type II alveolar cells (A) leads to lack of pulmonary surfactant production and the development of respiratory distress in the neonate and is a risk for premature babies. Gestational diabetes (B), placental insufficiency (C), and renal agenesis (D) all lead to a reduction in the volume of amniotic fluid, oligohydramnios.

22. E ★ ★ ★   OHMS 2nd edn → p675

Fig. 12.3 is a schematic diagram of the fetal face at around 6 weeks of development. Each medial nasal process (E) fuses with the other medial nasal process to form the intermaxillary process, which forms the median part of the nose, the philtrum, and the primary palate. The medial and lateral nasal processes grow around the paired nasal placodes. These invaginate forming the nasal pits, which will form the nasal cavities.

Label A is the 2nd branchial or pharyngeal arch which will contribute to the ear and neck, since part of the hyoid bone forms from this arch. The major contribution that the 2nd arch makes to the face is that the muscles of facial expression are all derived from this arch. B is the largest part of the 1st branchial/pharyngeal arch. This is the mandible, which forms the lower jaw. C is the smaller part of the 1st arch, the maxilla. The maxilla will fuse with the lateral nasal processes of the frontonasal process to form the cheeks. D is the lateral nasal process, which fuses with the maxilla and forms the lateral sides of the nose.

23. A ★   OHMS 2nd edn → p676

The answer is arrested descent of the kidneys. Three different, paired kidney structures arise from intermediate mesoderm in a cranial to caudal sequence during embryonic development. These are termed pronephros, mesonephros and metanephros (plura-nephroi). Each pronephros forms in the cervical region and is transient and non-functional. The mesonephroi are the embryonic kidneys and also contribute to the male genital system. Each mesonephros develops in the lower thoracic and lumbar region and is connected to a mesonephric duct. This duct persists in the male as the ductus deferens and epididymis. In females the mesonephros regresses almost completely (B).

The metanephroi develop in the lower lumbar and sacral regions. The ureteric bud (E) arises as an outgrowth from the caudal end of the mesonephric duct. The ureteric bud grows into the metanephric blastema (C). The two tissues stimulate each other to develop into the definitive kidney and collecting ducts. After formation in the sacral region of the embryo the kidneys ascend to their adult position in the lumbar region. This ascent is due to differential growth rates of the abdominal walls and the kidneys and the regression of the enlarged suprarenal glands. A horseshoe kidney develops because the kidneys become so close during their ascent that their lower poles fuse and ascent is arrested by the inferior mesenteric artery around the level of the lower lumbar vertebrae. Sometimes, as in this case, the kidneys are fully functional and cause few problems. In some cases they can cause pressure on the inferior vena cava, producing oedema of the lower limbs.

Renal dysplasia (D) occurs when the developing kidneys fail to form normal tubules and collecting ducts. It is a major cause of end-stage renal failure in children.

24. C ★ OHMS 2nd edn → pp678–9

In the female, the paramesonephric ducts give rise to the uterus, Fallopian (uterine) tubes and, where the ducts open into the peritoneal cavity, the fimbriae. The inferior ends of the paramesonephric duct meet in the midline and fuse to form the uterus.

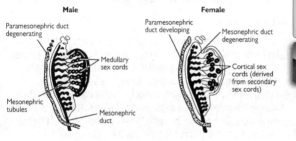

Male

Paramesonephric duct degenerating

Medullary sex cords

Mesonephric tubules

Mesonephric duct

Female

Paramesonephric duct developing

Mesonephric duct degenerating

Cortical sex cords (derived from secondary sex cords)

Fig. 12.7

Initially, there are two pairs of genital ducts in both the male and female: the mesonephric and paramesonephric ducts. In the male the mesonephric duct becomes the ductus deferens and epididymis, while the male paramesonephric duct regresses (see Fig. 12.7). In the female the mesonephric duct normally regresses, but a small remnant persists as the epoophoron (B). This may contain 10–15 transverse small ducts that lead to the Gartner's duct. It is located in the mesosalpinx—the area of broad ligament that stretches from the uterine tube to the level of the ovary. The broad ligament (A) is a wide fold of peritoneum that connects the sides of the uterus to the pelvis. The fibrous ovarian ligament (D) connects each ovary to the lateral aspect of the uterus. The vagina (E) arises from the sinuvaginal bulb and the vaginal plate. The plate is initially solid and is later canalized to form the vaginal lumen. The vaginal lumen remains separated from the urogenital sinus by a thin plate of tissue, which is the hymen.

Extended Matching Questions

1. I ★

Progesterone is secreted by the corpus luteum in the secretory phase of the menstrual cycle, which coincides with the luteal phase of the ovarian cycle. It optimizes conditions for implantation and placental formation within the uterus.

2. D ★

Human chorionic gonadotrophin (hCG) is responsible for the maintenance of the corpus luteum following fertilization so that it does not regress and can continue to secrete progesterone required for the normal pregnancy. hCG is present in the maternal urine approximately 2 weeks after ovulation and is detected by pregnancy tests to confirm pregnancy. In disease, hCG is secreted by trophoblastic tumours, such as gestational mole or choriocarcinoma, and can be detected in the plasma of affected patients to aid diagnosis.

3. M ★

The main testicular androgen, testosterone, requires both FSH and LH for its synthesis by the Leydig cells of the testes, and this process is regulated by the negative feedback loop within the hypothalamic–pituitary–gonadal axis. Low testosterone levels stimulate the hypothalamus to secrete gonadotrophin-releasing hormone, which acts on the anterior pituitary to secrete FSH and LH into the systemic circulation. On reaching the testis, these two hormones act on the Leydig cells to bring about secretion of the testosterone.

4. H ★

The milk 'let-down' reflex during lactation is a process by which milk is moved from the alveoli of the mammary gland to the nipple. This occurs in response to oxytocin secreted by the posterior pituitary during suckling.

5. F ★

The gonadotrophin luteinizing hormone (LH) is secreted by the anterior pituitary and plays an important role in the cyclical activity of the ovaries. A sharp rise in circulating levels of LH that takes place during the preovulatory stage of the ovarian cycle leads to ovulation. Following ovulation, in the second half of the ovarian cycle, LH is responsible for the formation of the corpus luteum, which secretes progesterone to ensure implantation.

General feedback on 1–5: OHMS 2nd edn → pp631, 634–41

CHAPTER 13

HEAD AND NECK AND NEUROSCIENCE

Two apparently separate areas of medical science, head and neck and neuroscience, are often combined in the early phases of undergraduate medical education. Perhaps an obvious reason for this is that the brain, together with the organs of special sense—eyes, ears, nose, and taste buds—are located in the head. Head and neck injuries can therefore be serious and are commonly life-threatening. Another reason is embryological. The development of the head and the central nervous system (CNS) are closely intertwined. The whole CNS is essentially a segmented structure, with a pair of spinal (or cranial) nerves arising in each body segment. For the spinal cord and spinal nerves, each segment is marked by its own vertebra. The situation is more complex in the head, where the developing brain undergoes cervical, cephalic, and pontine flexures. These folds in the growing neural tube, plus the development of a protective cranium, obscure the underlying segmental pattern, but each segment of the brain still bears its pair of cranial nerves.

The organization of the CNS and peripheral nervous system is complex but ordered, and neurological disorder can often be diagnosed by a process of clinical reasoning if the structural and functional properties of the system are sufficiently well understood. Neurological disorders commonly present as alteration in, or loss of, sensation or disturbance of motor function. Knowing which areas of skin (the dermatomes) and which muscles are innervated by each cranial or spinal nerve, together with understanding the characteristic deficiencies produced by abnormality, will often allow the neurologist to use clinical reasoning skills to localize a lesion with considerable accuracy, before radiological or other investigation is undertaken. The diagnostic process is assisted by specific neurological tests, performed during the physical examination, which investigate the integrity of various neural pathways.

Disorders of the CNS can involve alterations of sensory perception, motor performance, emotion, overt behaviour, consciousness, and perceptions of self. Some diagnoses may be made with neurological techniques, others by psychiatric techniques, and in many instances the recognition of characteristic patterns of altered perception, performance, or behaviour may be important clues.

In addition to its close relationship with the brain, cranial nerves, and special senses, the anatomy of the head and neck is important for other reasons. Apart from the non-neural structures associated with the special sense organs, the processes of eating, swallowing, voice production, and facial expression are located in this region, as are endocrine secretion by pituitary, thyroid, and parathyroid glands and exocrine secretion of the salivary glands. Finally, the neck contains some large and important blood vessels and a complex articulation linking head and trunk. Head and neck and neuroscience contain some of the most difficult and complex medical science encountered by the student of medicine. Not surprisingly, there is a correspondingly large number of complex clinical conditions to be mastered as well. ■

SINGLE BEST ANSWERS

1. A 19-year-old man falls from his motorbike whilst not wearing a helmet. He lands on his head and loses consciousness. He is rushed to hospital where a CT scan, Fig. 13.1, shows a convex lens-shaped haemorrhage in the left temple region. Which single vascular structure is most likely to have been injured? ★

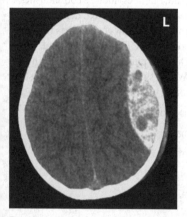

Fig. 13.1

A Cavernous sinus

B Middle cerebral artery

C Middle meningeal artery

D Superficial temporal artery

E Transverse sinus

2. A 24-year-old woman, who has suffered a laceration on her scalp from a car accident, subsequently develops severe swelling of the eyelids and periorbital ecchymosis. Through which single layer of the scalp do the inflammatory fluid and extravasated blood travel? ★

A Connective tissue

B Epicranial aponeurosis

C Loose areolar tissue

D Pericranium

E Skin

3. A 20-year-old woman falls and sustains a blunt trauma to the head, but does not lose consciousness. The following day she presents to the A&E department with a severe headache. She is drowsy and starts to vomit. A computerized tomography (CT) scan of her head appears normal, but lumbar puncture shows blood in the cerebrospinal fluid. Which single condition is the most likely cause of these observations? ★ ★

A Cerebral venous sinus thrombosis

B Extradural haematoma

C Intracerebral haemorrhage

D Subarachnoid haemorrhage

E Subdural haematoma

4. Submandibular resection is a surgical procedure for removal of a submandibular gland, often performed because of multiple recurrent calculi which block the duct lumen. Which single vessel would the surgeon most need to avoid damaging in this procedure? ★

A External jugular vein

B Facial artery

C Lingual artery

D Maxillary artery

E Retromandibular vein

5. A 47-year-old man, who has recently been suffering from headaches, becomes hoarse. He starts to have difficulty swallowing, and examination reveals deviation of the uvula from the midline. He is diagnosed with a skull base tumour. Which single nerve is most likely to be compressed by the tumour? ★

A Ansa cervicalis

B Glossopharyngeal nerve (CNIX)

C Hypoglossal nerve (CNXII)

D Mandibular nerve (CNV3)

E Vagus nerve (CNX)

6. A 12-year-old girl ruptured her tympanic membrane after inserting a nail file into the external acoustic meatus, in an attempt to remove ceruminous (ear) wax. Her doctor is concerned that she may also have damaged a nerve in this area. Which single function should be tested to demonstrate that an important nerve has not been damaged? ★ ★

A Balance

B Hearing

C Lacrimation (tear production)

D Taste sensation over anterior two-thirds of the tongue

E Salivation at parotid duct

7. A 23-year-old woman with a history of epilepsy dies after a prolonged seizure (status epilepticus). Post-mortem histological analysis of the brain shows a reduction in the number of a particular neuronal type. Which single neurone type is most likely to have been reduced in this case? ★ ★

A Chandelier cells

B Horizontal cells

C Purkinje cells

D Pyramidal cells

E Spiny stellate cells

8. A 32-year-old woman with a history of multiple sclerosis (MS) complains of persistent weakness such that she is confined to a wheelchair and is unable to walk. An MRI scan of the lumbar spinal cord reveals plaques. Which single glial cell type is most likely to produce the plaques? ★

A Astrocytes

B Ependymal cells

C Microglia

D Oligodendrocytes

E Schwann cells

9. CNS neurotransmission is achieved through the actions of excitatory and inhibitory neurotransmitters. Some neurotransmitters may also be neuromodulators. Which single neurotransmitter is the most common inhibitory neurotransmitter in the spinal cord? ★

A Acetylcholine

B GABA

C Glutamate

D Glycine

E Noradrenaline

10. The somatosensory pathway for discriminative touch and conscious proprioception from the body (excluding the head) decussates within the central nervous system. Which is the single most likely location of the decussation? ★

A At the level of the diencephalon

B At the level of the medulla

C At the level of the pons

D At the level of the spinal cord

E It does not decussate

11. This ascending pathway conveys information regarding the discriminative aspect and location of a noxious stimulus impinging on the surface of the body. Which single name best describes this pathway? ★

A Anterior (palaeo)spinothalamic tract

B Dorsal column medial lemniscus

C Lateral (neo)spinothalamic tract

D Spinocerebellar tract

E Spinoreticular tract

12. The retina has a highly ordered structure in which ten separate histological layers can be identified. The overall arrangement is curious in that light actually passes through the neurones of the retina before it reaches the photoreceptors. Rod and cone photoreceptors have an outer segment with membrane specializations (invaginations of the cell membrane in cones and intracellular membranous discs in rods) where phototransduction takes place. The outer segment is connected by a cilium-derived structure to an inner segment which contains the nucleus and mitochondria. Which single layer of the retina contains the inner segments of the photoreceptors? ★

A Ganglion cell layer

B Inner plexiform layer

C Inner nuclear layer

D Outer plexiform layer

E Outer nuclear layer

13. A 63-year-old man visits his optometrist because of difficulties with his sight. Confrontation testing reveals bitemporal hemianopsia. Which single point in the visual pathway is the most likely location of the problem? ★ ★

A Optic nerve

B Optic chiasm

C Optic tract

D Optic radiation

E Primary visual cortex (striate cortex)

14. The vestibular system contains sense organs capable of measuring various aspects of head and body motion and orientation with respect to gravity. One of these structures is responsible for detecting linear acceleration/deceleration in the medio lateral and anteroposterior directions. Which single vestibular structure is responsible for this? ★ ★

A Anterior semicircular canal

B Horizontal semicircular canal

C Posterior semicircular canal

D Saccule

E Utricle

15. A 21-year-old male motorcyclist is brought into A&E following a road traffic accident. He complains of constant, 'crushing, burning pain' and an inability to move his arm properly. His right arm biceps, triceps, and supinator tendon reflexes are absent. Two-point discrimination, joint position sense, and vibration and pinprick sensations are all absent but he is able to flex his fingers on voluntary command. Sensory and motor nerve conduction tests on peripheral nerves are normal. From the information in the scenario, identify the single most likely location of the pathology. ★ ★

A Dorsal root

B Ventral root

C Spinal nerve

D Neuromuscular junction

E Peripheral nerve

16. A 65-year-old man with a left-sided cerebrovascular accident is found to have difficulties initiating movements on the right side of his body. His reflexes are normal and there is no muscle weakness. Which single area of the cerebral cortex is most likely to have been damaged? ★ ★

A Posterior parietal cortex

B Prefrontal cortex

C Premotor cortex

D Primary motor cortex

E Supplementary motor cortex

17. Fig. 13.2a shows a coronal section of normal cerebral hemispheres. Identify the nucleus indicated by the arrow. ★

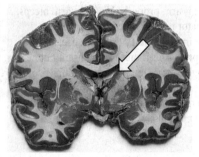

Fig. 13.2a

A Caudate

B Globus pallidus externa (GPe)

C Globus pallidus interna (GPi)

D Putamen

E Substantia nigra

18. Fig. 13.3a shows a sagittal cross-section of the cerebellum. Which single structure is indicated by the arrow? ★ ★

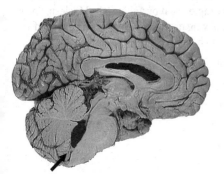

Fig. 13.3a

A Anterior lobe

B Flocculus

C Nodulus

D Posterior lobe

E Tonsil

19. A 65-year-old man complains of 'freezing' when starting to walk. His wife notices that at a pedestrian crossing, he hesitates to cross even though the light is green and does not start to cross until the light changes to amber. He is diagnosed with Parkinson's disease. In the neuronal control of locomotion, failure of which single CNS structure best accounts for this symptom? ★

A Basal ganglia

B Cerebellum

C Parietal cortex

D Premotor cortex

E Primary motor cortex

20. A 30-year-old woman complains of falling asleep inappropriately during the daytime. She undergoes sleep studies, which reveal the simultaneous occurrence of elements of rapid eye movement (REM) sleep and non-rapid eye movement (NREM) sleep. She is diagnosed as having narcolepsy. Which single type of rhythm is most characteristic of REM sleep? ★ ★

A Alpha rhythm

B Beta rhythm

C Delta rhythm

D Gamma rhythm

E Theta rhythm

21. A 70-year-old man with a suspected stroke is brought into A&E. On examination, he does not respond to verbal comments and moans in response to pain. His eyes are closed and do not move. He withdraws his arms from painful stimulation. Which single state of consciousness best describes this patient? ★ ★

A Coma

B Lethargy

C Locked-in syndrome

D Persistent vegetative state

E Stupor

22. A 21-year-old motorcyclist has been involved in a road traffic accident. When assessed at A&E, he withdraws his arm in response to painful stimuli. He subsequently opens his eyes and moans incoherently. Which single number best describes his Glasgow Coma Scale (GCS) score? ★ ★

A 6

B 7

C 8

D 9

E 10

23. A 75-year-old man with a history of chronic alcoholism and associated thiamine deficiency has learning and memory problems. On mental state examination, he is disorientated in time, place, and person and cannot remember the name of the physician who sees him on a daily basis. His long-term memory appears intact in that he can clearly remember events that occurred several years ago. Which single limbic structure associated with memory processing is most likely to be damaged in this patient? ★ ★ ★

A Amygdala

B Cingulate cortex

C Hippocampus

D Hypothalamus

E Mamillary body

24. A 55-year-old man suffering from Huntington's disease is unable to work out how to ride a bike. On further questioning, he correctly defines what a bike is and recollects his favourite childhood bike routes. When asked how to unlock his bike, he tells you where he keeps the padlock key. Which single type of memory is most likely to be affected in this patient? ★ ★ ★

A Declarative

B Episodic

C Procedural

D Semantic

E Working

25. Four months after being involved in a serious road traffic accident, a 30-year-old woman starts to experience nightmares and flashbacks. She is unable to work, feels emotionally numb, and has no interest in future life. A diagnosis of post-traumatic stress disorder (PTSD) is made. Which single brain structure, associated with emotion, plays the most important role in the pathophysiology of this condition? ★ ★

A Amygdala

B Anterior cingulate cortex (ACC)

C Cerebellum

D Hypothalamus

E Prefrontal cortex (PFC)

EXTENDED MATCHING QUESTIONS

Cranial nerves

Which single cranial nerve (or nerve division) from the option list is described in each of the following? Each option may be used once, more than once, or not at all.

A Abducens (CNVI)

B Accessory (CNXI)

C Facial (CNVII)

D Glossopharyngeal (CNIX)

E Hypoglossal (CNXII)

F Oculomotor (CNIII)

G Olfactory (CNI)

H Optic (CNII)

I Trigeminal (ophthalmic division, CNV1)

J Trigeminal (maxillary division, CNV2)

K Trigeminal (mandibular division, CNV3)

L Trochlear (CNIV)

M Vagus (CNX)

N Vestibulocochlear (CNVIII)

1. This nerve can be tested by asking a patient to bare the teeth, puff out the cheeks, or wrinkle the forehead. ★

2. Damage to this nerve produces a drooping eyelid and causes the pupil to deviate downwards and outwards. ★

3. Asking the patient to protrude the tongue and move it rapidly from side to side are clinical tests for this nerve. ★

4. This is the only cranial nerve to exit from the dorsal surface of the brainstem. ★

5. Sensory afferents of this cranial nerve innervate the posterior third of the tongue, the eustachian tube, middle ear, carotid body, and sinus. ★

Psychopharmacology

For each of the following, choose a single drug from the option list which best fits the drug properties described. Each option may be used once, more than once, or not at all.

A Acamprosate

B Alcohol

C Amitriptyline

D Bromocriptine

E Chlorpromazine

F Clozapine

G Cocaine

H Diazepam

I Disulfiram

J Fluoxetine

K Methadone

L Paroxetine

M Phenelzine

N Phenobarbital

O Selegiline

6. This tricyclic antidepressant is a non-selective inhibitor of monoamine transporters. ★

7. This monoamine oxidase inhibitor does not interact with food containing tyramine. ★

8. This neuroleptic is a postsynaptic dopamine D2 receptor antagonist. ★

9. This addictive drug potentiates the effects of GABA$_A$ receptor by increasing the duration of chloride (Cl$^-$) channel opening. ★

10. This alcohol aversion therapy drug is an inhibitor of aldehyde dehydrogenase. ★

Single Best Answers

1. C ★   OHMS 2nd edn → p684

The answer is middle meningeal artery. The pterion is the junction between 4 bones at the temple (squamous temporal, greater wing of sphenoid, parietal, and frontal) and is the weakest part of the skull. It may be fractured either by a direct blow, or through an indirect impact of sufficient force to injure this weakest point. The middle meningeal artery is closely related to the pterion and can be ruptured by a fracture here. This leads to a build-up of blood between the skull and the dura mater, which is an extradural haematoma. This can cause increased intracranial pressure leading to unconsciousness and death.

Extradural haematomas are arterial and so evolve rapidly, whereas subdural haematomas, where blood gathers between the dura mater and the arachnoid mater, are normally venous and therefore evolve more slowly. The superficial temporal artery (D) ascends over the temple superficial to the skull. A cerebral aneurysm of the middle cerebral artery (B) would lead to a subarachnoid haemorrhage. The cavernous sinus (A) and transverse sinus (E) are parts of a system of venous sinuses that drain blood from the internal and external veins of the brain and also collect cerebrospinal fluid. Head trauma can lead to dural venous thrombosis—a rare type of stroke.

2. C ★

The answer is loose areolar tissue. Each of the five layers of the scalp corresponds to a letter of the word scalp. The first 3 layers, the **s**kin (E), the **c**onnective tissue (A), and the epicranial **a**poneurosis (B) are firmly connected and move together. Blood vessels are found in the connective tissue layer, also called the superficial fascia. The fibrous nature of this layer prevents vasoconstriction of injured vessels, resulting in profuse bleeding from a small wound. The aponeurosis is the tendinous layer of the occipitofrontalis, which has an anterior belly over the forehead and the posterior belly over the occipital bone: these are responsible for wrinkling and smoothing the forehead respectively. If a cut is made through all three superficial layers, including the aponeurosis, the wound will gape and require suturing.

The **l**oose areolar connective tissue of the scalp allows infection and fluid (blood or pus) to travel through it. Infections in this area can pass into the cranial cavity via emissary veins. Because the frontalis muscle attaches into the skin and subcutaneous fascia and does not attach on to the frontal bone, fluid can descend into the connective tissue in the eyelids and around the eyes causing them to swell and bruise. The **p**ericranium (D) is the periosteum of the skull bones.

http://en.wikipedia.org/wiki/Scalp

3. D ★★   OHMS 2nd edn → pp690–1; OHCM → pp482–3

The subarachnoid space surrounds the brain and the spinal cord, between the arachnoid membrane and the pia mater. It is the cavity in which cerebrospinal fluid (CSF) is contained and is the interface between the vasculature and the CSF. A subarachnoid haemorrhage (SAH), which is a form of stroke, is bleeding into this space. SAH may occur as a result of a head injury, but more commonly occurs due to a ruptured cerebral aneurysm, particularly around the circle of Willis. SAH symptoms include a severe headache, which can have a very rapid onset ('a thunderclap headache'). Other symptoms can include vomiting, an altered state of consciousness, and, sometimes, seizures.

A head CT scan will correctly diagnose an SAH in the majority of cases and so should be performed immediately. If the CT is negative and an SAH is suspected, a lumbar puncture is performed. The arachnoid layer and subarachnoid space are continuous throughout the spinal cord, and so CSF sampled from the lumbar puncture can show evidence of haemorrhage.

Cerebral venous sinus thrombosis (A) is a clot within the dural sinuses. In CT scans, an extradural haematoma (B) is normally seen as a convex lens-shaped depression between the skull and the dura mater. The subdural space is not continuous around the spinal cord. An intracerebral haemorrhage (C) occurs when blood leaks directly into the brain. Subdural haematomas (E) collect between the outer meningeal layers (the dura and the arachnoid mater).

4. B ★   OHMS 2nd edn → pp692–3

The facial artery, which is the major superficial arterial supply to the face, branches from the external carotid artery in the carotid triangle of the neck adjacent to the hyoid bone. Medial to the ramus of the mandible, it wraps around the posterior part of the submandibular gland, and then ascends over the anterior border of the masseter where its pulse can be felt.

The external jugular vein (A) is superficial and runs between ear lobe and mid-clavicle; it does not form part of the submandibular triangle of the neck. The lingual artery (C) arises from the external carotid immediately proximal to the facial artery (sometimes as one common linguofacial trunk). This artery travels deep to the angle of the mandible and passes deep to the hyoglossus. The maxillary artery (D) is one of the terminal branches of the external carotid. It lies posterior to the neck of the mandible and provides the blood supply to the infratemporal fossa and the superior and inferior dentition, and gives rise to the middle meningeal artery. The retromandibular vein (E) runs posterior and deep to the ramus of the mandible. The facial vein is closely related to the facial artery and passes close to the angle of the mandible (see Fig. 13.4).

Salivary stones occur most commonly in the submandibular gland because the saliva produced by this gland is thicker than that produced by the parotid gland.

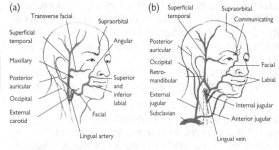

Fig. 13.4

5. E ★   OHMS 2nd edn → pp702–5

The vagus nerve (CNX), via the pharyngeal plexus, provides the motor supply to the muscles of the palate and the pharynx (except for the tensor veli palatini supplied by CNV3, and the stylopharyngeus by CNIX). The muscles of the larynx are also supplied by the vagus nerve via the superior and recurrent laryngeal nerves. Lesions of the vagus nerve can therefore lead to dysphagia (difficulty in swallowing) and dysphonia (voice impairment).

In the scenario, the tumour is on the posterior skull base near the jugular foramen. Involvement of the cranial nerves is due to either compression or infiltration. It would be rare for the vagus nerve to be involved in isolation because both the accessory nerve and the glossopharyngeal nerve accompany the vagus through the jugular foramen. However, the symptoms listed are all related to vagus nerve lesions. The headache would be due to the tumour spreading into the posterior cranial fossa, leading to raised intracranial pressure.

The ansa cervicalis (A) is the motor component of the cervical plexus of nerves and is motor to the infrahyoid strap muscles, which are responsible for depressing the hyoid bone during swallowing. The part of the glossopharyngeal nerve (B) that forms the pharyngeal plexus with the vagus is sensory to the oropharynx. It is therefore the afferent limb of the gag and swallowing reflexes. The hypoglossal nerve (C) is motor to the muscles of the tongue. A lesion in this nerve would lead to tongue wasting and deviation towards the side of the lesion. The mandibular division (D) of the trigeminal nerve is motor to the muscles of mastication and leaves the middle cranial fossa through the foramen ovale.

6. D ★★   OHMS 2nd edn → pp708–9

The chorda tympani nerve, which provides taste sensation for the anterior two-thirds of the tongue, branches from the facial nerve (CNVII) in the temporal bone. It runs superiorly across the tympanic membrane and can be damaged by a large tympanic perforation. Any incisions, for example to release pus from a middle ear abscess, must be made inferiorly through the tympanic membrane to avoid this nerve and the vasculature. The chorda tympani also contains parasympathetic secretomotor fibres, which synapse in the submandibular ganglion and innervate the sublingual and the submandibular salivary glands.

The vestibular branch of the vestibulocochlear nerve (VIII) travels to the utricle, the saccule, and the semicircular ducts, providing for sensations of equilibrium and motion that contribute to balance (A). These nerves and receptors are positioned in the inner ear.

Although hearing (B) may be impaired by damage to the tympanic membrane, the cause is mechanical, not neural. The greater petrosal nerve, which is also a branch of the facial nerve, supplies the lacrimal gland (C) with secretomotor parasympathetic fibres. This nerve arises from the geniculate ganglion located in the facial canal. The nerve does not continue through the middle ear and it does not traverse the tympanic cavity, but exits to the middle cranial fossa where it is joined by the sympathetic deep petrosal nerve, which travels to the pterygopalatine ganglion.

The parotid gland (E) receives its secretomotor innervation from the glossopharyngeal nerve (CNIX) via a very convoluted route. The tympanic nerve is a branch of CNIX, which enters the middle ear through the petrous temporal bone. Its sensory fibres supply the middle ear. The parasympathetic fibres form the tympanic plexus, which is on the medial labyrinthine wall of the middle ear. This gives rise to the lesser petrosal nerve, which penetrates the roof of the tympanic cavity and travels to the otic ganglion. The fibres of CNIX are therefore not on the lateral side of the middle ear and so will not be damaged if the tympanic membrane is ruptured. Salivation can, however, be affected due to recurrent middle ear infections (otitis media).

7. A ★★   OHMS 2nd edn → pp717–18

Epilepsy may be caused by an imbalance of excitatory and inhibitory neurotransmission. Chandelier cells are inhibitory interneurones in the cerebral cortex that regulate the activity of the excitatory pyramidal cells (D). Chandelier cells are lost in epilepsy.

Purkinje cells (C) are the inhibitory output neurones of the cerebellum, whilst spiny stellate cells (E) are interneurones found in the cerebral cortex and basal ganglia. Horizontal cells (B) are found in the retina and are involved in lateral inhibition of retinal ganglion cells.

8. A ★   OHMS 2nd edn → p720

The answer is astrocytes. MS is an autoimmune disease that causes destruction of the myelin sheath of CNS axons. Myelination in the CNS is the primary function of oligodendrocytes (D). However, they are not the glial cell responsible for the formation of the plaque. Demyelination produces an influx of other immune cells and activation of microglia (C) to remove the dying and degenerating axons. Axonal loss ensues and a scar is formed where the astrocytes replace the lost myelin and axons. The number and extent of the plaques correlate with the amount of disability. Ependymal cells (B) are found lining cavities in the CNS which contain cerebrospinal fluid. Schwann cells (E) also provide myelin sheaths for axons but are only found in the peripheral nervous system.

9. D ★   OHMS 2nd edn → p723

Of the options, only GABA and glycine are inhibitory neuro-transmitters; GABA (B) is the main inhibitory neurotransmitter in the brain whilst glycine is the main inhibitory neurotransmitter in the spinal cord. Acetylcholine (A), glutamate (C), and noradrenaline (E) are excitatory neurotransmitters in the spinal cord.

10. B ★   OHMS 2nd edn → p742

The answer is at the level of the medulla. The dorsal column medial lemniscus pathway (DCML) carries information from various peripheral receptors associated with discriminative touch (vibration, light touch, brush, pressure, and proprioception). Sensory afferents enter the spinal cord and send collaterals to the grey matter of the cord at the segment of entry. The axon ascends in the ipsilateral dorsal funiculus to the dorsal column nuclei in the medulla. From here information is transferred to the medial lemniscus pathway, which decussates to the contralateral side and ascends in the medial lemniscus to the ventroposterior lateral nucleus of the thalamus. From there it ascends to the primary sensory cortex. Therefore all second-order neurone axons in this pathway have crossed before the level of the pons (C) and diencephalon (A). Fibres of the anterolateral spinothalamic tracts decussate at the level of the spinal cord (D). The only sensory ascending pathway that does not decussate (E) is the dorsal spinocerebellar tract (see Fig. 13.5).

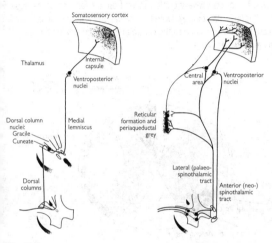

Fig. 13.5

11. C ★   OHMS 2nd edn → pp744–5

The answer is lateral (neo)spinothalamic tract. The spinothalamic tract transmits information about noxious stimuli to the brain. Two stimulus aspects are encoded in the pain percept: fast pain, which allows identification of stimulus type and location (i.e. discriminative aspects of pain), and slow pain, which allows an emotional tag to be placed upon the stimulus. Fast pain travels via the lateral spinothalamic tract (C) via the ventroposterior nuclei of the thalamus to the primary somatosensory cortex. Slow pain travels by the anterior spinothalamic (A) tract to the brainstem reticular formation (the intralaminar thalamic nuclei) and from there to the limbic lobe (cingulate, insula, and amygdala) and ventromedial hypothalamus.

The dorsal column medial lemniscus pathway (B) conveys information about discriminative touch from low threshold cutaneous mechano-receptors and muscle spindle afferents (conscious proprioception), while the spinocerebellar tract (D) is associated with unconscious proprioception and giving information about body position with respect to balance and gravity. Recent evidence suggests that this pathway may also convey pain associated with mechanical hyper-algesia (heightened pain sensitivity) and allodynia (pain resulting from a normally non-painful stimulus). The spinoreticular pathway (E) is thought to convey information about visceral nociception to produce autonomic responses. It is located close to the lateral spinothalamic tract. See Fig. 13.6, which is a diagrammatic cross-section of the spinal cord in the cervical region showing ascending sensory nerve tracts. The tracts conveying information from the left side of the body are shaded in darker grey. Note that lateral and anterior spinothalamic tract fibres have crossed to the contralateral (right) side within the spinal cord. See also Fig. 13.5.

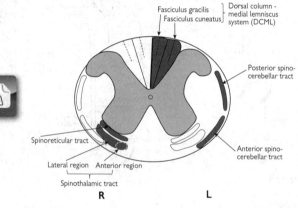

Fasciculus gracilis
Fasciculus cuneatus ⎱ Dorsal column -
medial lemniscus system (DCML)

Posterior spino-
cerebellar tract

Spinoreticular tract

Anterior spino-
cerebellar tract

Lateral region   Anterior region

Spinothalamic tract

R   L

Fig. 13.6

Michael-Titus, AT, Revest, P, & Shortland, P (2010). *The Nervous System*, Chs 4 and 5. London: Churchill Livingstone.

12. E ★   OHMS 2nd edn → p750

The answer is outer nuclear layer. There are three neurones in the pathway from photoreceptor to optic nerve: the photoreceptors (rods and cones), the bipolar cells and the ganglion cells. See Fig. 13.7, which is a diagrammatic representation of the layered structure of the retina, showing major cell types and regions of synaptic interaction.

Synaptic interactions between photoreceptor, bipolar, and horizontal cell dendrites occur in the outer plexiform layer (D) and between bipolar cell, ganglion cell, and amacrine cell dendrites in the inner plexiform layer (B). The ganglion cells are the output cells whose axons form the optic nerve; their cell bodies are located in the ganglion cell layer (A), the layer closest to the lens of the eye. The inner nuclear layer (C) contains bipolar cell axons and the cell bodies of the amacrine, bipolar, and horizontal cells, whereas the outer nuclear layer contains the inner, nucleus-containing segments of the rod and cone photoreceptors.

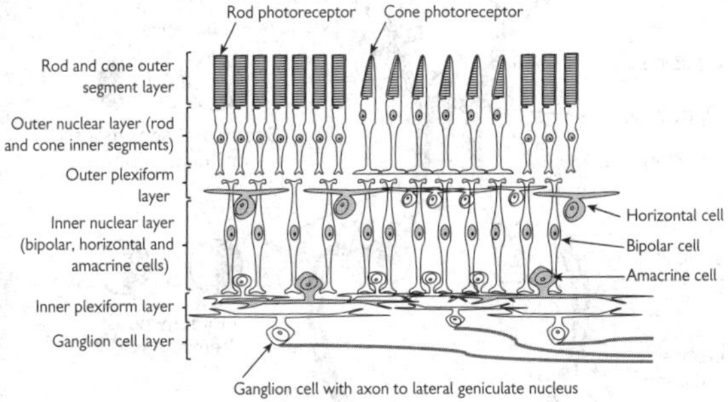

Fig. 13.7

---

13. B ★ ★   OHMS 2nd edn → p754

Tunnel vision (bitemporal hemianopsia) is caused by lesions or compression of the optic chiasm e.g. by upward pressure of a pituitary adenoma. The optic chiasm is a partial decussation. Ganglion cell fibres from the nasal halves of both retinae cross over, while those from the temporal halves do not. The pituitary gland is located in the midline, immediately inferior to the optic chiasm. Enlargement of the pituitary, such as occurs in a pituitary adenoma, creates upward pressure on the chiasm; initially this damages the most medial fibres, which cross from one side to the other. These are the ganglion cell fibres which originate in the nasal halves of each retina and view the temporal or lateral parts of the visual field. This leads to bitemporal hemianopsia, also called 'tunnel vision'.

All lesions in front of the chiasm (optic nerve and retina) produce unilateral, ipsilateral field defects (scotomas, monocular blindness) as they only affect one optic nerve. All lesions post-chiasm (to the optic radiation and striate cortex) produce bilateral, contralateral, homonymous (same side) hemianopsia (+/– macula-sparing). Homonymous hemianopsia implies that information from either the left or right field of both eyes is lost. The optic tract (C) refers to the whole pathway of visual information through the brain to the primary visual cortex and is not the single best answer. See Fig. 13.8, which illustrates the visual pathway from the eyes to the visual cortex of the brain and indicates the effects on the visual fields of damage to the pathway at various points.

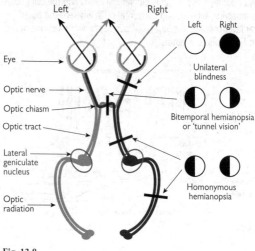

Fig. 13.8

14. E ★★   OHMS 2nd edn → pp762–3

The answer is utricle. The vestibular system measures linear acceleration and angular acceleration/deceleration. The three semicircular canals (A, B, C) are arranged at right angles to each other and contain endolymph fluid. They are, therefore, anatomically suited to the measurement of angular acceleration or deceleration produced by rotational movements of the head. The utricle (E) and the saccule (D) are otolith organs, containing heavy otoconia crystals which rest on a viscous gel layer. These are designed to sense linear acceleration and deceleration. The saccule (D) detects changes in the orientation of the head with respect to the pull of gravity. It is the utricle that detects the forward and backward (anterior–posterior) and side-to-side (mediolateral) accelerations associated with head tilting.

15. A ★★   OHMS 2nd edn → pp748–9

The answer is dorsal root. The man presents with sensory loss only. The normal sensory and motor nerve conduction tests rule out the ventral root (B), spinal (C), and peripheral (E) nerves as possible sites of injury. The ability to flex the fingers indicates that the connection between the corticospinal tract and the motor neurones is intact, as

312

are the lower motor neurone connections to the muscles and neuromuscular junctions (D). The absence of the various stretch reflexes indicates that the input to these monosynaptic reflexes is absent. Coupled with the other information, this means that the lesion must be at the level of the dorsal roots.

16. E ★ ★ OHMS 2nd edn → pp726–7

The answer is supplementary motor cortex. The primary motor cortex (D) lies in the precentral gyrus and produces isolated fine movements on the contralateral side of the body. Focal, small damage to the motor cortex alone does not result in permanent paralysis of limbs, but it may produce subtle impairment, such as weakness or fatigue.

The posterior parietal (A) and the prefrontal (B) cortices represent the highest level of integration in the motor control hierarchy. The posterior parietal cortex (A) receives somatosensory, proprioreceptive, and visual information in order to assess the context in which the voluntary movements are being made. It produces internal models of the movement to be made prior to the involvement of the premotor and motor cortices. Anterior to the primary motor cortex lies Brodmann's area 6, which is divided into a medial, supplementary motor cortex (E) and lateral, premotor cortex (C). These are implicated in the planning and rehearsal of movements before being performed. Unilateral lesions of the supplementary motor cortex, also known as medial area 6, result in the impaired initiation of movement (akinesia) on the contralateral side of the body. Bilateral lesions result in total akinesia, including akinesia for speech initiation. Lesions of the premotor cortex, lateral area 6, impair motor responses to visual or other sensory information. Damage to large parts of area 6 leads to the clinical syndrome of apraxia whereby patients have normal reflexes and no muscle weakness, but have difficulty performing complex tasks, such as brushing their teeth.

17. A ★ OHMS 2nd edn → pp728–9, 739, Fig. 11.45, Fig. 11.53

The coronal section shows 4 of the 5 nuclei associated with the motor loop of the basal ganglia. The caudate nucleus (arrowed) forms the lateral wall of the lateral ventricle. The globus pallidus externa (B) is sandwiched in between the globus pallidus interna (C) medially and the putamen (D) laterally. These are spatially separated from the caudate by the internal capsule. The substantia nigra (E) is found in the midbrain and this is not shown in this specimen.

See Fig. 13.2b showing a labelled coronal section of normal cerebral hemispheres.

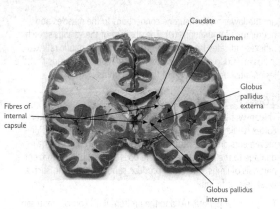

Fig. 13.2b

18. E ★★   OHMS 2nd edn → pp729, 739, Fig. 11.45

The tonsil (arrowed in Fig. 13.2a) lies on the inferior surface of the cerebellum above the medulla of the brainstem. This structure may herniate on to the medulla in instances of raised intracranial pressure in the posterior fossa. In this image, above the tonsil is the anterior lobe (A), with just a small portion of the posterior lobe (D) visible also. The flocculus (B) and the nodulus (C) form the flocculonodular lobe, with the flocculus placed laterally and the nodulus in the midline. These last two are not visible in the labelled specimen of a sagittal cross-section of the cerebellum shown in Fig. 13.3b.

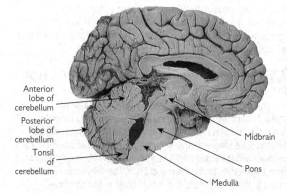

Fig. 13.3b

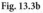

19. A ★   OHMS 2nd edn → pp739–40, 795

Parkinson's disease is a progressive neurodegenerative disorder in which dopaminergic nigrostriatal neurones are lost from the basal ganglia. These neurones are part of the basal ganglia loop involved in the production of movement. The main features of Parkinsonism are tremor at rest, rigidity, bradykinesia, and postural instability. Bradykinesia (slowness of movement) produces difficulties with planning, initiation, and execution of movement.

Movement initiation begins in the parietal cortex (C) and acts via the premotor cortex (D) which feeds signals into the basal ganglia—the area responsible for the onset and offset of movement sequences. Output from the basal ganglia then travels via the thalamus to the primary motor cortex (E) and thence to the spinal cord and the muscles via direct corticospinal tracts and extrapyramidal pathways. The cerebellum (B) is mainly involved with comparing the outflow of the motor commands (a so-called efference copy) with proprioceptive feedback for muscles and joints to provide feedback control and precision of movement. It also plays a role in memorizing movements. Some motor control resides within the brainstem and spinal cord in the form of neuromuscular and proprioceptive reflexes and motor pattern generators, responsible for repetitive movement.

20. D ★ ★   OHMS 2nd edn → pp768–70

On electroencephalography (EEG), electro-oculography (EOG) and electromyography (EMG) two types of sleep are identified: REM and NREM sleep. On the EEG, REM sleep shows 'awake-like' activity that is characterized by low-amplitude, high-frequency gamma waves (30–80Hz), rapid eye movements in the EOG, and reduced muscle tone. NREM sleep is predominantly associated with slow delta wave (C) activity interspersed with higher frequency 'sleep spindles'. Theta waves (E) are low frequency (4–7Hz) and together with delta waves (<3.5Hz) are seen in reduced levels of arousal. Higher frequency (8–13Hz) alpha waves (A) are characteristic of the EEG of the awake but resting brain. Beta waves (B) are associated with mental activity and have a higher frequency (>13Hz).

Narcolepsy is a rare neurological disorder characterized by the tendency to fall asleep inappropriately during the daytime, particularly during sedentary or non-stimulating activities, despite adequate sleep. Narcoleptics have unique sleep cycles because they are unable to keep the normal boundaries of wakefulness, NREM sleep, and REM sleep. They enter the REM sleep quickly after falling asleep, whereas most people take about 90 minutes to enter REM sleep. Characteristically, in these patients, EEG and EMG studies show the simultaneous occurrence of elements of NREM sleep (e.g. sleep spindles) and REM sleep (e.g. rapid eye movements, sawtooth waves and muscle atonia).

Hobson, JA (2005). Sleep is of the brain, by the brain and for the brain. *Nature* 437: 1254–6.

Mahowald, MW, & Schenk, CH (2005). Insights from studying human sleep disorders. *Nature* 437: 1279–85.

21. E ★★   OHMS 2nd edn → p771

Consciousness is a state in which a person is awake and aware of his/her surroundings. It requires the function of the midbrain reticular formation in the brainstem (for the state of wakefulness) and the cerebral cortex (for the state of awareness). In stupor, as in the case of the suspected stroke patient in the scenario, the patient will speak only following painful stimuli, and voluntary movements are nearly absent. The eyes are closed with very little spontaneous movement.

Clinically, there are different states of consciousness, of which stupor is one. Others are lethargy (B), where the patient's speech and voluntary movements, including eye movements, are preserved, and coma (A), where the continuously unconscious patient does not speak, has closed eyes, and painful stimuli result in reflexes at the most. Locked-in syndrome (C) is a condition in which the patient is aware and awake. However, due to an almost complete paralysis of voluntary muscles, except for being able to move the eyes, the patient cannot move or speak. This is usually caused by damage to the ventral part of the pons. In persistent vegetative state (D), the patient has a functional reticular formation, but a dysfunctional cerebral cortex. The patient is awake with open eyes, but cannot respond to stimuli, such as verbal commands or pain, due to lack of awareness.

Snell, RS (2009). *Clinical Neuroanatomy for Medical Students*, 7th edn. London: Lippincott Williams and Wilkins.

22. C ★★   OHMS 2nd edn → p772; OHCM → p802

The answer is 8. The GCS is used to assess consciousness in adults. It includes three parameters: motor function (6 grades), verbal response (5 grades) and eye opening (4 grades). A total score is the sum of the individual scores from each parameter. A score of 8 or less indicates severe injury, a score of 9 to12 is associated with moderate injury, and a score of 13 to15 implies minor injury. The lowest possible score is 3, while the highest is 15.

Table 13.1 The Glasgow Coma Scale (adapted from *Oxford Handbook of Medical Sciences*)

	1	2	3	4	5	6
Motor	No response to painful stimulus	Extensor posturing to painful stimulus (a *decerebrate* response)	Abnormal flexor response to painful stimulus (a *decorticate* response)	Withdraws limb away from painful stimulus	Localizing movements in response to painful stimulus	Obeys commands
Verbal	None	Incomprehensible speech	Inappropriate speech	Confused, conversation	Oriented	Not applicable
Eyes	No eye opening	Eyes open in response to pain to limbs	Eyes open in response to speech	Spontaneous eye opening	Not applicable	Not applicable

Head and Neck and Neuroscience

In the case scenario, the GCS would be as follows: the best motor response—'Withdraws to pain' scores 4; the best verbal response—'Incomprehensible speech' scores 2; and eye opening—'Eye opening in response to pain' scores 2. Therefore, the overall score is 8, which indicates severe injury. Table 13.1 (overleaf) gives more detail of the GCS parameters.

Teasdale, G, & Jennett, B (1974). Assessment of coma and impaired consciousness. A practical scale. *Lancet* **2**: 304(7872): 81–4.

23. E ★ ★ ★   OHMS 2nd edn → pp774–5

This patient probably suffers from Werncike–Korsakoff syndrome, seen in chronic alcoholism and other conditions. It results from damage to the mamillary bodies due to thiamine deficiency. Clinically, this presents as difficulties with memory of recent events, while memories from before the damage occurred remain intact. This is known as anterograde amnesia.

The limbic system is involved with emotions and the basic drives needed for survival, such as eating, drinking, and sex. It comprises a number of structures in the brain, including the amygdala (A), the cingulate cortex (B), the hippocampus (C), the hypothalamus (D), the septum pellucidum, and the septal nuclei. The hippocampus and mamillary bodies are the main players in memory processing. The hippocampus controls data acquisition and recall. Lesions in the hippocampus interfere with consolidation of memory, i.e. transfer to long-term storage, and tend to produce not only anterograde amnesia but also retrograde amnesia in which long-established memories cannot be recalled.

There are two mamillary bodies, located on the underside of the brain, one at each end of the anterior arches of the fornix.

Naish, J, Revest, P, & Syndercombe Court, D (2009) *Medical Sciences*, pp444–7. London: Elsevier.

24. C ★ ★ ★   OHMS 2nd edn → pp776–7

Memory is divided into declarative (explicit) and non-declarative (implicit) memory. Procedural memory, a type of non-declarative memory, is implicated in the acquisition of skills and habits. In Huntington's disease, damage to the striatum impairs the procedural memory of motor task learning (e.g. the ability to ride a bike without working out how to do it) without affecting declarative memory. Declarative memory (A) refers to the formation and retrieval of explicit past memories of facts and events. It is divided into episodic and semantic memory. Episodic memory (B) refers to the recollection of specific events occurring at a particular time and place (e.g. recollection of the bike route). Semantic memory (D) refers to the memory of meanings, understanding, and general knowledge unrelated to specific experiences (e.g. knowledge that a bike is for riding). Working memory (E) is a form of memory used for the short-term retention of information important for problem-solving or reasoning (e.g. that the padlock key is in the garage).

25. A ★★   OHMS 2nd edn → p780

The amygdala (A), the anterior cingulate cortex (ACC) (B), the hypothalamus (D), the prefrontal cortex (PFC) (E), and their interactions influence the processing of emotion. In particular, the amygdala is critical for processing emotional content and significance of stimuli, and is implicated in post-traumatic stress disorder (PTSD). Research has shown that exposure to traumatic stimuli can lead to fear-conditioning with resultant activation of the amygdala and associated structures, such as the hypothalamus, locus ceruleus, periaqueductal grey, and parabrachial nucleus. These interactions produce many of the symptoms of PTSD, due to the activation of autonomic neurotransmitters and endocrine stimulation such as the release of stress hormones.

Dalgleish T (2004). The emotional brain. *Nature Reviews Neuroscience* 5: 583–9.

Extended Matching Questions

1. C ★

The five peripheral branches of the facial nerve innervate the muscles of facial expression. Each branch can be tested by asking a patient to perform a specific test. It is important to note that the forehead muscles receive bilateral input from the corticobulbar upper motor neurones whereas the muscles below the eye receive only a contralateral input from the corticobulbar upper motor neurones. Thus forehead wrinkling may remain symmetrical despite a unilateral upper motor neurone lesion.

2. F ★

The eye moves down and out due to the unopposed actions of the lateral rectus (CNVI) and superior oblique (CNIV) muscles. The eyelid droops due to the unopposed action of the orbicularis oculi (CNVII). Cranial nerve III (F) moves all the other extraocular eye muscles and the levator palpebrae superioris.

3. E ★

The hypoglossal nerve innervates the intrinsic and extrinsic tongue muscles. Injury to CNXII paralyses the ipsilateral half of the tongue, producing ipsilateral deviation on protrusion. Also, some time after injury, the tongue may appear shrunken and wrinkled.

4. L ★

Eleven of the twelve cranial nerves exit from the ventral surface of the brainstem. Trochlear nerve CNIV is the only one to leave on the dorsal surface of the mid-brain. It crosses over and then descends to the ventral side to travel along the clivus towards the superior orbital fissure.

5. D ★

The special sensory fibres of glossopharyngeal nerve CNIX provide taste sensations from the posterior third of the tongue. Other somatic sensory fibres innervate the oropharynx. The carotid sinus nerve supplies the carotid sinus (baroreceptors) and the carotid body (chemoreceptors) to detect changes in blood gases. This nerve also contains parasympathetic fibres to the parotid gland and motor fibres to the stylopharyngeus.

6. C ★

Tricyclic antidepressants (TCAs) are one of the main antidepressant drug groups, which facilitate monoaminergic (noradrenaline and serotonin) transmission. Amitriptyline is a TCA, which non-selectively inhibits monoamine transporters, thereby increasing the levels of monoamine transmitters. Fluoxetine is also an antidepressant drug but acts by selective serotonin re-uptake inhibition (SSRI), which selectively inhibits serotonin transporters.

7. O ★

Selegiline is a selective inhibitor of monoamine oxidase-B (MAO-B), an enzyme which terminates the actions of dopamine. Selegiline therefore raises dopamine availability. This forms the rationale for its use in the treatment of early-stage Parkinson's disease. Unlike non-selective MAO inhibitors, used in the treatment of depression, selegiline does not interact with food containing tyramine due to its selective action on MAO-B.

8. E ★

Neuroleptics, such as chlorpromazine, are used in the treatment of schizophrenia. Their anti-psychotic actions are mainly due to the blockade of dopamine D_2 receptors. By blocking D_2 receptors, they increase prolactin secretion and this results in side-effects, such as breast development and lactation. Bromocriptine is a dopamine receptor agonist, which is used to suppress prolactin secretion by tumours of the pituitary gland.

9. N ★

The GABA$_A$ receptor operates a ligand-gated chloride ion channel. The conductance of such channels is the product of channel open time and frequency of channel opening. Barbiturates, such as phenobarbital, facilitate GABA$_A$ action by increasing the duration of chloride channel opening, whereas benzodiazepines, such as diazepam, increase the frequency of channel opening.

10.I ★

Disulfiram is used to make alcohol consumption unpleasant. It acts through inhibition of aldehyde dehydrogenase, one of the enzyme steps in the metabolism of alcohol. Inhibition of the enzyme leads to acetaldehyde accumulation, leading to nausea. Disulfiram is therefore used in alcohol aversion therapy. Note that acamprosate reduces alcohol craving, but the mechanism of action is unknown.

General feedback on 1–10: OHMS 2nd edn → pp702–5, 782–92

CHAPTER 14

INFECTION AND IMMUNITY

A key outcome in medical education is the training of doctors to acquire the knowledge and understanding of the basic science that underpins clinical practice.

'The doctor as a scholar and a scientist

The graduate will be able to apply to medical practice biomedical scientific principles, method and knowledge relating to: anatomy, biochemistry, cell biology, genetics, immunology, microbiology, molecular biology, nutrition, pathology, pharmacology and physiology.' (Tomorrow's Doctors 2009, GMC, UK).

In this, the last of the themed chapters of questions that map to the *Oxford Handbook of Medical Sciences*, we will test knowledge of infectious diseases and the host immune responses that counteract them. Despite the shift of the world health problem to non-communicable diseases in recent times (*Global status report on non-communicable diseases 2010*, World Health Organization), infectious diseases remain a major health problem in many parts of the world. Even in developed countries, epidemics and outbreaks of infections are not infrequent events, pandemics sporadically crop up at the least expected times. In addition, microorganisms constantly evolve to escape the host immune response and to develop resistance to treatments that have been developed. Therefore, we have no choice but to keep up our knowledge and to develop new treatments. ■

SINGLE BEST ANSWERS

1. In a small Indian village, 20 children ranging from age 2 to 6 are suffering from severe watery diarrhoea and vomiting which developed over a period of 3 days. There had been heavy rains and flooding 2 weeks previously, and at its worst, the village had been submerged under 0.6m of water for at least 3 days. What is the single most likely mechanism underlying their symptoms? ★ ★

A Cell damage by virus

B Neurotoxin

C Pre-formed toxin

D Tissue invasion by bacteria

E Toxin production *in vivo*

2. A 63-year-old man with COPD has been on multiple courses of broad-spectrum antibiotics. He develops persistent diarrhoea, with abdominal pain and fever. The diarrhoea has persisted despite stopping the broad-spectrum antibiotics. What is the single most appropriate drug to treat him with now? ★ ★

A Ceftazidime

B Ciprofloxacin

C Colistimethate sodium

D Gentamicin

E Metronidazole

3. A 67-year-old man is in hospital for a hernia repair. He develops a wound infection, which is shown to be caused by a multi-resistant strain of *Staphylococcus aureus*. What is the single most effective treatment for this infection? ★

A Ceftazidime

B Ciprofloxacin

C Gentamicin

D Metronidazole

E Vancomycin

4. There are two types of MHC proteins, both of which are important for T-cell activation. These are classified into Class I and Class II. Which single cell type does not display MHC type I proteins on its surface? ★

A B-cell

B Dendritic cell

C Endothelial cell

D Erythrocyte

E Macrophage

5. The human immunodeficiency virus (HIV) is a blood-borne, sexually transmissible retrovirus belonging to the lentivirus family, and is subdivided into two genetically distinct but similar forms—HIV1 and HIV2. The hallmark of the acquired immunodeficiency syndrome (AIDS) caused by HIV infection is profound immunosuppression, mainly due to loss of cell-mediated immunity (CMI) caused by tropism of the virus for the CD4 molecule present on T-cells, monocytes/macrophages, and dendritic cells. Which single clinical manifestation is most likely to signify depleted CMI in patients with HIV/AIDS? ★ ★

A Autoantibody-mediated nephrotic syndrome

B CNS demyelination with oligoclonal bands in CSF

C Delayed-type hypersensitivity reaction (e.g. positive tuberculin skin test)

D Neutropenic sepsis and invasive *Aspergillus* infection

E Varicella-Zoster virus (VZV) reactivation (shingles)

6. A 9-month-old, previously well boy who was weaned at 6 months has developed severe, recurrent upper respiratory tract infections in the past 6 weeks. Investigations reveal low (essentially immeasurable) plasma IgA levels, and persistent inability to produce IgAs is suspected. Which single property of secretory IgA is most important in its role as the major antibody present in mucosal secretions and breast milk? ★ ★

A Dimeric structure

B Long half-life (23 days)

C Monomeric structure

D Pentameric structure

E Short half-life (2 days)

7. Antibodies (immunoglobulins) are produced by B-cells and can be secreted or membrane-bound. Which single antibody is the first to be produced following infection or immunization? ★

A IgA

B IgD

C IgE

D IgG

E IgM

8. An 18-month-old girl is given a peanut butter sandwich and immediately vomits after taking a few bites. She develops hives on her face and trunk and her face begins to turn red. She starts to cough and has difficulty in breathing. The emergency paramedics give her intramuscular adrenaline at the scene. Which single immunoglobulin is responsible for this reaction? ★

A IgA

B IgD

C IgE

D IgG

E IgM

9. The histological section in Fig. 14.1 (see Plate 7) is taken from a lymphatic organ which plays an important role in the maturation of T-lymphocytes. Which single important autoimmune condition may be associated with tumours or hyperplasia of this organ?

A Aplastic anaemia

B Graves' disease

C Histocytic necrotizing lymphadenitis (Kikuchi–Fujimoto disease)

D Immune thrombocytopenic purpura (ITP)

E Myasthenia gravis

10. A 72-year-old man receives intravesical bacille Calmette-Guérin (BCG) (normally used to vaccinate individuals against tuberculosis) as part of his treatment for high-risk superficial bladder cancer (carcinoma *in situ*). He later develops a febrile illness with enlarged cervical lymph nodes, and fine-needle aspiration of one of these lymph nodes reveals necrotizing granulomatous inflammation, from which acid-fast bacilli are isolated (see Fig. 14.2 (a) and Fig. 14.2 (b), Plate 8, Papanicolaou and Ziehl–Neelsen stains). Which single type of vaccine does BCG represent? ★

A Conjugated polysaccharide vaccine

B Live attenuated vaccine

C Recombinant DNA vaccine

D Toxoid vaccine

E Whole inactivated vaccine

11. A 32-year-old man undergoes an open lung biopsy as part of investigation into subacute onset of cough and shortness of breath. Histology of the lung biopsy is shown (see Fig. 14.3 (a) and Fig. 14.3 (b), Plate 9). Which single infective agent is the most likely to be associated with this pattern of inflammation? ★ ★ ★

A Cytomegalovirus (CMV)

B *Mycobacterium tuberculosis*

C *Pneumocystis jiroveci*

D *Streptococcus pneumoniae*

E *Strongyloides stercoralis*

12. Inflammation is the body's response to a variety of stimuli, including trauma and infection, and is closely linked with the process of repair. Although fundamentally a protective response, inflammation may be associated with significant systemic effects, for example, the systemic inflammatory response syndrome (SIRS). Features include pyrexia (temperature>38°C), tachycardia, hypotension, coagulation abnormalities, and end-organ dysfunction. Which single mediator is the most likely to exert direct vasodilator effects contributing to hypotension and shock in SIRS? ★ ★

A Complement fragment 5a (C5a)

B Interleukin-1 (IL-1)

C Leukotriene C_4

D Nitric oxide

E Platelet-activating factor (PAF)

13. A 27-year-old man had been treated at a GUM clinic for a chlamydial infection 5 weeks previously. He now presents with a swollen left knee, which appeared suddenly 2 days ago. He also has a raised temperature, conjunctivitis, and generally feels unwell. A blood sample shows a raised ESR, raised C-reactive protein, plus IgA antibodies specific for *Chlamydia*. Which single type of hypersensitivity reaction is likely to have developed in this patient? ★ ★

A Type I

B Type II (macrophage-mediated)

C Type II (complement-mediated)

D Type III

E Type IV

14. A 52-year-old man suffered a myocardial infarction (MI). Two weeks after the MI he develops a persistent low-grade fever with pericardial effusion with a pericardial rub. There is an elevated ESR. Dressler's syndrome is diagnosed and the patient is prescribed non-steroidal anti-inflammatory (NSAID) medication. Which single pathogenesis is the most likely to underlie the autoimmune reaction seen in this case? ★ ★ ★

A Dendritic cell apoptosis

B Drug-induced lupus

C Epitope spreading

D Exposure of hidden antigens

E Molecular mimicry

15. Autoimmune diseases can be broadly divided into conditions that affect a single organ or those that affect the whole body, depending on whether the antigen is present in a specific organ or is more widespread. In most cases the autoantibodies are destructive, causing damage to the organ. However, in a few cases the autoantibody is stimulatory. Which single autoimmune disease is the best example of stimulatory antibody production? ★ ★

A Addison's disease

B Coeliac disease

C Graves' disease

D Hashimoto's thyroiditis

E Myasthenia gravis

16. Transplantation of organs and tissue (such as bone marrow) has now become a common treatment for the failure of individual organs, or replacement of the bone marrow after leukaemia and chemotherapy and radiotherapy treatments. However, preventing the rejection of a new organ by the host's immune system is a major difficulty. Patients have to take immunosuppressant drugs for the rest of their lives and may still develop host-versus-graft rejection. Another complication can be the development of graft-versus-host disease, when the transplanted cells mount an immune attack on the host. Which single transplant procedure is most likely to produce graft-versus-host disease? ★ ★

A Bone marrow transplant

B Heart transplant

C Kidney transplant

D Liver transplant

E Lung transplant

17. A 27-year-old man is declared dead after being involved in a road traffic accident. He is carrying an organ donor card, and his family are happy for the use of his organs for transplants. Recipients are identified for his heart, lungs, cornea, kidneys, and liver. Which single donated tissue is least likely to be rejected by the host's immune system? ★

A Cornea

B Heart

C Kidney

D Liver

E Lung

18. A 31-year-old man had an unremarkable past medical history until 9 years ago when he developed chickenpox, from which he made a full recovery. However, ever since then he has suffered recurrent infections, mainly ENT infections but also urinary tract infections. He has also suffered three episodes of viral hepatitis. Combination antibiotic therapy has treated most of the infectious episodes successfully. Analysis of a blood sample for immunoglobulins showed undetectable IgM and IgA, and very low IgG. The B- and T-cell counts showed a slight increase in B-cell numbers and slightly fewer T-cells. His parents and one brother and one sister have no significant medical history. Which is the single most likely diagnosis in this patient? ★ ★

A Acquired hypogammaglobulinaemia

B Hyper-IgM syndrome

C Selective immunoglobulin deficiency

D Transient hypogammaglobulinaemia

E X-linked agammaglobulinaemia

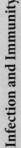

19. A 3-year-old girl had suffered severe neonatal hypocalcaemia and a persistent ductus arteriosus. Since then she has had numerous opportunistic infections, including recurrent *Candida* infections, which have been treated with antibiotics and antifungals. She was born at term, by normal vaginal delivery, to an intravenous drug user. Her birth weight was 3.5kg, and it had been noted that she had micrognathia, low-set dysplastic ears, hypertelorism, and a long philtrum. On investigation, she was found to have a deletion on chromosome 22 (q11.2). Which single deficiency of CMI is most likely to present in this girl? ★ ★ ★

A Chronic mucocutaneous candidiasis

B Congenital thymic aplasia

C Functional T-cell defects

D Secondary defects in T-cell function due to HIV

E Secondary defects in T-cell function due to immunosuppressant therapy

20. A 12-month-old boy, whose parents are first-degree cousins, is referred to hospital with a history of frequent severe chest infections, chronic diarrhoea, and failure to thrive. The parents had lost two children previously at 6 and 9 months of age due to severe combined immunodeficiency disease (SCID). In order to assess the mutation causing SCID in this family, genomic DNA was analysed. This showed a mutation in an enzyme involved with purine metabolism. Flow cytometry was also performed to analyse the quantities of B-, T-, and natural killer (NK) cells. The results showed that lymphocytes were almost completely absent (2% of the white blood cells). T-cells formed 88% of the sample, B-cells 5%, and natural killer cells 7%. Which single type of SCID is the most likely diagnosis in this patient? ★ ★ ★ ★

A Adenosine deaminase deficiency (ADA)

B Bare lymphocyte syndrome

C Mutation in JAK3 tyrosine kinase

D Mutations in the RAG genes (Omenn syndrome)

E X-linked severe combined immunodeficiency

21. A 27-year-old woman is referred to the haematology department because of a history of recurrent infections. She reports recurrent episodes of mouth ulcerations and tonsillitis, for which she had undergone tonsillectomy 2 years previously but with no improvement in the recurrent mouth and throat infections. A prior blood test taken by her GP had revealed marked neutropenia. A more detailed history revealed that there is a regular interval of 3–4 weeks between bouts of infections. At the time of presentation, another blood sample reveals a near-normal level of neutrophils. Which is the single most likely diagnosis in this patient? ★ ★

A Chédiak–Higashi syndrome

B Chronic granulomatous disease

C Cyclical neutropenia

D Job's syndrome

E Myeloperoxidase deficiency

22. A 25-year-old man from Nigeria has sickle-cell anaemia, which caused autosplenectomy when he was 4 years of age. He has recently returned from a visit to his relatives in Nigeria. He presents to his local A&E with a 5-day history of fever. On examination he has a temperature of 38.4°C and is hypotensive (90/60mmHg). On further questioning and investigation, he also has macroscopic haematuria, thrombocytopenia, and renal insufficiency. He normally takes prophylactic penicillin daily to prevent infection by encapsulated bacteria, but his supply ran out while abroad and he has not taken any antibiotics for 2 weeks. He has been fully immunized against encapsulated bacteria. Which single infectious organism is the most likely cause of his illness? ★ ★ ★

A *Babesia microti*

B *Haemophilus influenzae*

C *Neisseria meningitides*

D *Plasmodium falciparum*

E *Streptococcus pneumoniae*

EXTENDED MATCHING QUESTIONS

Infection and immunity

Choose from the option list the single cell type that is described in each of the scenarios below. Each option may be used once, more than once, or not at all.

A Antigen-presenting cells

B B lymphocytes

C CD4 T-lymphocytes

D CD8 T-lymphocytes

E Eosinophils

F Immature T-cells

G Kupffer cells

H Macrophages

I Mast cells

J Natural killer cells

K Neutrophils

L Plasma cells

1. Langerhans cells are normally found in the epidermis of the skin and lymph nodes and are part of the immune system. Langerhans cell histocytosis is a relatively rare condition where there is clonal proliferation of Langerhans cells. This causes severe skin rashes and lymph node enlargement with more systemic effects such as non-specific inflammation. What is another name for a Langerhans cell? ★

2. A 45-year-old man has a 25-year history of heavy alcohol consumption. He needs a liver transplant because of cirrhosis of the liver. He has abstained from alcohol for 12 months now, and a donor liver has been identified for him. A liver biopsy showed extensive cirrhosis and aggregates of this cell type, which has been implicated in the production of pro-inflammatory cytokines such as TNFα, which stimulates the stellate cells to produce collagen. What is the name of these stellate cells? ★ ★

3. A 34-year-old woman attends the miscarriage clinic following 8 consecutive miscarriages over the last 5 years. All miscarriages occurred between 8 and 10 weeks of gestation. She had no significant medical, surgical, obstetric, or gynaecological history other than the repeated miscarriages. There were no abnormalities in her hormone levels and the viral screen was negative, as was the autoimmune screen. A karotype screen of the last fetus was also normal. A mid-luteal phase endometrial biopsy was taken and showed very high levels of this cell type. What is the single most likely cell type in the biopsy? ★ ★ ★

4. A 22-year-old intravenous drug user diagnosed with HIV attends the haematology department for a blood test that monitors the numbers of this cell. Which cell type is most likely to be monitored? ★

5. A 27-year-old woman presents with a 1-week history of watery diarrhoea. She also had intermittent fevers, muscle and joint pain, and periorbital oedema is noted. She has returned from living and working in the Philippines. A blood test is taken and confirms a diagnosis of trichinosis. Which immune cell would be greatly increased in the blood test? ★

ANSWERS

Single Best Answers

1. E ★ ★   OHMS 2nd edn → pp802–3

The answer is tissue invasion by bacteria. The outbreak of severe watery diarrhoea, classically painless, in a setting where there is likely to be poor sanitation, suggests that the cause of the gastroenteritis is *Vibrio cholera*. *V. cholera* is a flagellated bacterium that produces toxins once it reaches the small intestine. The toxin, in turn, is responsible for the diarrhoea. One of the commonest cause of childhood gastroenteritis is rotavirus, but these cases are usually sporadic and the diarrhoea is accompaned by vomiting and a low-grade fever. Viruses infect and damage the epithelial cells of the small intestine (A). Shellfish may contain neurotoxins that give diarrhoeal symptoms (B). Food poisoning caused by *Staph. aureus* or *C. botulinum* is due to pre-formed toxins (C). *Salmonella* and *Shigella* may cause bloody diarrhoea by invasion of the bowel mucosa and toxin production. All the other causes are less likely to account for the epidemiology of the outbreak.

2. E ★ ★   OHMS 2nd edn → pp247, 806–7

The answer is metranidazole. Chronic use of broad spectrum antibiotics is one of the major risk factors for developing *Clostridium difficile* colitis. *C. difficile* is a normal commensal in a small proportion of adults. The use of antibiotics can alter the balance of bacteria in the gut, thereby allowing *C. difficle* to proliferate and produce toxins that cause diarrhoea. Although the history and symptoms are typical, stools should be tested for *C. difficile* toxin in this patient. In mild cases, discontinuation of the broad-spectrum antibiotics is sufficient to manage the condition. In more severe cases, vancomycin or metronidazole may be used and both are effective within 3 days of treatment.

3. E ★   OHMS 2nd edn → pp806–7

The answer is vancomycin. Although meticillin-resistant *Staph. aureus* first developed in hospital, an increasing number of cases are now community-acquired; up to 10% of normal individuals carry the bacteria and, in effect, self-infect. Many hospitals carry out pre-operative screening, and carriers are treated with disinfectant washes with chlorhexidine prior to admission. MRSA is resistant to most of the antibiotics to which *Staph. aureus* is usually susceptible, including beta-lactams and cephalosporins.

4. D ★   OHMS 2nd edn → p825

As the MHC class I proteins are displayed on nearly all nucleated cells in the body, the correct answer is the non-nucleated erythrocyte. Exceptions to the rule include nucleated syncytiotrophoblast cells in the placenta and neurones which lack MHC class I molecules. The class I MHC proteins are recognized by cytotoxic CD8 T-cells. The role of the class I MHC proteins is vital as they signal to cytotoxic T-cells that infectious microorganisms are hidden with the cells of the body. The class I protein is made within the cell and then binds to an 8–9 amino acid peptide produced by the cell which is either 'self' or 'foreign'. The loaded class I MHC protein is then transported to the plasma membrane. In this way, virally infected and cancerous cells are recognized. The class II MHC proteins are expressed on antigen-presenting cells.

5. E ★★   OHMS 2nd edn → pp822, 825–31;
OHCM → pp408–15

CMI is an immune response involving antigen-specific cytotoxic T-lymphocytes, macrophages, and natural killer cells, which all act under the influence of various cytokines. VZV reactivation in the dorsal root ganglion causes neuronal necrosis and a typical painful, dermatomal, vesicular skin rash (shingles). The loss of VZV-specific CMI accounts for this process (which is not seen with increased frequency in hypogammaglobulinaemia, for example, which represents a loss of humoral immunity). Nephrotic syndrome (A) does occur in HIV nephropathy, but this is not an autoimmune-mediated process, but rather is thought to be a direct effect of viral infection in the kidney. Progressive multifocal leukoencephalopathy (PML) is a demyelinating CNS condition associated with HIV/AIDS. It is due to oligodendrocyte injury caused by the JC polyomavirus and is thought to be determined by a cell-mediated (type IV) hypersensitivity reaction against myelin protein, with resultant oligoclonal bands in CSF (B); this may lead to a misdiagnosis of multiple sclerosis. Loss of cutaneous delayed-type hypersensitivity (DTH) (C) would be expected in advanced HIV infection, and therefore TB skin tests would be negative. Neutropenia (D) can occur in HIV infection, either through the effects of the virus, antiviral therapy, or associated malignancies (e.g. lymphoma). Neutrophil polymorphs are phagocytes which are one of the principal effectors of innate immunity.

6. A ★ ★ OHMS 2nd edn → pp834–5

IgA exists in two forms: secretory and intravascular (serum). The intravascular form exists as a monomeric structure (C), but the secreted form has an extra protein chain (J chain) giving rise to a dimeric structure, which renders the antibody resistant to proteolytic enzymes present in secretions. IgA's half-life is intermediate (6 days), as opposed to IgG's which is long-lasting (23 days as in B) and IgE's which is short-lived (2 days as in E). IgM is the first antibody to appear in response to antigen and exists as a pentameric structure (D), which means it is highly avid for antigen and is also able readily to bind complement.

Selective IgA deficiency is regarded as the commonest primary immunodeficiency syndrome and is associated with recurrent sinopulmonary infections, autoimmune disease, allergies (particularly potentially life-threatening reactions to blood or blood products) as well as gut and lymphoid malignancy. A large number of affected individuals are, however, asymptomatic.

7. E ★ OHMS 2nd edn → pp834–5

IgM is the initial antibody produced and secreted by plasma cells during an infection or immunization. It has a half-life of around 5 days. It exists as a pentameric structure with 5 immunoglobulin units bound by a J chain, forming a large antibody. It is able to bind to specific antigens even in the absence of prior immunization, making it responsible for clumping (agglutination) of red blood cells after a non-compatible blood transfusion. This is because it is able to bind to A and B antigens on the red blood cells.

> IgA (A) is the major immunoglobulin in the gut and respiratory tract and in combination with lysozyme is bactericidal but is unable to activate complement.
>
> IgD (B) acts to signal to B-cells to be activated. It is attached to the surface of the B-cell where it functions as an antigen receptor of the B-cell.
>
> IgE (C) is important for the host defence against parasites such as worms. It also mediates atopy and as such, is important for allergic reactions.
>
> IgG (D) is produced later but comprises the majority of serum immunoglobulins and also has the longest half-life.

8. C ★ OHMS 2nd edn → pp834–5

IgE plays an important role in defence against parasites, but in people with an allergy it binds to basophilic granulocytes and mast cells, associated with epithelial cells in the mucosal lining of the bronchial and gastrointestinal tract, causing mast cell degranulation and release of histamine. The histamine causes the hives and reddening of the face and will cause swelling in the upper airways that leads to the difficulty in breathing. The appropriate action in an acute allergic reaction is to administer adrenaline rather than antihistamines. The adrenaline shuts off the mast cell mediator release, thus preventing any further release of histamine. Adrenaline also promotes general vasoconstriction (reducing the fall in systemic arterial blood pressure) and bronchodilation, counteracting the histamine effects. Antihistamines may be given to help resolve the itching and hives but they have no anti-anaphylactic properties.

- IgA (A) is the major immunoglobulin in the gut and respiratory tract and in combination with lysozyme is bactericidal but is unable to activate complement.

- IgD (B) acts to signal to B-cells to be activated. It is attached to the surface of the B-cell where it functions as an antigen receptor of the B-cell.

- IgG (D) is produced later but forms the majority of serum immunoglobulins and also has the longest half-life.

- IgM (E) is the initial antibody produced and secreted by plasma cells during an infection or immunization. It has a half-life of around 5 days and exists as a pentameric structure with 5 immunoglobulin units bound by a J chain. It is able to bind to specific antigens even in the absence of prior immunization, making it responsible for clumping (agglutination) of red blood cells after a non-compatible blood transfusion. This is because it is able to bind to A and B antigens on the red blood cells.

9. E ★ ★   OHMS 2nd edn → pp264, 828, 836

The answer is myasthenia gravis. The histological section is from normal thymus (small lymphocytes and a Hassall's corpuscle are shown), where immature T lymphocytes from the bone marrow undergo maturation (genetic rearrangement of T-cell receptors) and positive selection. A significant proportion of patients with myasthenia gravis also have thymic hyperplasia or thymic tumours (thymoma) and may benefit from thymectomy. Aplastic anaemia (A) is a form of bone marrow failure which may be congenital, but in most cases it is acquired (about 80%). Clinical and laboratory observations suggest that some of the acquired, idiopathic forms of aplastic anaemia are autoimmune in nature. Graves' disease (B) is an autoimmune thyroid condition characterized by hyperthyroidism due to circulating autoantibodies. Kikuchi–Fujimoto disease (C) is a condition of unknown aetiology affecting lymph nodes which may have an autoimmune basis (it is sometimes associated with systemic lupus erythematosus, SLE). Immune thrombocytopenic purpura (D) is caused by increased peripheral platelet destruction, usually caused by antibodies against specific platelet membrane glycoproteins, and may be improved by splenectomy.

10. B ★ OHMS 2nd edn → p837

BCG is an example of a live attenuated vaccine which is prepared from a weakened strain of *Mycobacterium bovis* in order to prevent tuberculosis. It is also used as a form of immunotherapy to treat high-risk superficial bladder cancer, which is rarely complicated by disseminated mycobacterial infection ('BCGosis'), as in this case. Conjugated polysaccharide vaccines (A) use more immunogenic proteins linked to poorly immunogenic polysaccharides (e.g. *Haemophilus influenzae*) in order to improve the immune response. Recombinant protein vaccines (C) are usually produced in yeast cells, allowing purification of specific viral surface antigens (e.g. hepatitis B virus), while toxoid vaccines (D) are highly immunogenic vaccines made by inactivating toxins produced by organisms themselves (e.g. tetanus). Whole inactivated vaccines (E) are made from previously virulent organisms which are inactivated by chemicals or heat (e.g. influenza vaccine).

11. E ★★★ OHMS 2nd edn → p848

The answer is *Strongyloides stercoralis*. The histological sections show diffuse filling of alveolar spaces by eosinophils, recognized by the bright, eosinophilic cytoplasmic granules and bilobed nuclei (eosinophilic pneumonia). Parasitic worm infestation is an important differential diagnosis in this case, but other causes to consider include idiopathic hypereosinophilic syndrome, Churg–Strauss syndrome, drug reactions, hypersensitivity reactions to *Aspergillus* fungi, collagen vascular disease, etc. CMV (A) is more often associated with interstitial inflammation (lymphocytic) and typical intranuclear and cytoplasmic inclusions in infected cells (pneumocytes and endothelial cells), while TB (B) is associated with necrotizing granulomatous inflammation. *Pneumocystis* infection (C) typically causes a foamy intra-alveolar exudate with lymphocytes and plasma cells in the interstitium. *Streptococcus pneumoniae* (D) would more likely be associated with suppurative inflammation (neutrophils).

12. D ★★ OHMS 2nd edn → pp810, 838–9, 846–9

Nitric oxide is an important signalling molecule and causes vasodilation, circulatory collapse, and consequent tissue damage. C5a (A) is an anaphylatoxin and has an important role in chemotaxis, neutrophil-activation, and release of histamine from mast cells (and may therefore cause vasodilation indirectly), while IL-1 (B) plays a role in the development of fever. IL-1 and tumour necrosis factor (TNF) are endogenous pyrogens. Leukotriene C_4 (C) is derived from arachidonic acid and has effects on vascular permeability and bronchial smooth muscle (bronchoconstriction). Platelet-activating factor (E)—PAF—mediates (amongst others) platelet aggregation, endothelial permeability, and bronchoconstriction (the latter probably via the production of leukotrienes). Furthermore, PAF may have secondary effects on the circulation, which are mediated via histamine and nitric oxide.

13. D ★ ★   OHMS 2nd edn → pp856–9

Type III hypersensitivity occurs when the levels of antigens and antibodies are present in roughly equal amounts, leading to extensive cross-linking. It is different from type II hypersensitivity because the antigens are soluble rather than bound on to the surface of the cell. The relatively small immune complexes are not cleared by macrophages and can insert themselves into small blood vessels, joints, and glomeruli, causing symptoms. Examples are post-bacterial infection glomerulonephritis or reactive arthritis, as in this case.

Type I hypersensitivity (A) is an immediate reaction. Some allergens (antigens) can induce the formation of IgE antibodies in people who have a predisposition. The IgE antibodies bind via the Fc receptors to mast cells and if the person is re-exposed to the allergen, cross-linkage of the membrane-bound IgE occurs. This leads to the immediate release of histamine, causing vasodilation and bronchial smooth muscle contraction, mucus secretion, oedema, and blistering of the skin. Most of the allergens are small proteins that can easily diffuse through the skin or mucosa.

Type II hypersensitivity is an antibody-mediated cytotoxic reaction. This can be mediated by macrophages (B) binding to the tails of specific antibodies, which have bound to antigens on a host cell. The macrophage could phagocytose the antigen-covered cell, or a natural killer cell could induce its death. Alternatively, the mechanism is mediated by complement (C), which binds to the tails of the specific antibody, and either leads to the formation of the membrane attack complex and lysis of the cell or attraction of neutrophils by the C3b component. An example of type II (complement-mediated) hypersensitivity is seen when a fetus with Rhesus-positive blood antigen develops in a Rhesus-negative mother who has had previous exposure to Rhesus-positive antigen from an earlier pregnancy, resulting in her producing Rhesus antibodies. The maternal antibodies can cross the placenta into the fetal circulation, where they bind to the surface of the fetal red blood cells and start the complement cascade, resulting in lysis of the fetal red blood cells. Several autoimmune conditions, such as

Graves' disease, are also classified as a type II hypersensitivity reaction.

Type IV (E) hypersensitivity is known as delayed hypersensitivity as the reaction takes 2–3 days to develop and is a cell-mediated response rather than antibody-mediated. The antigenic complex is presented to T-cells by specific types of macrophages. The T-cells clonally expand and, when the antigen is encountered, it is again recognized by these T-cells.

14. D ★ ★ ★   OHMS 2nd edn → pp824–33, 860; OHCM → p712

Some tissues in the body are not patrolled by the immune system or they are found within sealed compartments. The latter is the case with myocardial cell proteins, which are found, sealed off, within the pericardial cavity. However, after an MI or heart surgery, the proteins are released and the previously hidden antigens are exposed and induce an immune reaction. This is usually 2–8 weeks after the MI.

Dendritic cells (A) present antigens to active lymphocytes. Dendritic cells that are defective in apoptosis can lead to the inappropriate activation of lymphocytes and a decline in self-tolerance. Drug-induced lupus erythematosus (B) is an autoimmune disorder, caused by the chronic use of certain drugs, such as hydralazine, procaninamide, or isoniazid. The symptoms of drug-induced lupus typically present as myalgia and arthralgia. Generally, once the drugs are stopped, the symptoms also decline. Epitope spreading (C), or epitope drift, occurs when the immune reaction changes from targeting the primary epitope to also targeting other epitopes. Unlike molecular mimicry, the new epitopes that are recognized do not have to be structurally similar to the primary epitope. Molecular mimicry (E) can occur when an exogenous antigen shares structural similarities with certain host antigens. This means that any antibody produced against the exogenous antigen could also bind to the self-antigens and mount an immune response. An important example is rheumatic fever, in which infection with group A beta-haemolytic streptococci can generate antibodies that cross-react with heart valve tissue, leading to, for example, aortic or mitral stenosis.

15. C ★ ★   OHMS 2nd edn → p860; OHCM → pp208, 210, 218, 516, 555

Graves' disease is unusual in that the autoantibody is stimulatory rather than destructive. This autoantibody binds to the thyroid-stimulating hormone receptor on thyroid epithelial cells, stimulating the production of thyroxine, and thus causing hyperthyroidism.

Addison's disease (A) is also known as chronic adrenal insufficiency or hypocortisolism. The adrenal glands do not produce normal levels of steroid hormones such as glucocortocoids. Autoimmune adrenalitis can cause Addison's disease by destroying the adrenal cortex. This is the result of antibodies against the 21-hydroxylase enzyme—a common cause of Addison's in teenagers and adults. Coeliac disease (B) is an autoimmune condition that affects the small intestine and is associated with sensitivity to dietary gluten. Antibodies to transglutaminase are found in the majority of cases. The autoimmunity develops because gliadin (a gluten protein) cross-links gluten peptides to produce a new epitope that triggers the immune response to form autoantibodies against tissue transglutaminase. Hashimoto's thyroiditis (D) is a form of hypothyroidism that develops because the thyroid gland is destroyed by a variety of cell- and antibody-mediated immune processes. Various autoantibodies may be present against thyroid peroxidize, thyroglobulin and TSH receptors. Activated lymphocytes may also destroy the epithelial cells of the thyroid gland. Myasthenia gravis (E) is an autoimmune condition where antibodies are produced that attack the nicotinic acetylcholine receptor (nAChR) at the neuromuscular junction. Some antibodies impair acetylcholine binding to the receptor while other antibodies destroy the receptor itself. Both types reduce neuromuscular transmission causing weak, easily fatiguing, skeletal muscle contraction.

16. A ★ ★ OHMS 2nd edn → p861

Transplantation of bone marrow can result in a reversal of the usual transplant rejection scenario, where the host immune system rejects the transplanted tissue. When a bone marrow transplant is undertaken, the transplanted cells are replacing the host's immune system and can therefore mount a graft-versus-host reaction as the new immune system does not recognize the host as 'self'.

Even with good tissue matching, heart (B), kidney (C), liver (D), and lung (E) transplants may all be vulnerable to host-versus-graft rejection.

17. A ★ OHMS 2nd edn → p861

Every individual has a large number of different antigens that are expressed on their cells. The major challenge with transplantation is to prevent the new host from rejecting the organ by an immune process. The only organs that would not be rejected without immunosuppressant therapy are those organs that came from a site that does not have immune surveillance, such as the cornea. The cornea is avascular and so does not suffer from the same problems as most other transplants, as it does not require immunosuppressant therapy or tissue-typing to be as stringent as for other transplants. For all other transplants, a number of methods need to be employed to prevent rejection. These include matching the blood group type and HLA types as far as possible. Using immunosuppressive therapy, the new organ is monitored for its function, and any immunosuppressive therapy can be adjusted based on the results from these tests.

18. A ★★ OHMS 2nd edn → p862

Acquired hypogammaglobulinaemia is much more common than congenital immune deficiency. The pathogenesis of the disorder is unknown, and diagnosis is usually based on the absence of infections in the 1st decade of life followed by recurrent pyogenic infections together with hypogammaglobulinaemia, as in this case.

Hyper-IgM syndrome (B) is characterized by high IgM levels and low IgA, IgG, and IgE. Selective immunoglobulin deficiency (C) most commonly causes selective reduction of IgA levels, while levels of IgG and IgM remain normal. Transient hypogammaglobulinaemia (D) can appear after birth, leading to a reduction in the level of IgG and sometimes IgA and IgM as well. It is usually self-limiting, and usually resolves by the age of 2 years. X-linked agammaglobulinaemia (E), also called Bruton syndrome, is a rare X-linked genetic disorder where patients do not form mature B-cells. There are low levels of all classes of antibodies.

19. B ★★★ OHMS 2nd edn → p863

Because of the other anomalies, such as the facial and heart conditions plus the hypocalcaemia and genetic deletion, this girl has congenital thymic aplasia. She has DiGeorge syndrome, in which there is a developmental defect in the third pharyngeal pouch, and often the fourth as well. The third pharyngeal pouch gives rise to the thymus gland and so these children have severe dysplasia or aplasia of the thymus gland. The condition is autosomal dominant. Since there is no thymus gland, there is a complete absence of (or very few) mature T-cells. The number of B-cells is normal but there is a defective response to T-cell-dependent antigens. The third pouch also gives rise to the inferior parathyroids, while the superior parathyroids arise from the fourth pouch. Absence of the parathyroids results in hypocalcaemia. Approximately 80% of cases are caused by a chromosomal deletion on chromosome 22 of a 300 megabase region at q11.2 which contains around 30–50 genes. There are also defects in the other pouches, which account for the facial anomalies, and heart defects due to lack of neural crest integration into the outflow tract.

Chronic mucocutaneous candidiasis (A) is a selective defect involving a response to *Candida* species. There are recurrent or persistent skin infections, usually with *Candida albicans*. There is some evidence of alterations in cytokine production in response to *Candida* antigens, with decreased levels of interleukin-2 and interferon-gamma levels, but increased interleukin-10. Patients who lack normal T-cell immunity, such as those with DiGeorge syndrome, or HIV, are more at risk of developing this condition. In functional T-cell defects (C) there are normal numbers of T-cells but they have mutations in the TCR complex or ZAP-70 tyrosine kinase, which impair interaction with Nuclear Factor Kappa B (NF-kB). Secondary defects in T-cell function constitute a large, heterogeneous group of conditions, including HIV infection (D), where T-cell function is severely impaired or the consequence of chronic immunosuppressant drug treatment (E).

20. A ★ ★ ★ ★ OHMS 2nd edn → p864

Adenosine deaminase deficiency is the second most common form of SCID after the X-linked form of the condition. It is an autosomal recessive condition and accounts for 10–20% of all cases of SCID. Adenosine deaminase is necessary for the breakdown of purines; lack of the enzyme causes an accumulation of deoxyATP, which inhibits the activity of ribonucleotide reductase. The effectiveness of the immune system depends on lymphocyte proliferation and hence deoxynucleoside triphosphate synthesis. Without functional riboncleotide reductase, the proliferation of lymphocytes is compromised. Infants with the condition are lymphopaenic and have severe deficiencies in T- and B-cell numbers and functions. The fact that the parents are first cousins is consistent with an autosomal recessive condition.

In bare lymphocyte syndrome (B) the MHC class II is not expressed on the surface of all antigen-presenting cells. The number of T- and B-cells is normal. Mutations in Janus kinase 3, JAK3 (C), have also been reported, and this enzyme mediates the downstream transduction of the common gamma chain. So the mutation causes similar symptoms to those of the X-linked SCID.

Omenn syndrome (D) is also autosomal-recessive in its inheritance pattern. For immunoglobulin production, recombinase enzymes derived from recombination-activating genes (RAG1 and RAG2) are required.

X-linked SCID (E) is recessive and the most common form of SCID. It is most often due to a mutation in the common gamma chain coded by the IL-2 receptor gamma gene. The common gamma chain is shared by the receptors for interleukin-2, 4, 7, 9, 15, and 21. These interleukins are involved in the development and differentiation of T- and B-cells. There is near-complete failure of the immune system with low or absent T- and natural killer cells, and, while B-cells are present, they are non-functional.

21. C ★ ★ OHMS 2nd edn → pp864–5

Cyclical neutropenia is a form of neutropenia that occurs usually every 3–4 weeks and lasts for 3–6 days. The fact that the patient intermittently has low and near-normal neutrophil counts suggests a cyclical pattern to the disease. Such patients often have recurrent oral infections and on detailed history show periods free of infection, with bouts of more severe infections. Cyclical neutropenia also makes them more prone to post-operative infections if the operation coincides with their neutropenia. They are treated by injections of granulocyte colony-stimulating factor (G-CSF).

Chédiak–Higashi syndrome (A) is a rare autosomal recessive disorder that affects lysosome degranulation within phagosomes. There is mutation within the lysosomal trafficking regulator gene (LYST). This causes the formation of large lysosomes within polymorphonuclear (PMN) leukocytes, as they do not release their contents and phagocytosed bacteria are not destroyed. Chronic granulomatous disease (B) covers a diverse group of hereditary diseases that are both X-linked and autosomal recessive. The defect is in components of the NADPH oxidase which catalyses $NADPH + 2O_2 \rightarrow NADP^+ + 2^{\cdot}O_2 + H^+$. Phagocytes require the oxygen free radicals ($2^{\cdot}O_2$) to destroy bacteria after they have phagocytosed them. Therefore, in affected individuals, their phagocytic cells are unable to kill the organisms that they engulf. Symptoms include recurrent bouts of infection due to decreased capacity of the immune system to fight off pathogenic organisms. The most common infections are pulmonary, skin, and bone infections. The failure of the phagocytes leads to the formation of granulomata in the organ infected.

Job's syndrome (D) is due to abnormal neutrophil chemotaxis because of decreased production of interferon gamma by T-lymphocytes. There are very high concentrations of IgE in the serum of patients with this condition, which leads to it also being referred to as hyperimmunoglobulin E syndrome. Myeloperoxidase deficiency (E) is a common genetic condition where either the quantity or the functioning of myeloperoxidase is deficient. This enzyme is found in certain phagocytic cells, especially PMN leukocytes. Myeloperoxidase deficiency presents in a similar way to chronic granulomatous disease. It is usually clinically silent, suggesting that myeloperoxidase is redundant to other mechanisms of killing phagocytosed bacteria.

22. D ★ OHMS 2nd edn → p866

The answer is *Plasmodium falciparum*. Because of the narrow vessels within the spleen and its role in clearing defective red blood cells, the spleen is a major target during a sickle-cell crisis. It is usually infarcted before the end of childhood and this eventually leads to autosplenectomy. The lack of a spleen increases the risk of infections from encapsulated organisms. Treatment for this condition involves prophylactic antibiotics, with immunization against encapsulated bacteria, and is considered essential for asplenic patients. Immunizations are available for *H. influenzae* (B), *N. meningitides* (C), and *S. pneumoniae* (E).

The other infections that cause problems in these patients are parasitic infections, especially with *Babesia microti* (A) and *Plasmodium* spp. *Babesia* is a protozoan parasite of the blood that causes a haemolytic disease (babesiosis), *Babesia microti* is most common in the Americas; *B. divergens* is the predominant strain in Europe. *Plasmodium falciparum* is also a protozoan parasite that causes malaria in humans; it is responsible for 98% of malarial infections in Africa and is especially prevalent in sub-Saharan Africa. Loss of the spleen increases the susceptibility and severity of the malaria infection. As this individual has been immunized against most encapsulated bacteria, and even though he has been without penicillin, the infectious organism is unlikely to be bacterial. Having travelled to relatives in West Africa, he is more likely to have malaria.

Extended Matching Questions

1. A ★

Langerhans cells are antigen-presenting cells that are normally present in the stratum spinosum layer of the epidermis and in lymph nodes. They can be found in other locations associated with histocytosis. When there is a skin infection, the local Langerhans cells take up and process the microbial antigens and become fully-functional antigen-presenting cells. After they have taken up the antigen, they migrate to the regional lymph nodes where they activate naive T-cells and B-cells.

2. G ★ ★

Kupffer cells are specialized macrophages that are found within the liver and line the walls of sinusoids. The Kupffer cell is also part of the innate immune system as it also expresses the complement receptor of the immunoglobulin family. When alcohol or hepatic viruses activate Kupffer cells, they are responsible for liver injury and damage. The activation of the Toll-like receptor 4 and CD14 receptors expressed by the Kupffer cells internalize endotoxin. This activates the transcription of pro-inflammatory cytokines such as TNFα and superoxides, which stimulate Kupffer cells to synthesize collagen that leads to the fibrosis seen in cirrhosis.

3. J ★ ★ ★

Natural killer (NK) cells are effectors of the innate response and are especially important for antiviral responses. NK cells are large granular lymphocytes that do not contain T-cell receptors and they do not require prior stimulation. They express killer-cell inhibitory receptors (KIR) on their surface. These receptors bind the MHC class

I antigens, which prevent death of the cell. When there is viral infection of a cell, the MHC class I may be down-regulated and thus there is no signalling via the KIR, and the NK cell kills the target by lysis or apoptosis. In the normal endometrium there are normally 0.5–9.5% NK cells. NK cells in the female uterine endometrial lining are unusual and differ from NK cells in peripheral blood by being CD16 negative. The number of uterine NK cells will vary with menstrual cycle phase and between first and third pregnancy semesters. In patients with idiopathic miscarriage, it has been shown that patients are more likely to have higher levels of NK cells (up to 31%). The endometrium contains an unique subset of NK cells (uNK), and women with a high number of these uNK cells are more likely to suffer miscarriages.

4. C ★

HIV can infect a variety of different immune cells such as macrophages and microglial cells in the nervous system; however, the CD4+ T-cells are probably the first cells the virus infects. HIV-1 entry into the CD4+ cell is mediated via gp120 and chemokine receptors. Once infected, the CD4+ cell migrates to the lymphoid tissue where the virus replicates and releases the new viral particles that infect more CD4+ cells. As the infection progresses, the number of CD4+ cells declines producing immunosuppression. CD4+ cell count is therefore used as an indicator of the severity of the disease.

5. E ★

Eosinophils are part of the immune system that attacks multicellular parasites. Their cytoplasmic granules contain cationic proteins, which can kill worms (and other cells) by binding to the cell surface. Eosinophilia has a wide variety of causes, including allergic reactions, skin diseases, and even use of certain medications.

Trichinosis is a parasitic disease caused by eating raw or undercooked pork or wild game. While the incidence in the United Kingdom has been reduced by meat inspection, there are still a number of cases per year in people returning from eastern Europe or Asia. A large population of adult worms in the intestines causes nausea and diarrhoea 2–7 days after infection. The next stage is parenteral, where the larvae migrate from the intestines to other tissues, causing inflammatory responses. Larval stages can enter the muscles causing myalgia, and periorbital oedema is a classic sign.

General feedback on 1–5: OHMS 2nd edn → pp826, 828–35, 844–5; OHCM → pp408–9

MEDICAL SCIENCES IN CLINICAL REASONING

CHAPTER 15

CLINICAL APPLICATION OF MEDICAL SCIENCES

This chapter comprises a mixture of questions overlapping in content with those in the preceding 14 chapters, but often at a higher level, testing the understanding and application of basic science in clinical medicine. As such, students in the earlier years of the medicine course should leave this section until you have attempted questions in most of the other chapters. However, senior medical students or newly qualified doctors who may be using this book to revise for postgraduate examinations should feel more confident in this section.

Since the questions are a mixture, and represent a sample of many areas of basic science, we will use it to show how an exam paper is set. Of course, students should realize that there may be some variation between medical schools, but some broad principles will still apply.

The team or person organizing the exam will initially design an exam blueprint. The blueprint is determined by the learning objectives and skills to be tested, and the relative importance of each, expressed as relative percentages or number of questions. Usually, these are proportional to the amount of time allocated to the topics in the curriculum. This will ensure that there is adequate coverage and sampling of the learning objectives. The blueprint consists of a table showing the content and allocation of questions.

The table may be very detailed, in which case there will not be many questions in each category, or it may be rather more broad. In an integrated medical exam, the contents usually reflect body systems and tasks or skills. Some blueprints may also include traditional subject areas such as anatomy, pathology, and pharmacology to make sure that these are not under-represented.

An example is shown overleaf.

	Mechanisms of disease	Investigation of disease and data interpretation	Diagnosis	Patient management, including therapeutics	
CVS					16%
RS					13%
GIT					7%
LIVER & PANCREAS					8%
GU inc KIDNEY					11%
GYNAE & BREAST					6%
CNS inc PNS					13%
LYMPHORET					5%
EYES EARS THROAT					5%
ENDO					11%
SKIN BONE JOINTS					5%
	20%	25%	30%	25%	

Some of the categories are somewhat artificial as they are intimately related. For example, some questions that are entered under 'diagnosis' require 'interpretation of laboratory data'. Some questions that test management require a student to make the diagnosis beforehand.

Once the blueprint is set, question writers are then directed to populate the question paper accordingly.

At the end of this section, the questions contained herein will be displayed according to how they are divided in a blueprint (see Table 15.1). Since the answers will be given, please refrain from peeping at pages 415 and 416, or it will reduce the educational value and spoil your fun! ∎

SINGLE BEST ANSWERS

1. A 39-year-old man presents with malaise and weight loss of 6kg over the last 3 months. Clinical examination does not reveal any abnormality. Of note, his grandfather and one of his uncles had colorectal carcinoma. He is referred to a gastroenterologist. On investigation, he is found to have several nodules in the liver, confirmed to be metastatic adenocarcinoma. Colonoscopy and biopsy show an adenocarcinoma of the caecum. What is the single most likely mechanism underlying his malignancy? ★ ★

A BRAF mutation

B Loss of cell senescence

C Loss of e-cadherin

D MLH-1 germline mutation

E Over-expression of Indian Hedgehog signalling

2. A 60-year-old man presents with a 6-month history of malaise and weight loss. On examination, he has cervical and axillary lymphadenopathy. His full blood count shows Hb 9.2g/dL, white cell count 90×10^9/L, and platelet count 100×10^9/L. Examination of the peripheral blood film shows large numbers of myeloid blasts, as does the bone marrow aspirate. What is the single most likely genetic abnormality behind the disease? ★ ★

A Deletion in short arm of chromosome 7

B JAK1 mutation

C Translocation from chromosome 7 and chromosome 14

D Translocation of Abl gene on chromosome 9 to Bcr gene on chromosome 22

E Trisomy 12

3. A 53-year-old woman presents with a 3-month history of fatigue. She also complains of nausea and vague abdominal pain. Examination does not show any abnormality. Her GP performs some screening blood tests, including a full blood count and serum biochemistry. The only abnormality found is adjusted serum calcium concentration of 3.0mmol/L. What is the single most likely mechanism accounting for the hypercalcaemia? ★ ★

A Autonomous secretion of parathyroid hormone

B Compensatory secretion of parathyroid hormone

C Extra-renal production of Vitamin D

D Secretion of parathyroid-hormone-related peptide

E Vitaminosis D

4. A 22-year-old woman sees her GP complaining of vague symptoms. These include tiredness, chronic low-grade diarrhoea alternating with constipation, and two missed periods in the last 6 months. She appears pale, and her Hb is 8g/dL . Her GP suspects coeliac disease, but wishes to perform another blood test before referring her to a gastroenterologist. What is the most appropriate test to confirm coeliac disease? ★ ★

A Anti-cardiolipin antibody

B Anti-endomysial antibody

C Anti-mitochondrial antibody

D Anti-nuclear antibody

E Anti-smooth-muscle antibody

5. A 66-year-old woman attends a follow-up breast clinic for her annual check-up since she had a mastectomy for breast cancer 7 years ago. She complains of pain in her back and the side of her chest. This is worsened when she bends to pick up objects. There is some tenderness over the lateral chest wall. A skeletal survey shows a few lytic lesions in her ribs. Her initial investigations show Hb 8g/dL, white cell count 11.0×10^9/L and platelet count 95×10^9/L. Serum urea concentration is 35mmol/L and creatinine 580μmol/L. The serum calcium is 2.9mmol/L. Examination of a biopsy of a rib lesion shows numerous plasma cells. These exhibit light chain restriction for kappa. What is the single most likely diagnosis? ★ ★ ★

A Metastatic breast carcinoma

B Myeloma

C Non-Hodgkin lymphoma

D Paget's disease

E Renal bone disease

6. A 62-year-old man presents with poor stream, nocturia, and urinary frequency. The symptoms started a year ago, and have worsened, especially the nocturia, which disrupts his sleep. On rectal examination, the prostate is moderately enlarged and has a smooth contour and firm consistency. His serum prostatic-specific antigen concentration is 1.2ng/mL (<1.5ng/mL). What is the single most appropriate management? ★ ★

A α-Antagonist

B α-Reductase inhibitor

C No management

D Radical prostatectomy

E Trans-urethral resection of prostate

7. A 26-year-old woman developed urinary frequency associated with dysuria. Urinalysis shows traces of protein and blood. She had similar symptoms lasting for a week 6 months ago, but they resolved without treatment. What is the single most appropriate management? ★

A Co-amoxiclav

B Co-trimoxazole

C Oral fluids

D Gentamicin

E No treatment indicated

8. A 53-year-old man has proteinuria of 2g/24h associated with serum albumin of 28mmol/L. There are red blood cells detected in the urine. His blood pressure is 160/90mmHg. Serum urea concentration is 30mmol/L and creatinine is 510mmol/L. Histological examination of the renal biopsy shows normal glomeruli and tubules, but the interstitium is filled by numerous lymphocytes and scanty eosinophils. No immune complexes are detected. What is the single most appropriate management? ★ ★

A Albumin replacement

B Azathioprine

C Colchicine

D Prednisolone

E Ramipril

9. An 18-year-old man presents with bilateral ankle oedema. He is found to have proteinuria of 10g/24h, associated with serum albumin of 18mmol/L. There are no casts or red blood cells detected in the urine. His blood pressure is 140/80mmHg. Serum urea concentration is 20mmol/L. Histological examination of the renal biopsy shows normal glomeruli, tubules, and interstitium. No immune complexes are detected. What is the single most appropriate management? ★

A Albumin replacement

B Azathiaprine

C Colchicine

D Prednisolone

E Ramipril

10. A 67-year-old woman reports a 2-year history of numbness and burning pain in both feet to her GP. The numbness started in her toes but has now spread up to her knees and fingers. On examination there was diminished sensitivity to pinprick and heat over both feet and up to the knees. There was also diminished pinprick sensation of her distal fingertips. Vibratory sensitivity was reduced at the great toes but normal at the ankles. She underwent a 2-h oral glucose tolerance test (OGTT) which showed a borderline normal fasting glucose at 7mmol/L and a 2-h glucose level that was elevated at 10mmol/L. Which single mechanism is the most likely to be responsible for these symptoms? ★

A Alcohol abuse

B Hyperglycaemia

C Lumbar spinal nerve root compression

D Syringomyelia

E Vitamin B$_{12}$ deficiency

11. A 52-year-old woman is referred to a rheumatologist for an acutely painful left ankle. She has a history of hypertension, which she takes bendroflumethiazide. There is no family history of arthritis, and she reports that she has been in good health until the development of the recent monoarthritis. On examination, she has marked swelling and erythema of her left ankle, which she reports as being very painful. There is nothing further of significance on physical examination. An X-ray showed no bony deformity but did show soft tissue swelling of the joint. The synovial fluid aspirated from the joint was cloudy with many leukocytes, with around 75% of them being neutrophils. Which is the single most likely cause of disease in this case? ★ ★

A Articular cartilage degeneration

B Bacterial infection

C Formation of microbial antigens

D Overproduction of TNFα

E Uric acid excess

12. An 80-year-old woman has been virtually housebound for the last 4 years following an ischaemic stroke, which has restricted her ability to walk. She has no family and has a nurse who comes in to see her every day. One day the nurse comes in to find her on the kitchen floor, unable to move, and calls for an ambulance. In hospital, the woman is lucid and able to answer questions. She reports generalized bone pain and muscle weakness that had gradually increased over the last 2–3 years, which she attributed to the stroke. She has kyphosis and scoliosis, which has developed over the last year. A blood sample was taken and X-rays taken of the hip and spine.

The blood results are:

- Serum 25(OH)D$_3$ 6ng/ml
- Serum 1,25(OH)$_2$D$_3$ 20pg/ml
- Serum Ca^{2+} 2mmol/L
- Serum PO$_4^{3-}$ 0.4mmol/L
- Alkaline phosphatase   250iu/L

The X-rays showed a fractured hip and multiple vertebral fractures. Which is the single most likely diagnosis of the woman's underlying problem? ★ ★

A Osteoarthritis

B Osteomalacia

C Osteopenia

D Osteoporosis

E Paget's disease

13. An 82-year-old woman stumbled on a stair a few days previously and has been limping since then. When an X-ray is taken, it shows an intracapsular fracture of the left femoral neck. She undergoes surgery to stabilize the fracture. Which of the following would be the single most appropriate treatment to be started in this woman? ★

A Bisphosphonate

B Calcitriol

C Hormone replacement therapy

D Strontium ranelate

E Teriparatide

14. A 25-year-old sexually active woman attends a cervical smear clinic. Her last menstrual period was 7 days ago and her only complaint is a scant, white, curd-like vaginal discharge. She recently completed a course of antibiotics for an episode of cervicitis. Microscopic examination of her cervical smear shows severe dyskaryosis and presence of fungal pseudohyphae. She is referred to a colposcopy clinic and undergoes a cervical biopsy, which is reported as cervical intraepithelial neoplasia III (CIN III). Which of the following organisms is most single likely cause of the dysplasia? ★ ★

A *Candida albicans*

B *Chlamydia trachomatis*

C Herpes simplex virus

D Human papillomavirus

E *Trichomonas vaginalis*

15. A 45-year-old woman has experienced progressive fatigue and generalized pruritus for the past 6 months. On physical examination she appears jaundiced and has numerous scratch marks on her body. There is no hepatomegaly. Her full blood count is normal, but serum biochemistry shows: albumin 33g/L, bilirubin 40μmol/L, AST 41U/L, ALT 32iu/L, and alkaline phosphatase 300iu/L. Test results for antimitochondrial antibody are positive, but antinuclear and perinuclear antineutrophil cytoplasmic antibodies (pANCA) are negative. Which of the following is the single most likely diagnosis? ★ ★

A Autoimmune hepatitis

B Haemochromatosis

C Primary biliary cirrhosis

D Primary sclerosing cholangitis

E Wilson's disease

16. A 39-year-old woman with a recent history of trauma to the left breast presents with an ill-defined 1cm nodule in the outer lower quadrant. The overlying skin is normal. There is no nipple discharge. No axillary lymphadenopathy is detected. She attends a rapid access breast clinic and undergoes a fine-needle aspiration of the nodule. Cytological examination reveals abundant foamy macrophages in a 'dirty' lipidic background. Which of the following is the most likely diagnosis? ★ ★

A Duct ectasia

B Fat necrosis

C Fibroadenoma

D Intraductal papilloma

E Radial scar

17. A 50-year-old woman presents with a firm 1cm irregular mass in the outer upper quadrant of the left breast for the past 4 months. The overlying skin and nipple are normal. No axillary lymphadenopathy is detected. Mammography confirms the presence of an irregular density with scattered calcifications. She undergoes a wide local excision with axillary node clearance. Histopathological examination of the excised breast tissue shows an infiltrating ductal carcinoma that is positive for oestrogen and progesterone receptors. The immunohistochemistry of the breast lesion is negative for HER2 protein. All retrieved lymph nodes are free of malignancy. Which of the following additional treatment options is most likely to be used in this patient? ★ ★

A Isoflavone

B Lapatinib

C Tamoxifen

D Teicoplanin

E Trastuzumab

18. A 45-year-old man presents with rapid mental decline over the past 5 weeks. On physical examination he has weakness of the left arm and ataxia. Magnetic resonance imaging (MRI) shows multifocal white-matter lesions in the parieto-occipital regions and the cerebellum with sparing of the optic nerves and spinal cord. Immunohistochemistry of the biopsied brain tissue shows JC polyoma virus in oligodendrocytes. Which single laboratory test result is this patient most likely to have? ★ ★ ★

A High serum glucose

B High serum triglycerides

C Low CD4 count

D Low serum sodium

E Oligoclonal bands in CSF

Clinical application of medical sciences

365

19. A 66-year-old man is admitted for investigation of chronic cough, leg swelling, poor effort tolerance, and inability to lie flat due to breathlessness. The chest radiograph shows an enlarged heart and features of pulmonary oedema, and because of a modest pancytopaenia he has a bone marrow trephine. This shows increased numbers of plasma cells. He suffers an acute arrhythmic cardiac arrest, from which he could not be resuscitated. A consented hospital post-mortem examination is performed and histology of the myocardium is shown in Fig. 15.1 (a) and Fig. 15.1(b) (see Plate 10). Which gross pathological finding would you expect to see at autopsy? ★ ★ ★

A Heavy, firm heart with brownish, waxy cut myocardial surface

B Heavy, flabby heart with dilation of all chambers and wall thinning

C Severe coronary artery atheroma with dense myocardial scarring

D Severe left ventricular hypertrophy with disproportionate thickening of the interventricular septum

E Thickened, fused aortic valve leaflets with marked concentric left ventricular hypertrophy

20. A 75-year-old man complains of increasing shortness of breath and right-sided chest pain on deep inspiration. He worked for many years in a shipyard. The right hemithorax is dull to percussion and breath sounds are markedly reduced on that side. The chest radiograph is shown in Fig. 15.2. Which is the single best pathophysiological alteration to explain the clinical findings in this patient? ★ ★ ★

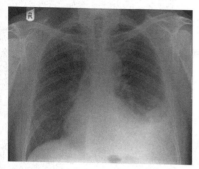

Fig. 15.2

A Decreased colloid osmotic pressure

B Decreased lymphatic drainage

C Increased intrapleural negative pressure

D Increased vascular permeability

E Increased venous hydrostatic pressure

21. A previously fit and well 82-year-old woman is brought into A&E complaining of central abdominal pain. She has atrial fibrillation, with a heart rate of 140bpm and her blood pressure is 90/60mmHg. On examination her abdomen is tender centrally with no other abnormal findings. What is the single most likely diagnosis? ★ ★

Results of blood tests are:

- Hb: 17.1g/dL
- MCV 84f
- Platelets 325 x 10⁹/L
- WCC 14.1 x 10⁹/L

- Na+ 146mmol/L
- K+3.9mmol/ L
- Creat 151μmol/ L
- Urea 8.2mmol/ L
- Amylase 201U/dL
- Lactate 5.4mmol/L
- Liver function tests normal.

Arterial blood gas on air shows:

- pH 7.29
- PO₂ 12.2kPa
- PCO₂ 4.7kPa
- Base excess −8.7
- Abdominal X-ray normal

A Acute cholecystitis

B Acute mesenteric ischaemia

C Acute pancreatitis

D Perforated bowel

E Ruptured abdominal aortic aneurysm

22. A 33-year-old woman sees her GP as she is complaining of dyspepsia. She has been advised to try over-the-counter antacid medication but this has not helped. The GP performs a urease breath test which is positive. What is the single best next treatment to be initiated? ★ ★

A Continue antacids for a further 4 weeks

B Lansoprazole, amoxicillin, and metronidazole

C Omeprazole

D Ranitidine bismuth citrate

E Sucralfate, clarithromycin, and metronidazole

23. A 27-year-old man visits his GP as he is feeling unwell. He tells his GP he had a sore throat about a month ago, from which he thought he had recovered but he is now feeling generally unwell. The GP performs blood tests which show renal impairment, and urine dip shows proteinuria and haematuria. What is the single most likely diagnosis? ★ ★ ★

A Anti-glomerular basement membrane disease

B IgA nephropathy

C Minimal change glomerulonephritis

D Proliferative glomerulonephritis

E Rapidly progressive glomerulonephritis

24. A 76-year-old woman who moved from India to the UK 12 months ago visits her GP as she is feeling very lethargic. The GP does some blood tests that show a low calcium level. What is the single most likely diagnosis? ★ ★

A Primary hyperparathyroidism

B Pseudopseudohypoparathyroidism

C Sarcoidosis

D Secondary hyperparathyroidism

E Tertiary hyperparathyroidism

25. A 24-year-old woman who is known to have asthma attends her GP because she has noticed that she is coughing at night. She has a blue 'reliever' (short-acting β-2 agonist) that she occasionally uses during the day, but is not on any other medication. What would be the single most appropriate management decision? ★ ★

A Add in a long-acting β-2 agonist

B Add in an anticholinergic

C Add in an inhaled steroid

D Advise more frequent use of her reliever

E No change

26. A 65-year-old man who has never smoked is complaining of breathlessness. His lung function results are shown in Fig. 15.3. These data are a part of the analysis produced using CareFusion Spirometry PC software. What is the single most likely diagnosis? ★ ★ ★

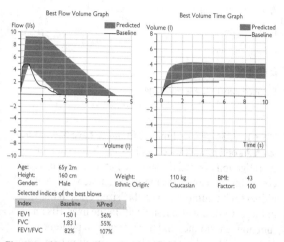

Age:	65y 2m				
Height:	160 cm	Weight:	110 kg	BMI:	43
Gender:	Male	Ethnic Origin:	Caucasian	Factor:	100

Selected indices of the best blows

Index	Baseline	%Pred
FEV1	1.50 l	56%
FVC	1.83 l	55%
FEV1/FVC	82%	107%

Fig. 15.3 Abbreviations: 'FEV1' – Forced expiratory volume in first second of expiration; 'FVC' – forced vital capacity. 'Baseline' is the patient's data, '%Predict' is the percentage of predicted value (predict) obtained with the patient's 'best blow'. 'BMI' is body mass index.

A Kyphoscoliosis

B Muscular dystrophy

C Obesity hypoventilation syndrome

D Previous pulmonary radiotherapy

E Pulmonary fibrosis

27. A 48-year-old woman attends A&E as she has a very painful red eye and blurring of her vision. On examination her pupil is not responding to light and her cornea is noted to be hazy. What is the single most likely diagnosis? ★ ★

A Acute glaucoma

B Acute iritis

C Conjunctivitis

D Keratitis

E Subconjunctival haemorrhage

28. A 54-year-old man is found to have haematuria on an insurance medical and is referred for investigation of renal disease. He has an elevated serum creatinine, and an ultrasound scan shows very enlarged kidneys with numerous, variably sized cysts in both kidneys. Cysts are also noted within the liver. His renal function deteriorates and he is started on peritoneal dialysis, with a plan for renal transplantation later. Some months later he collapses suddenly during a friendly football match and dies. A coroner's post-mortem is performed. What is the single most likely autopsy finding explaining the cause of sudden death in this patient? ★ ★ ★

A Acute bacterial peritonitis and sepsis

B Acute retroperitoneal haemorrhage from a ruptured renal cyst

C Intrathoracic haemorrhage from ruptured aortic dissection

D Severe mitral valve stenosis and left atrial dilation

E Subarachnoid haemorrhage from ruptured berry aneurysm

29. A 36-year-old Afro-Caribbean man who has been diagnosed recently with sarcoidosis complains of excessive thirst, polydipsia, and polyuria. Biochemical investigations show the following:

- Fasting blood glucose = 5.8mmol/L   Haemoglobin A$_{1c}$ = 5%

- Sodium = 149 mol/L   Urea = 3mmol/L

- Chloride = 108mmol/L   Creatinine = 57mmol/L

- Potassium = 3.9mmol/L   Calcium (total) = 2.2mmol/L

- Plasma osmolality = 309mOsmol/kg   Urine osmolality <200mOsmol/kg

A water deprivation test is performed. The urine osmolality remains low during the test and upon administration of subcutaneous vasopressin, it increases by more than 50%. Which is the single most likely explanation for the symptoms and biochemical findings? ★ ★

A Granulomatous inflammation of the anterior pituitary gland

B Granulomatous inflammation of the hypothalamus

C Granulomatous inflammation of the kidneys

D Granulomatous inflammation of the pancreas

E Granulomatous inflammation of the posterior pituitary gland

30. A 27-year-old man has endoscopy of the upper GIT for persistent symptoms of bloating, diarrhoea, and mild iron-deficiency anaemia. A duodenal biopsy reveals villous atrophy and increased intra-epithelial lymphocytes. Serology identifies circulating antigliadin and anti-endomysial antibodies. He then develops a pruritic, blistering skin rash on the extensor surfaces of his arms, knees, and buttocks. A punch biopsy of peri-lesional and lesional skin is taken. Histology of the blister is shown in Fig. 15.4 (see Plate 11). Immunofluorescence (IMF) shows granular IgA deposition along the dermo-epidermal junction. What is the single most likely cause of his skin rash and gastrointestinal symptoms? ★ ★ ★

A Drug reaction

B Gluten sensitivity

C Malignant lymphoma

D Strongyloidiasis

E Porphyria

31. A 45-year-old woman complains of weakness, polyuria, and paraesthesia. She is hypertensive. Investigations reveal a serum K$^+$ of 2.9mmol/L. A secondary cause of the hypertension is suspected. Which is the single most appropriate initial investigation? ★ ★ ★

A Abdominal CT scan

B Renal angiography

C Renal ultrasound scan

D Serum aldosterone : renin ratio

E Urine collection for catecholamines

32. Neurodegenerative diseases are characterized by progressive neuronal loss in cortical or subcortical grey matter due to the deposition of aggregates of abnormal proteins, which are resistant to normal cellular mechanisms of degradation and ultimately result in neuronal death. A consented hospital post-mortem examination is performed on a 72-year-old man who died of a neurodegenerative disorder. The neuropathologist reports the presence of pallor of the substantia nigra (SN) with histological loss of pigmented neurones and the presence of Lewy bodies in many of the remaining SN neurones. Which is the single most likely abnormal protein responsible for this condition? ★ ★ ★

A α-synuclein

B Beta amyloid

C Huntingtin

D Prion protein

E Tau

33. A 23-year-old woman attends her GP complaining of headaches, malaise, fever, and dry cough over the preceding week. Examination was unremarkable and she is prescribed bed rest and antipyretic medication for presumed viral infection. Ten days later she attends the A&E department with acute onset of confusion, headache, nausea, and vomiting. A history of recent travel to India is elicited. She is febrile and a generalized tonic–clonic seizure is observed in the emergency room, after which she remains drowsy and irritable. A VIth cranial nerve palsy is present and MRI demonstrates basilar meningeal thickening and a ring-enhancing lesion in the right parieto-occipital region. An HIV test is negative, and other test results are given below.

CSF examination:

- Raised CSF opening pressure and fibrinous 'webs' noted within the fluid
- CSF Protein 1.6g/L (reference range 0.15–0.45g/L)
- CSF Glucose 1.2mmol/L (blood glucose 6.5mmol/L)
- Cell count 425 cells/mm^3 (reference range $\leq$ 5 lymphocytes/mm^3), mainly lymphocytes

Which single test result would you most likely expect in this scenario? ★ ★ ★

A Detection of JC virus genome fragments in CSF

B Malignant lymphoid cells present on cytological examination of CSF

C Positive CSF cryptococcal latex agglutination test

D Positive CSF fluorescent treponemal antibody absorption (FTA-ABS) test

E Positive CSF *Mycobacterium tuberculosis* PCR

EXTENDED MATCHING QUESTIONS

CVS drugs

For each of the following clinical scenarios, select the most appropriate drug. Each option may be used once, more than once, or not at all.

A Adenosine

B Adrenaline

C Amiodarone

D Atenolol

E Bendroflumethiazide

F Digoxin

G Doxazosin

H Furosemide

I Glyceryl trinitrate

J Irbesartan

K Lidocaine

L Methyldopa

M Nifedipine

N Ramipril

1. A 73-year-old man who has type II diabetes mellitus is is found to be hypertensive and has microalbuminuria. He is started on medication by his GP. Four weeks later he returns to his GP as he is not sleeping, due to a dry irritating cough. The GP stops the new drug and changes to another. What is the drug he should be switched to? ★ ★ ★

2. A 69-year-old woman is being treated for heart failure and has noticed her ankles are becoming progressively more swollen. Before starting medication she has her renal function checked and is found to have mild renal impairment. What medication should she be started on? ★ ★

3. A 74-year-old man was started on medication several years ago by a cardiologist. He visits his GP as he is becoming increasingly short of breath. On examination there are fine inspiratory bibasal crepitations, and spirometry reveals a restrictive picture. The clinician decides to discontinue one of his medications. Which one? ★ ★ ★

4. A 32-year-old woman is brought into A&E resus as she is complaining of palpitations and her ECG shows a supraventricular tachycardia rate of 150BPM. Having tried carotid massage and the Valsalva manoeuvre, there is no resolution of the tachycardia. Which treatment should she be given now? ★ ★

5. A 27-year-old pregnant woman is found to be hypertensive and her obstetrician recommends that she starts treatment. Which drug is safe to use in pregnancy? ★ ★

Management of diabetes

For each of the clinical scenarios, select the most appropriate management for the patient. Each option may be used once, more than once, or not at all.

A Amitriptyline

B Bendroflumethiazide

C Ezetimibe

D Gliclazide

E Intravenous antibiotics

F Lifestyle advice

G Long-acting sub-cutaneous insulin plus short-acting insulin depending on meals and activity

H Losartan

I Metformin

J Once daily sub-cutaneous insulin

K Oral antibiotics

L Pioglitazone

M Ramipril

N Repaglinide

O Simvastatin

6. A 17-year-old is newly diagnosed with type I diabetes mellitus. This is explained to her fully and she has good understanding of the disease. She is currently undertaking her A levels and wants to go to university to study sports science. In her spare time, she is a competitive runner. ★ ★

7. A 65-year-old man has an oral glucose tolerance test performed. His fasting glucose is 6.7mmol/L and his 2-h glucose is 7.7mmol/L. ★ ★

8. A 54-year-old businessman is admitted to hospital following a myocardial infarct. He undergoes primary angioplasty and makes a good recovery. The cardiologists start him on the regular secondary prevention medication and perform a fasting blood glucose, which is found to be elevated at 9.3mmol/L. ★ ★

9. A 73-year-old woman with type II diabetes sees her chiropodist as she has noticed that she has a hot red area surrounding the ulcer on her foot which is getting bigger. The chiropodist organizes an X-ray which shows evidence of osteomyelitis. ★

10. An 82-year-old woman with type II diabetes sees her GP as she cannot sleep at night due to a burning sensation in her feet. Her GP checks her HbA1c which is 7.4%. ★ ★

Diagnosis of diseases of liver and pancreas

For each of the clinical scenarios, select the single most likely diagnosis. Each option may be used once, more than once, or not at all.

A α_1-antitrypsin deficiency

B Acute pancreatitis

C Alcoholic hepatitis

D Ascending cholangitis

E Autoimmune hepatitis

F Carcinoma of pancreas

G Cholangiocarcinoma

H Chronic pancreatitis

I Gilbert's syndrome

J Haemochromatosis

K Hepatocellular carcinoma

L Liver adenoma

M Metastatic carcinoma

N Pancreatic pseudocyst

O Primary biliary cirrhosis

P Von Meyenburg complex

11. A 26-year-old man develops a strange orange tinge to his skin following a recent bout of flu. When questioned by his GP, he reports that he had a similar colour change when he had flu-like illness a few years previously. On examination, he is mildly jaundiced. He is otherwise well and shows normal physical and mental development. Liver function tests are performed. These show:

- Alkaline phosphatase 83iu/L
- Alanine aminotransferase (ALT) 15iu/L
- Aspartate aminotransferase (AST) 28iu/L
- Bilirubin 43μmol/L
- γ-Glutamyltransferase (GGT) 11iu/L ★ ★

12. A 56-year-old man presents with severe upper abdominal pain which radiates to the back. This came on a few hours ago and has worsened. He also feels nauseous. His blood pressure is 110/60mmHg and pulse 100/min. On examination, his abdomen is rigid. Three days ago he had an ERCP (endoscopic retrograde chloangiopancreatogram) to investigate a raised serum bilirubin and alkaline phosphatase, but no bile duct obstruction was found. ★ ★ ★

13. A 63-year-old man presents to his GP with upper abdominal pain. He has had this on and off for 12 months, and it is not relieved by antacids. In the last 2 months, the pain has increased in severity and is almost persistent. It worsens after meals and alcohol. He also reports that his stools have become paler. On questioning, he admits to drinking 5–6 pints of beer each day and up to half a bottle of whisky at weekends. He has not lost his appetite, but has lost 10kg in the last 6 months. There is no significant finding on clinical examination. Urine dipstick is positive for glucose. Liver function tests are performed, and these show: ★ ★ ★

- Alkaline phosphatase 350iu/L
- Alanine aminotransferase (ALT) 15iu/L

- Aspartate aminotransferase (AST) 28iu/L
- Bilirubin 36μmol/L
- γ-Glutamyltransferase (GGT) 107iu/L

14. A 38-year-old Buddhist monk from Thailand on sabbatical in London presents with vague upper abdominal pain experienced for the last 3 months. He is mildly jaundiced. On examination, he has hepatomegaly. No ascites is detected. The abdominal ultrasound shows a nodular mass in the left lobe of liver, measuring 18cm in diameter. A biopsy is performed and the histological diagnosis is made. ★ ★ ★

15. A 48-year-old man has a check-up when applying for life insurance for a new mortgage as his family with two young children have outgrown their two-bedroom flat. No abnormality is found on clinical examination. Urinalysis does not reveal any abnormality. In view of his age, some screening blood tests are performed. These show: ★ ★

- Hb 11.8g/dL
- White cell count 4.0×10^9/L
- Platelet count 285×10^9/L
- Alkaline phosphatase 259iu/L
- Aspartate aminotransferase (AST) 62iu/L
- Alanine aminotransferase (ALT) 72iu/L
- Bilirubin 26μmol/L
- γ-Glutamyltransferase (GGT) 53iu/L
- Albumin 22g/L

A liver ultrasound is then performed, and this suggests cirrhosis.

Diagnosis in CNS disorders

For each of the following clinical scenarios, choose the most likely diagnosis from the list below. Each option may be used once, more than once, or not at all.

A Arteriovenous malformation

B Bacterial meningitis

C Basal ganglia haemorrhage

D Cavernous malformation

E Cerebral contusion

F Cerebral venous thrombosis

G Choroid plexus papilloma

H Ependymoma

I Extradural haematoma

J Glioma

K Herpes simplex encephalitis

L Hydrocephalus

M Pontine haemorrhage

N Progressive multifocal leukoencephalopathy

O Ruptured berry aneurysm

P Subdural haematoma

16. A 30-year-old man complains of headaches, nausea, and vomiting for the past 3 months. He is afebrile, and physical examination elicits no focal neurological deficits. Magnetic resonance imaging shows sharply demarcated fourth ventricular lesion with heterogenous enhancement and cyst formation. ★ ★

17. A 70-year-old woman hits her head with a cupboard door while reaching for tea bags and sustains a bruise. Over the next month she develops headaches, becomes forgetful, and has difficulty with coping at home. ★

18. A 30-year-old previously healthy man presents with sudden onset of mental confusion and has a seizure. A lumbar puncture yields colourless cerebrospinal fluid under normal pressure. Analysis of cerebrospinal fluid shows abundant white blood cells, scanty red blood cells, and normal glucose and protein. Magnetic resonance imaging shows swelling of the left temporo-parietal region with haemorrhagic areas. ★ ★

19. A 30-year-old previously healthy woman develops a sudden, severe headache and loses consciousness. An urgent head computer tomography scan shows extensive subarachnoid haemorrhage at the base of the brain. ★

20. A 30-year-old previously healthy man presents with seizures of new onset. Magnetic resonance imaging shows abnormal collections of large and tortuous blood vessels in the temporo-parietal region, and cerebral angiography demonstrates a high flow character of the shunts. ★ ★

Differential diagnosis of solitary pulmonary nodule

A solitary pulmonary nodule (SPN) is defined radiologically as a single, well-defined pulmonary opacity, <3cm in size and not accompanied by adenopathy or atelectasis. The differential diagnosis is broad, and the implications of missing malignancy are severe. Computed tomography (CT) and positron emission tomography (PET) scans with or without percutaneous CT-guided biopsy or open biopsy and intra-operative frozen section (IOFS) diagnosis are important tools used in evaluating SPNs.

From the list , choose the option that corresponds best to each scenario. Each option may be used once, more than once, or not at all.

A Amyloidosis

B Aspergilloma

C Bronchogenic cyst

D Carcinoid tumour

E Cryptococcal granuloma

F *Histoplasma* granuloma

G Lung abscess

H Metastatic adenocarcinoma

I Pulmonary hamartoma

K Schwannoma

L Silicotic nodule

M Small cell carcinoma

N Solitary fibrous tumour

O Squamous cell carcinoma

21. The patient is a 55-year-old woman, non-smoker with 2cm, rounded SPN with popcorn calcification; PET-CT scan (see Fig. 15.5a) shows increased FDG uptake (i.e. metabolically active), and therefore wedge biopsy is performed. Histology reveals a circumscribed nodule composed of a combination of cartilage, fat, and invaginations of respiratory epithelium seen at IOFS (see Fig. 15.5b, Plate 12). ★ ★ ★

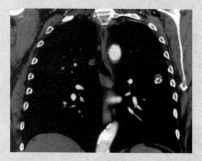

Fig. 15.5a

22. A 72-year-old woman, non-smoker with slowly enlarging left lower lobe SPN had a nephrectomy 25 years previously. CT-guided biopsy shows sheets and cords of epithelial cells with abundant clear cytoplasm, supported by rich capillary network. ★ ★

23. A 62-year-old man, smoker, lived for many years in the eastern United States. Incidental upper lobe SPN is detected on chest radiograph. Histology of open-wedge biopsy (see Fig. 15.6 (a), Plate 13) shows a well-defined lesion composed of a rim of dense fibrous tissue, beneath which is a layer of palisaded histiocytes and multinucleated giant cells surrounding a central core of necrotic debris. Silver stains (see Fig. 15.6 (b), Plate 13) reveal budding yeasts within this necrotic material. ★ ★ ★

24. A 67-year-old woman, heavy smoker, presents with sensory neuropathy and is found to have SPN on chest radiography. CT-guided fine-needle aspiration cytology of the nodule shows necrotic debris, with loose sheets of round-to spindle-shaped cells displaying dispersed nuclear chromatin, inconspicuous nucleoli, frequent apoptotic bodies, and mitotic figures. Histology of the corresponding core biopsy is also shown (see Fig. 15.7 (a) and (b), Plate 14). ★ ★ ★

25. A 37-year-old male, alcoholic, presents with fever and cough productive of purulent sputum. The chest radiograph demonstrates solitary rounded opacity with air-fluid level. Sputum culture reveals mixed aerobic and anaerobic bacterial growth. Fig. 15.8 shows a CT scan of the chest. ★ ★

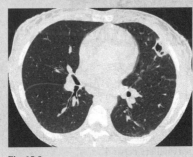

Fig. 15.8

Infectious conditions of the eyes, ears, and throat

From the list above, choose the single most appropriate drug to use in each scenario outlined below. Each option may be used once, more than once, or not at all.

A Aciclovir

B Adrenaline

C Amphotericin

D Ceftazidime

E Clindamycin

F Co-trimoxazole

G Flucloxacillin

H Ganciclovir

I Indinavir

J Metronidazole

K Oseltamivir

L Pentamidine

M Salbutamol

N Terbinafine

O Vasopressin

26. A 68-year-old woman complains of paroxysmal, deep-seated right ear pain for 2 days and then attends her GP with an erythematous, vesicular rash involving the right external auditory canal, pinna, and soft palate. She is unable to elevate the right corner of her mouth. ★ ★

27. A 72-year-old man is seen by his GP for a 1-week history of severe, progressive left-sided ear pain and purulent discharge from that side. He has insulin-dependent diabetes mellitus (IDDM) and lives for part of the year in the Seychelles. He is apyrexial. Examination reveals granulation tissue in the external ear canal at the osseocartilaginous junction and an intact tympanic membrane. The left corner of his mouth droops. ★ ★ ★ ★

28. A 43-year-old male with poorly controlled diabetes mellitus presents to the A&E department with a 3-day history of feeling unwell. He complains of cough, fever, and severe frontal headache. There is marked tenderness over the maxillary and frontal sinuses, and a mild left-sided proptosis is seen. An urgent CT scan shows opacification of the left paranasal sinuses associated with bony destruction of the roof of the left maxillary sinus. There are changes reported as suspicious for cavernous sinus thrombosis. ★ ★ ★

29. A 2-year-old boy is brought into the emergency department with recent onset of fever, 'barking' cough, and difficulty breathing, which was preceded by a short period of mild upper respiratory tract symptoms. The child appears restless and mildly tachypnoeic, and there is inspiratory stridor. He is not cyanotic or 'toxic', and there is no drooling. ★

30. An 8-year-old girl wakes up with swelling around her right eye. Her father notices two puncture marks on her eyelid and is concerned about a spider bite. He takes

her to see their GP who prescribes an antihistamine. Three days later they return to the practice. The child's eye is more swollen and erythematous, eye movements are painful, and she has a fever. There is conjunctival chemosis and she complains of decreased visual acuity on that side. She has a history of penicillin allergy. ★ ★ ★

ANSWERS

Single Best Answers

1. D ★★   OHMS 2nd edn → pp876–8

The answer is MLH-1 germline mutation. The young age of the patient and strong family history of colorectal carcinoma (CRC) suggests that the man has a hereditary non-polyposis colorectal carcinoma (HNPCC). This is an autosomal dominant condition with a germline mutation in one of several DNA mismatch repair proteins, MLH-1, MSH-2, MSH-6, or PSM-2. While BRAF mutations (A) are common (5–40%) in sporadic CRC, they are absent in HNPCC. Loss of cell senescence (B) is a tumour suppressor mechanism involved in many tumours, but not in CRC. Over-expression in Hedgehog signalling (E) has been found in basal cell carcinomas.

2. D ★★   OHCM → p352

The results of the haematology investigations suggest that the man has chronic myeloid leukaemia. Genetic abnormalities are important in understanding the pathogenesis of leukaemias, in developing treatment, and in prognosis, including elucidation of treatment-resistant cases. The Philadelphia chromosome is formed as a result of translocation of the Abl gene on chromosome 9 to the Bcr gene on chromosome 22. The abnormal gene product Abl-Bcr leads to overproduction of tyrosine kinase, which is the driver of neoplastic proliferation of the cells in chronic myeloid leukaemia. CML treatment consists of tyrosine kinase inhibitors. Translocations between chromosome 7 and chromosome 14 (C) are common in acute myeloid leukaemia. Trisomy 12 (E) is common in chronic lymphocytic leukaemia. JAK1 mutation (B) is uncommon, but confers poor prognosis in acute lymphoblastic leukaemia.

3. A ★★   OHMS 2nd edn → pp876–8

In the context of a patient without renal disease or metastatic carcinoma, the most common and likely cause of hypercalcaemia is a parathyroid adenoma, resulting in autonomous secretion of parathyroid hormone. Hypocalcaemia will cause compensatory secretion of parathyroid hormone (B). Some tumours, for example lung carcinoma, may cause hypercalcaemia by production of parathyroid-hormone-related peptide (D). Extra-renal production of Vitamin D (C) is thought to be the mechanism of sarcoidosis-related hypercalcaemia. Excessive ingestion of Vitamin D is uncommon (E), but may result in hypercalcaemia.

4. B ★★ OHCM → pp280, 555

Anti-tissue transglutaminase antibody and anti-endomysial antibody, if elevated, confirm the diagnosis of coeliac disease. Nevertheless, since the treatment involves lifelong dietary restriction of gluten, diagnosis will require a duodenal biopsy to demonstrate villous atrophy and increased intra-epithelial lymphocytes. Anti-cardiolipin antibody (A) is found in patients with systemic lupus erythematosus. Anti-nuclear antibody (D) is found in many autoimmune conditions, including systemic lupus erythematosus. Anti-mitochondrial antibody (C) and anti-smooth-muscle antibody (E) indicate primary biliary cirrhosis.

5. B ★★★ OHCM → p362

Although the patient's symptoms are vague, the definitive diagnosis of myeloma rests with demonstration of monoclonality of the plasma cells in the rib lesion. Multiple myeloma is also corroborated by the presence of lytic bone lesions, anaemia, hypercalcaemia, and impaired renal function. Further confirmatory tests would include demonstration of a monoclonal paraprotein in serum and Bence–Jones protein in urine, together with monoclonal plasma cells in bone marrow aspirate. While the bone lesions and hypercalcaemia may be observed with metastatic breast carcinoma (A), this is refuted by the histological findings. The other three options are less than likely as they are suggested by no more than one of the findings. For example, renal bone disease (E) is suggested by impaired renal function tests, and bone pain may be observed in Paget's disease (D), but the latter is usually accompanied by normal renal function tests and normocalcaemia, and enlargement of bones with areas of lucency and sclerosis.

6. A ★★ OHCM → p644

α-Antagonists are useful in the initial management of lower urinary tract symptoms in men. 5-α Reductase inhibitors (B) such as finasteride are effective in the management of moderate to severe benign prostatic hyperplasia, preventing acute retention and avoiding the need for surgery such as transurethral resection of prostate.

7. B ★   OHCM → p293

With the symptoms and urinalysis findings, this woman should be treated for a urinary tract infection. Before antibiotic treatment is commenced, a mid-stream urine specimen should be collected for culture and sensitivity. Co-trimoxazole is effective for most uncomplicated urinary tract infection. Even though her previous urinary tract infection resolved spontaneously, antibiotic treatment is advisable to prevent ascending infection including acute pyelonephritis. Fluids are encouraged, but are inadequate treatment on their own. Co-amoxiclav (A) is 2nd-line treatment and carries a risk of *Clostridium difficile* colitis.

8. D ★★   OHCM → p306

The answer is prednisolone. This man has proteinuria and haematuria associated with impaired renal function. The histological examination shows an acute interstitial nephritis. Many of these cases are caused by drugs such as non-steroidal anti-inflammatory drugs or antibiotics, but some cases are idiopathic. The normal glomeruli and tubules suggest that this is an acute process. The immediate treatment should involve discontinuation of the implicated aetiological agent. Steroids are also indicated to prevent damage to the tubules.

9. D ★   OHMS 2nd edn → p486, OHCM → pp296, 394

The clinical features and laboratory findings show that the patient has nephrotic syndrome, with normal blood pressure and renal function. Histology shows features of minimal change disease, This condition is highly responsive to steroid treatment. All the other treatments are inappropriate for minimal change disease, but choosing the correct treatment option is straightforward once the correct diagnosis is made.

10. B ★   OHCM → p508

The answer is hyperglycaemia. Peripheral neuropathies can develop in both type I and II diabetes, suggesting that there is a common aetiological mechanism based on chronic hyperglycaemia. Often, patients with type II diabetes have already developed neuropathy at the time of their diagnosis, as with this patient. The neuropathy is symmetrical, with negative symptoms including numbness, and positive symptoms including burning, prickling pain, and tingling. The distribution is classically called a 'stocking and glove distribution' as it starts distally in the toes, progresses up the legs, and later starts in the fingertips and moves up the arms. While the actual pathophysiology is not fully understood, the underlying cause is the hyperglycaemia. Hyperglycaemia causes increased levels of intracellular glucose in the nerves, which causes a saturation of the normal glycolytic pathway. The excess glucose is shunted into the polyol pathway where it is converted to sorbitol and fructose. The accumulation of sorbitol and fructose leads to a decrease in the nerves' myoinositol, decreased membrane NA+/K+ -ATPase activity, impaired axonal transport, and structural breakdown of the nerves, causing abnormal action-potential propagation. Excess glucose will also increase the oxidative stress of the axons, which causes further axonal damage.

Patients with alcoholic neuropathy (A) typically present with a history of alcoholism. Alcoholic neuropathy starts in the distal lower extremity with paraesthesias, dysaesthesias, or weakness. The most common symptom is a burning dysaesthesia, and patients may also have a history of gait ataxia and difficulty in walking. In advanced cases, there may be upper limb involvement. The classical symptoms are the same as for a diabetic neuropathy. However, there is no history of alcohol consumption, and the fasting glucose levels support the diagnosis of diabetes.

With lumbar spinal nerve root compression (C), the neurological symptoms are usually in the dermatomal distribution of the nerve root that is being compressed. In this case, there is also involvement of both the upper and lower extremities, which is unlikely to occur with nerve root compression. The pain begins slowly and is located in the lower back and posterior thigh. Therefore, the symptoms are more proximal than the distal location of the symptoms mentioned in this scenario.

Syringomyelia (D) is a fluid-filled cavity within the spinal cord; the causes of the cavity are varied and include Arnold–Chiari malformation, which obstructs the CSF circulation, and spinal cord injury. The sensory loss damages the spinothalamic tract fibres that mediate pain and temperature sensations, resulting in the loss of these sensations, while light touch and vibration sensations are still present. Therefore, the pattern of sensory loss does not match that in the scenario. In addition, syrinx are usually in the cervical spinal cord and the sensory loss is in a 'cloak-like' distribution.

Deficiency in vitamin B_{12} (E) has a prevalence of around 1.6% to10% in Europe and is more common in the elderly population and vegans. The neurological features are the result of damage to the posterior and lateral columns in the spinal cord. The symptoms are often a sensation of cold, numbness, or tightness in the tips of the toes and then in the fingertips. Vitamin B_{12} deficiency should be considered with neurological features such as paraethesia and sensory deficits. However, additional CNS symptoms such as urinary incontinence, dysarthria, and ataxia are usual in vitamin B_{12} deficiency, which this patient does not have.

This is a case of gout. It usually presents as an acute monoarthropathy. While over half of all cases present with monoarthritis in the metatarsophalangeal joint of the big toe, other joints that are commonly affected are the ankle, wrist, elbow, and knee. Gout is caused by the deposition of monosodium urate crystals within and around the joints. Causes include increased dietary purines, which when metabolized produce uric acid; excessive alcohol consumption; and the use of diuretics, especially thiazide diuretics as they compete with the same transporter as uric acid. While gout is 5 times more common in men than women, it can occur in women, as in this case. The increased number of leukocytes causes the cloudy synovial fluid. The presence of large, negatively birefringent crystals is confirmation of gout, but crystals are not always identified.

Articular cartilage degeneration (A) is the underlying cause of osteoarthritis. This is the most common condition to affect the joints; it typically starts after the age of 50 and has an insidious onset. It usually starts in the larger joints of the lower limb, such as the hip and knee. It can also affect the small joints of the hands, especially the distal and proximal interphalangeal joints of the hands, leading to Heberden's and Bouchard's nodes. On radiological examination, loss of joint space and development of osteophytes around the joint margins are seen, along with subchondral sclerosis and, in later stages, subchondral cysts. The synovial fluid is clear in osteoarthritis.

Bacterial infection (B) would be the underlying cause of septic arthritis. This also manifests as an acute monoarthritis. The synovial fluid would also be cloudy and filled with leukocytes, over 90% of which are neutrophils; the bacteria can be cultured to identify the organism causing the problem. There is often an underlying infection, possibly a sexually transmitted disease. In this case, there is no history of an infection, and commonly the joints affected by septic arthritis are the knee, hip, and shoulder, with few cases affecting the ankle.

Overproduction of TNFα (D) is the main cause of the damage to the joints in rheumatoid arthritis, along with other pro-inflammatory cytokines. Rheumatoid arthritis usually presents as a symmetrical arthritis of the small joints of the wrists and metacarpophalangeal joints. In rheumatoid arthritis, as well as the production of autoantibodies (i.e. rheumatoid factor), the abnormal production of numerous inflammatory mediators—especially TNFα—has been demonstrated. These pro-inflammatory cytokines cause proliferation of the synovial membrane, which creates the destructive pannus.

Reactive arthritis or Reiter's syndrome is an autoimmune condition that develops in response to an infection, particularly gastrointestinal and genitourinary infections. It normally develops 2–6 weeks after the primary infection, and the development of microbial antigens appears (C) to cross-react with self-proteins, stimulating a Th2-cell-mediated autoimmune response. The synovial fluid analysis would be clear and aseptic in this condition.

12. B ★ ★ OHCM → pp678, 698–9;
OHMS 2nd edn → p593

Osteomalacia (rickets in childhood) is due to poor mineral content but a normal amount of bone. Bone osteoid needs vitamin D for ossification to proceed normally. While dietary deficiency is rare, it can still occur in vegans. The most common cause now is lack of sunlight exposure, as in this case because of the woman being housebound for the last 4 years. The failure of the bones to ossify results in a softening of the bones. There is generalized bone pain and muscle weakness due to the low calcium levels. X-rays show pseudofractures (Looser's zones) which run at right angles to the cortex of the bone and usually match up to muscle attachment points as these are under more strain and the bone is turned over more quickly at these locations. The blood tests will show a mild decrease in the serum calcium, decreased phosphate, raised alkaline phosphatase, and low $25(OH)D_3$. If the parathyroid levels are measured, they will be raised. While the vertebral and hip fractures could indicate osteoporosis (D), the serum levels would be normal for all the parameters. In osteoporosis, there is normal mineralization but reduced bone mass.

Osteopenia (C) is an earlier stage of bone loss, prior to development of osteoporosis, and is often localized to specific locations. It is asymptomatic. Paget's disease (E) would show normal serum calcium and phosphate, with very high levels of alkaline phosphatase indicating increased bone turnover. In Paget's disease, there is generalized bone pain but localized enlargement of bone with cortical thickening.

Osteoarthritis (A) is usually the result of age-related degeneration of the articular cartilage, and this is not associated with abnormalities in serum biochemistry.

13. A ★ OHCM → pp696–7
Alendronate (a bisphosphonate) is the 1st-line treatment for women aged over 70 who have an independent clinical risk factor for a fracture or indicator of low bone mineral density, such as a femoral neck fracture caused by minor trauma, as in this case. A DEXA scan is not necessarily required before commencing treatment.

Strontium ranelate (D) is recommended as an alternative to alendronate in individuals where the prescription of bisphosphonates is contraindicated or who are intolerant to bisphosphonates.

Teriparatide (E), a recombinant parathyroid hormone, is useful in individuals who suffer further fractures, having been taking other treatments.

Calcium and vitamin D (calcitriol) supplementation (B) can reduce fracture risk but should be given in combination rather than on its own.

Hormone replacement therapy (C) was considered the 1st-line therapy but is no longer recommended in post-menopausal women. It is still used in peri-menopausal women, not only to help with the symptoms of the menopause, but also to prevent the development of osteoporosis.

14. D ★★ OHMS 2nd edn → pp872–3

Infections with human papillomavirus, in particular types 16 and 18, are associated with squamous epithelial dysplasia and carcinoma of the cervix. The most common cause of cervicitis in sexually active women is *Chlamydia* (B), which is treated with antibiotics. *Candida* infections (A) are common, and patients most likely develop iatrogenic candidiasis secondary to recent antibiotic use. Trichomonal infection (E) is caused by a protozoan. It manifests with frothy, green to yellow vaginal discharge and vulval itch. Herpes simplex virus (C) typically involves the external genitalia, but cervical or vaginal lesions also occur. It clinically presents as intensely painful vesicles on the skin in the perineal areas.

15. C ★★ OHCM → p555

This patient has an autoimmune condition, primary biliary cirrhosis. The disease occurs in middle-aged women and causes progressive destruction of bile ducts. Positivity for antimitochondrial antibody is found in more than 90% of patients. Pruritus, conjugated hyperbilirubinaemia, and markedly increased alkaline phosphatase levels are due to obstructive jaundice secondary to bile duct damage. Autoimmune hepatitis (A) is an unresolving inflammation of the liver of unknown aetiology. It typically affects young women and is characterized by the presence of the antinuclear antibody and raised transaminases. Haemochromatosis (B) is an autosomal recessive condition, in which there is excessive iron deposition in tissues. A raised serum ferritin raises suspicion of this condition. Primary sclerosing cholangitis (D) is an idiopathic condition, which may be associated with ulcerative colitis. It is characterized by destruction of intrahepatic bile ducts. Increased bilirubin and alkaline phosphatase levels are seen, but the antimitochondrial antibody is negative. A high prevalence of pANCA antibodies is seen in this condition.

Wilson's disease (E) is an inherited disorder of biliary copper excretion. Reduced serum caeruloplasmin is the typical screening test. Kayser–Fleischer rings in the eyes are a useful clinical clue.

16. B ★★ OHCM → p605

This patient has a condition known as fat necrosis, which typically develops following trauma and produces an ill-defined, palpable mass that mimics a carcinoma. Disrupted fat cells and lipid are phagocytosed by macrophages, and healing leaves a fibrous scar. Duct ectasia (A), also a mimic of carcinoma, forms from inspissated duct secretions that induce chronic inflammation and fibrosis. Fibroadenomas (C) are common and present as well-circumscribed, firm, mobile masses in young women. They are histologically composed of proliferation of fibrous stroma around compressed ductules. Intraductal papilloma (D) is a benign solitary lesion of a lactiferous sinus and presents with a bloody nipple discharge. Radial scar (E) is a rare lesion that appears as a stellate scar with fibroelastic core. It is not induced by trauma.

17. C ★★ OHCM → p604

This patient may benefit from hormonal treatment with tamoxifen, an oestrogen receptor antagonist because the tumour cells are positively staining with oestrogen and progesterone receptors. Isoflavone (A) (soy) is a type of complementary therapy that helps to reduce symptoms of menopause by exerting oestrogen-like effects. It is, however, not recommended for the treatment of menopausal symptoms in women with breast cancer. Lapatinib (B) is a new drug that blocks the effects of the HER2 protein. It is a tyrosine kinase inhibitor that is intended to benefit patients with HER2-positive advanced breast cancer that has progressed following treatment with trastuzumab (E). Teicoplanin (D) is an antibiotic and will not be effective against cancer. This patient is unlikely to benefit from treatment with trastuzumab (Herceptin®), a monoclonal antibody that blocks the effects of the growth factor protein HER2, as her tumour is negative for HER2/neu.

18. C ★★★ OHCM → p410

The JC polyoma virus causes progressive multifocal leucko-encephalopathy (PML),which is almost exclusively confined to immunosuppressed patients, such as AIDS patients. This patient is thus most likely to have a low CD4 count. The JC virus causes productive lytic infection in oligodendrocytes, rather than neurones, which leads to oligodendroglial cell loss and loss of myelin; hence the pattern of tissue damage is one of demyelination. This infection can mimic multiple sclerosis, which shows white-matter plaques of demyelination on MRI and oligoclonal bands in CSF (E). However, in JC polyoma virus infection, oligoclonal bands are absent in the CSF. Hyponatraemia (D) can lead to cerebral oedema, and rapid correction of sodium in hyponatraemic patients can give rise to osmotic demyelination syndrome. The syndrome tends to affect alcoholics and the malnourished. High glucose (A) may suggest diabetes mellitus, which is a risk factor for atherosclerotic cerebrovascular disease, but not for the JC polyoma virus infection. Similarly, hypertriglyceridaemia (B) is a risk factor for atherosclerosis, but not demyelinating disease.

19. A ★ ★ ★ OHMS 2nd edn → pp428–9, 438–9;
OHCM → pp128–31

The answer is heavy, firm heart with brownish, waxy cut myocardial surface. The clinical presentation is typical of congestive cardiac failure (CCF); the presence of a plasmacytosis within the bone marrow should raise suspicion of a plasma cell disorder and associated amyloidosis. The gross pathological findings are suggestive of cardiac amyloidosis and this is confirmed histologically—note the abnormal, amorphous pink material deposited around cardiac myocytes in the photomicrograph (see Plate 10). The amyloid protein stains a salmon-red colour with the Congo red stain, and shows 'apple green' birefringence under polarized microscopy (see Plate 10). Answer B describes the findings of a dilated cardiomyopathy which may be primary or secondary to a wide variety of conditions. Chronic ischaemic heart disease (C) is a common cause of congestive cardiac failure but the scenario still favours amyloidosis. Asymmetrical left ventricular hypertrophy (D) is a clue to hypertrophic cardiomyopathy, which would have a different appearance histologically (myocyte hypertrophy, fibrosis, and myocyte disarray). Finally, valvular heart disease (E) from any cause may present acutely with sudden cardiac death and/or CCF, but the lack of a history of rheumatic fever or of an older patient with a history of angina or syncope (senile calcific aortic stenosis) would be against this.

20. B ★ ★ ★ OHMS 2nd edn → pp360–1;
OHCM → pp184–5, 778–80

The clinical presentation and chest radiograph findings are fairly typical of a pleural effusion. The occupational history suggests asbestos exposure, and malignant mesothelioma would have to be top of the list of differential diagnoses. The exudative effusion resulting from this is best explained by lymphatic obstruction secondary to malignant infiltration of the pleura. Decreased colloid osmotic pressure secondary to hypoproteinaemia (A) (e.g. cirrhosis, nephrotic syndrome) would result in a transudate and the effusion is usually bilateral, while increased intrapleural negative pressure (C) would occur in the setting of a collapsed lung (atelectasis) e.g. bronchial obstruction by tumour or foreign body. There may also be an element of increased vascular permeability (D) contributing to the development of some malignant effusions, but usually this would be due to an infective or inflammatory condition such as TB, bacterial pneumonia, or rheumatoid arthritis. Finally, effusions due to raised venous hydrostatic pressure (E) are transudative in nature, often bilateral, and are seen commonly in congestive cardiac failure.

21. B ★★ OHCM → pp608, 622

Mesenteric ischaemia is a cause of acute abdominal pain that can be overlooked yet is serious and life-threatening. It typically presents with acute severe abdominal pain, non-specific abdominal signs, and shock. Atrial fibrillation and abdominal pain should always trigger the thought of mesenteric ischaemia as a possible diagnosis as AF is a common source of embolus. It is common to see a mild rise in amylase in this condition; in acute pancreatitis (C) the rise is more commonly > 3-fold the upper limit of normal. It is also common to get a rise in white cell count and lactate and a metabolic acidosis. Most patients require surgery to resect the segment of ischaemic bowel. The amylase level rules out acute pancreatitis, and the normal abdominal X-ray rules out perforated bowel (D). Acute cholecystitis (A) is unlikely to cause the hypotension, and a low haemoglobin would be expected with ruptured abdominal aortic aneurysm (E).

22. B ★★ OHCM → pp242–3

A positive urease breath test indicates this patient is *Helicobacter pylori* positive. The next step in management is *H. pylori* eradication. This involves giving a combination of proton pump inhibitor and antibiotics. The various regimens can be found in the BNF. Antacids (A) would not be appropriate given that the aetiology has been found. Omeprazole (C) and ranitidine (D) are similarly inappropriate for treating *H. pylori*.

23. D ★★★ OHCM → pp294–7

This is usually a post-streptococcal proliferative glomerulonephritis, occurring 1–12 weeks after a sore throat or skin infection. It normally presents with a nephritic syndrome (haematuria, proteinuria, hypertension, progressive oliguria, and renal impairment). Most typical cases do not require renal biopsy, treatment is supportive and 95% recover. IgA Nephropathy (B) is rarely associated with renal impairment. Minimal change glomerulonephritis (C) presents with a nephrotic syndrome, and renal impairment and haematuria are absent. Rapidly progressive glomerulonephritis (E) would present with a nephritic syndrome. In addition to renal impairment, proteinuria, and haematuria, the person might also be hypertensive. Note that nephritic syndrome should not be confused with nephrotic syndrome.

24. D ★★ OHCM → p214

In secondary hyperparathyroidism, there is an appropriate rise in PTH in response to low calcium levels. The latter may commonly be due to low vitamin D levels or chronic renal failure. Primary hyperparathyroidism (A), due to an adenoma, would be associated with hypercalcaemia.

Pseudopseudohypoparathyroidism (B) is a hereditary condition with characteristic features of hypoparathyroidism, but there are also associated skeletal and developmental abnormalities. As such, it is most unlikely to have an initial presentation in an elderly person. Serum calcium levels may be elevated or normal in sarcoidosis (C). In patients with chronic renal failure, the parathyroid undergoes hyperplasia and hypersecretion to compensate for the low calcium; in some cases an adenoma develops and this is then known as tertiary hyperparathyroidism (E).

25. C ★★ OHCM → pp174-5

The aim of asthma management is for patients to be symptom-free. Night-time cough is a common symptom of asthma that is not adequately controlled. It is recommended that patients who are using their short-acting beta-agonist more than once daily, or those who have night-time symptoms, should be started on an inhaled steroid and the dose titrated to response.

26. C ★★★ OHMS 2nd edn → p180; OHCM → pp156-7

If you calculate this patient's BMI, it is >40 and he is morbidly obese. His lung function shows a restrictive picture. Although all the possibilities mentioned in the option list cause a restrictive ventilatory defect, this patient is extremely obese and his lungs are most likely to be restricted by his weight. There is nothing else mentioned in his history that makes the other options more likely. Therefore, this is most consistent with obesity hypoventilation syndrome, which is becoming increasingly common.

27. A ★★ OHMS 2nd edn → p238; OHCM → p563

This is a typical presentation of glaucoma. Urgent referral to an ophthalmologist is necessary as permanent visual loss can rapidly occur if it is not treated. Acute iritis (B) is the main differential diagnosis but the pupil will still have some reaction to light, although it is often constricted and there is commonly ciliary injection causing redness. Conjunctivitis (C) tends to cause discomfort rather than pain and there is normally discharge from the eye. Keratitis (D) is corneal inflammation which may or may not be caused by infection; it may result in corneal opacification and astigmatism. Subconjunctival haemorrhage (E) is commonly caused by trauma and appears as bright red blood visible through the transparent conjunctiva. It usually can just be left to resolve.

28. E ★★★   OHCM → pp312–13

The answer is subarachnoid haemorrhage from ruptured berry aneurysm. Autosomal dominant (adult) polycystic kidney disease (ADPKD) is a hereditary disorder which may present with isolated haematuria, hypertension, urinary tract infection, renal colic, or end-stage renal disease. Gene mutations in PKD1 (85% of cases) and PKD2 (encoding polycystin-1 and polycystin-2) are responsible for the disease. Ruptured saccular ('berry') aneurysms of the circle of Willis account for death in about 4–10% of patients with ADPKD. Peritoneal dialysis may be complicated by infection, but the patient would be unlikely to be fit enough to play football with peritonitis (A)! ADPKD may be associated with hypertension which could theoretically predispose to acute aortic dissection (C), but this might not be the first thing you would think of in this scenario. Mitral valve prolapse (D) is also recognized in patients with ADPKD, but this is usually asymptomatic. (If this were the only pathological finding at autopsy, however, a case could be made for this as the cause of death.)

29. B ★★   OHMS 2nd edn → pp734–7; OHCM → pp232–3

The answer is granulomatous inflammation of the hypothalamus. Antidiuretic hormone (ADH) deficiency causes diabetes insipidus (DI) which may be either central (disorders affecting primarily the hypothalamus or suprasellar region) or nephrogenic (as a result of decreased renal tubular response to circulating ADH). Common causes of central DI include trauma, surgery, suprasellar tumours (e.g. craniopharyngioma), and various idiopathic and infiltrative disorders including Langerhans' histiocytosis and sarcoidosis. ADH is synthesized in the hypothalamus and stored in the posterior pituitary, and therefore inflammation of the anterior pituitary (A) should not affect ADH levels. Granulomatous interstitial nephritis (C) may be seen in sarcoidosis, and this could potentially result in nephrogenic DI; however, exogenous administration of vasopressin as part of the water deprivation test would not have an effect on urine osmolality in nephrogenic DI. Common causes of nephrogenic DI include drugs (especially lithium), chronic hypercalcaemia (which could potentially also result from sarcoidosis), acquired renal disease, and familial nephrogenic DI. Granulomatous pancreatic inflammation (D) is very unusual and is more likely to be related to infection (e.g. TB) or autoimmune disease (e.g. Crohn's) but may theoretically result in abnormalities in glucose metabolism (this patient's fasting blood glucose is normal). Disease of the posterior pituitary (E) rarely causes permanent DI because ADH can still be released from the hypothalamus into the circulation.

30. B ★ ★ ★ OHMS 2nd edn → p566; OHCM → p564

Dermatitis herpetiformis (DH) is an uncommon autoimmune blistering condition associated with gluten-sensitive enteropathy (coeliac disease), which affects men twice as often as women, usually in the second to fourth decades. Neutrophilic microabscesses are seen involving the tips of dermal papillae, and IMF shows deposition of IgA at the dermo-epidermal junction. Not all patients with DH have gastrointestinal symptoms but the majority will have endoscopic and histological evidence of enteropathy (as described in the above scenario).

Treatment is with dapsone and a gluten-free diet. Drug reactions have a wide range of skin manifestations, but the skin biopsy and IMF pattern in DH is characteristic. Dermatitis herpetiformis and coeliac disease may be associated with an increased incidence of non-Hodgkin lymphoma, in particular enteropathy-associated T-cell lymphoma (C). Parasites (D) may cause bowel and skin symptoms, and in the case of *Strongyloides stercoralis* infection, may cause partial villous atrophy, but one would expect to find peripheral eosinophilia (and not circulating autoantibodies); also the appearance of the larvae on small bowel biopsy is typical. Porphyrias (E) are disorders of haem metabolism of which there are several types, clinically divided into those associated with cutaneous, neuropsychiatric/liver, or mixed involvement. Porphyria cutanea tarda presents with cutaneous fragility and blistering of the hands and forearms, but not usually with abdominal symptoms (unlike acute intermittent porphyria).

31. D ★ ★ ★ OHMS 2nd edn → pp456–9; OHCM → pp220–1

The answer is serum aldosterone : renin ratio. The clinical features should raise concern for secondary hypertension due to hyperaldosteronism. Although an abdominal CT scan is likely to be useful in detecting adrenocortical adenoma or hyperplasia, raised serum aldosterone should be confirmed before adrenal imaging is undertaken (high incidence of incidental adrenal nodules). A good initial screening test for this is the serum aldosterone : renin ratio (ARR). Renal angiography (B) would be undertaken if high renin levels suggested renal artery stenosis. Renal ultrasound (C) is performed if the patient is suspected to have end-stage renal disease, and urine catecholamine collection (E) is used to ascertain whether the hypertension could be secondary to phaeochromocytoma, a tumour of the adrenal medulla.

32. A ★ ★ ★ OHMS 2nd edn → pp794–6

The gross and microscopic findings described above are typical of Parkinson's disease, hereditary forms of which have been found to be due to mutations in the gene encoding α-synuclein. Deposition of α-synuclein filaments in neurones, astrocytes, and oligodendroglial cells results in cell death and neuronal loss. Similar inclusions are seen in the cortical areas of patients with dementia with Lewy bodies (DLB). Beta amyloid (B) is the abnormal protein associated with Alzheimer's disease, and forms the central core within neuritic plaques seen especially in the hippocampus and amygdala.

Huntingtin (C), as the name suggests, is the protein associated with Huntington's disease, an autosomal dominant disorder resulting in progressive movement disorder (chorea) and dementia, and associated pathologically with striking atrophy of the caudate nucleus. Prion protein (D) is a normal neuronal protein which undergoes a conformational change and accumulation of which results in spongiform encephalopathy. The transmissible form of this is known as variant Creutzfeldt–Jakob disease (vCJD). Finally, accumulations of tau protein (E), an axonal microtubule-associated protein, is seen in Pick's disease, corticobasal degeneration, and frontotemporal dementia ('tau-opathies'). Abnormally phosphorylated forms of tau protein are also a major component of the neurofibrillary tangles seen in Alzheimer's disease.

33. E ★ ★ ★ OHMS 2nd edn → pp342–5, 690–1; OHCM → pp399, 832–3

The answer is positive CSF *Mycobacterium tuberculosis* PCR. TB meningitis (TBM) has a wide variety of clinical presentations, and a high level of suspicion is needed to arrive at the correct diagnosis. Treatment needs to be instituted promptly to avoid death or permanent neurological deficit. Seizures are common (especially in children and the elderly) and may be due to tuberculomas (suggested here by the ring-enhancing lesion), hydrocephalus, cerebral oedema, or hyponatraemia due to SIADH. Radiological mimics include cryptococcal meningitis, CMV encephalitis, meningeal metastases, lymphoma, and sarcoidosis.

The culture of *M. tuberculosis* from the CSF is the gold standard in diagnosis, but is insensitive and slow. Detection of acid-fast bacilli on a Ziehl–Neelsen stain is still one of the most effective and rapid diagnostic tests, but requires a sufficient volume of CSF (10ml is recommended) and a fastidious technician. PCR gives an answer more quickly. JC virus (test A) is the agent responsible for progressive multifocal leukoencephalopathy (PML), which is a demyelinating disorder seen more commonly in the setting of advanced HIV infection or other immunosuppressed state. Primary CNS lymphoma (test B) usually presents with focal signs indicative of a mass lesion (depending on immune status), but may present with non-specific changes in mental status or seizures. Cryptococcal meningitis (test C) (caused by the encapsulated yeast *Cryptococcus neoformans*) is once again usually associated with profound immunosuppression, often due to HIV/AIDS, but should be considered in the differential diagnosis as the clinical and radiological features may be very similar. Neurosyphilis (*Treponema pallidum*), (test D) is more likely to present insidiously with cognitive or personality changes, gait disturbance, or visual abnormality, but there is a spectrum of CNS involvement to be considered.

Extended Matching Questions

1. J ★★★

NICE guidelines recommend that type II diabetics with BP≥140/80 and microalbuminuria should be on either an ACE inhibitor or angiotensin II antagonist. In this case the patient had a dry cough after starting the first medication, which is a well-recognized side-effect of ACE inhibitors. The patient should therefore be switched to an angiotensin II antagonist such as irbesartan.

2. H ★★

Patients with fluid overload secondary to heart failure should receive either a loop- or thiazide diuretic. Thiazide diuretics can be useful in patients with mild heart failure and good renal function but in those with impaired renal function, loop diuretics (Furosemide) are preferred. Patients' renal function and electrolyte balance need to be carefully monitored.

3. C ★★★

Amiodarone, used as an antiarrhythmic agent, is known to be a cause of pulmonary fibrosis. If patients on amiodarone develop new or progressive shortness of breath or cough, they should be investigated for this possibility.

4. A ★★

If patients with SVT do not respond to carotid massage or Valsalva manoeuvres, adenosine is the drug of choice (if the patient is haemodynamically stable and not asthmatic). Adenosine is given in incremental doses until the SVT is terminated or maximal dose reached.

5. L ★★

Methyldopa is a centrally acting antihypertensive, and patients often experience side-effects when taking it. However, it is recognized as being safe for use in all trimesters of pregnancy.

General feedback on 1–5: OHCM → pp120, 203; BNF pp59, 102, 106, 110

6. G ★★

In this case, with a patient who has good understanding and has an active lifestyle, a flexible insulin regimen is most appropriate. One such as 'DAFNE' (dose adjustment for normal eating) would be appropriate.

7. F ★★

According to the WHO classification, this patient has impaired fasting glucose and should be given lifestyle advice.

8. G ★★

According to the DIGAMI study, patients who are post-MI and diabetic should be started on s/c insulin. In view of the fact that this patient is young and well, a flexible regimen would be most appropriate.

9. E ★

This patient has osteomyelitis and should be admitted for iv antibiotics and review by the surgeons.

10. A ★★

This woman has reasonably good blood sugar control with an HbA1c of 7.4; the burning sensation in her feet, particularly at night, is typical of a diabetic neuropathy. Amitriptyline is a recommended treatment for this.

General feedback on 5–10: OHCM → pp199, 201

11. I ★★

Gilbert's syndrome is not uncommon, but is generally not recognized by patients until adulthood. It is one of the mild forms of inherited glucuronyl transferase deficiencies, characterized by mild, persistent unconjugated hyperbilirubinaemia. Patients are asymptomatic and usually minimally jaundiced, but jaundice may be exacerbated by prolonged fasting, infection, alcohol ingestion, or surgery. The enzyme deficiency results in unconjugated hyperbilirubinaemia without any abnormality in liver function tests. However, it should be a diagnosis of exclusion, and the presence or causes of haemolysis should be excluded.

12. B ★★★

Acute pancreatitis following bile reflux along the pancreatic duct is a well-recognized complication of ERCP. The diagnosis can be confirmed by finding an elevated serum amylase or lipase.

13. H ★★★

Chronic pancreatitis is a difficult diagnosis to make clinically as the symptoms are vague and there is little to find on examination. The diagnosis is made by a triad of pancreatic calcification, steatorrhoea, and diabetes mellitus. The abdominal pain, which worsens with meals and alcohol, accompanied by glycosuria, should make one suspicious in a man with heavy alcohol consumption. An elevated fasting blood glucose and pancreatic calcification on abdominal X-ray will help to confirm the diagnosis.

14. K ★★★

Carriers of hepatitis B are at risk of developing hepatocellular carcinoma, and indeed this is one of the commonest tumours in parts of Asia and sub-Saharan Africa. Although this would not be the most likely diagnosis in a young Caucasian adult in the UK, hepatocellular carcinomas are not unusual in young adults in countries in which hepatitis B is endemic. Cholangiocarcinoma is also more common in the Far East, where it is associated with liver flukes. However, the mild jaundice and large size of the tumour makes this less likely. The size of the single nodule makes a liver adenoma unlikely. Von Meyenburg complexes are small sub-capsular bile duct hamartomas that are a relatively common incidental finding.

15. A ★★

α_1-antitrypsin deficiency is a relatively common inherited disorder and occurs at a frequency of 1 in 3500 to 1 in 5000 of the UK population. It is inherited in an autosomal dominant manner. α_1-antitrypsin, a protease inhibitor produced by the liver, is the natural protection against the action of neutrophil elastase. This is released by neutrophils during the course of inflammation, and hence contributes to the destruction of supporting tissue in alveoli, leading to emphysema or liver disease, when it is deficient. MM is the normal allelic version. The S allele results in moderately reduced α_1-antitrypsin and the Z allele in very low levels.

Individuals with MZ have a low risk of developing emphysema or cirrhosis, particularly if they smoke, and individuals with ZZ invariably develop respiratory or liver disease. Although α_1-antitrypsin deficiency is the cause of 10–20% of chronic liver disease in children, it may present as cirrhosis in adults. Asymptomatic cirrhosis may occur in the absence of respiratory disease. Haemochromatosis is also a relatively common inherited condition that may be unrecognized and present late. However, if the cirrhosis were due to haemochromatosis, then the patient might also be sterile and have diabetes mellitus, which are absent from the history and urinalysis.

General feedback on 11–15: OHCM → pp264, 270, 638, 714

16. H ★★

This is a typical presentation of an ependymoma—a CNS tumour that arises from the ependymal lining cells. Sharp demarcation from the surrounding brain parenchyma is typical for this tumour. Ependymomas are the third most common paediatric CNS tumours. They display a bimodal age distribution, with peak incidences at ages 6 and 30 to 40 years, respectively. Clinical signs and symptoms are related to hydrocephalus and increased intracranial pressure. Complete resection is generally curative, and prognosis in adults tends to be better than in children due to less malignant histology and more accessible tumour localization. Differential diagnosis of ependymoma includes glioma. Glioma, however, occurs most frequently in the cerebral hemispheres.

17. P ★

The clinical presentation is that of a subdural haematoma, which typically occurs after head trauma that damages the bridging veins from the dura to brain. Since venous bleeding is not brisk, blood collects over time, and onset of symptoms is variable. An extradural haematoma results from a blunt head trauma causing a tear in the middle meningeal artery, resulting in a collection of blood in the extradural space. There is a lucid interval followed by rapid decline and coma.

18. K ★★

This patient has herpes simplex virus (HSV) encephalitis, which is the most common sporadic form of viral encephalitis. Haemorrhagic lesions within the temporal lobe are characteristic of HSV encephalitis. Progressive multifocal leucoencephalopathy is caused by the JC polyoma virus and can be distinguished from HSV encephalitis by MRI findings of multifocal white-matter lesions. In bacterial meningitis, the CSF shows a high protein level and a low glucose concentration.

19. O ★

In this context, the most likely diagnosis is an acute subarachnoid haemorrhage due to ruptured berry aneurysm. Berry aneurysms are relatively common (1–2 in 100 persons) and affect women twice as often as men. They arise due to a congenital defect in the arterial tunica media, but manifest later in life with aneurysmal dilation and rupture. These aneurysms commonly involve the arteries of the circle of Willis, so that rupture with bleeding occurs into the subarachnoid space at the base of the brain.

20. A ★ ★

This patient suffers from arteriovenous malformations (AVMs). AVMs are a common form of vascular malformations in the brain and are of congenital aetiology. They affect young adults between the ages of 20 and 40 years. About 50% of patients with AVMs present with a cerebral haemorrhage, and seizures occur in 25% of patients. Patients are diagnosed using MRI and cerebral angiography. Cavernous malformations are non-arterial vascular abnormalities that on MRI show a characteristic compact lesion with a central 'core' of increased vascularity and a 'ring' of hypodensity. The ring corresponds to haemosiderin deposition in the adjacent brain tissue ('ferruginous penumbra').

General feedback on 16–20: OHCM → pp400, 482, 486, 502

21. I ★ ★ ★

Pulmonary hamartoma is one of the commonest benign causes of a solitary pulmonary nodule (SPN). Although still referred to as a 'hamartoma', it is likely to represent a benign neoplasm as SPNs have been shown to display distinctive clonal cytogenetic abnormalities. Multiple hamartomas may be part of Carney triad (pulmonary hamartoma, gastric gastrointestinal stromal tumour (GIST), and extra-adrenal paraganglioma.)

22. H ★ ★

Metastatic adenocarcinoma, including renal cell carcinoma (conventional or clear cell type in this case), may present many years after the primary tumour with isolated metastases. Metastatic tumours to the lung may mimic primary lung cancer in a number of ways, and therefore providing the pathologist with the correct clinical information may be vital to arriving at the correct diagnosis.

23. F ★ ★ ★

Histoplasma capsulatum is a dimorphic fungus which is endemic in certain parts of the United States and which often results in asymptomatic infection. Nodules may develop with chronic infection and are often identified on chest imaging for other reasons. Special histochemical stains for fungi and mycobacteria, in particular, should be routinely performed when necrotizing granulomatous inflammation is identified in surgical pathology specimens.

24. M ★★★

Less than 5% of small cell carcinomas present as an isolated pulmonary nodule without radiologically detectable pathological lymph nodes. Of all primary lung carcinomas, small cell carcinoma is the one most likely to present with a paraneoplastic syndrome, which includes neurological disorders and endocrine abnormalities.

25. G ★★

The chest radiograph demonstrates the typical findings of a lung abscess, for which predisposing conditions include aspiration of gastric contents (e.g. alcoholism, coma, and general anaesthesia), pneumonia (especially those due to necrotizing infections such as *Klebsiella* or *Staphylococcus*) and septic emboli (e.g. infective endocarditis).

General feedback on 21–25: OHCM 8th edn → pp170–1

Moran, CA, & Suster, S (2010) *Tumours and tumour-like conditions of the lung and pleura,* pp2–8. London: Elsevier Saunders.

26. A ★★

Ramsay Hunt syndrome (herpes zoster oticus) is defined as a varicella-zoster virus (VZV) infection involving the facial nerve and is thought to cause nearly 20% of Bell's palsies. Treatment includes oral aciclovir and corticosteroids in order to try and prevent permanent facial nerve damage.

27. D ★★★★

The scenario described should raise suspicion for malignant otitis externa, a more infection more commonly seen in elderly patients, especially those with diabetes or other form of immunocompromise. It involves the external auditory canal and temporal bone and may be associated with cranial nerve palsies (in this case CNVII), other intracranial complications, and death. *Pseudomonas aeruginosa* is the usual causative organism and therefore parenteral anti-pseudomonal cephalosporins (ceftazidime) are used together with oral/iv quinolones and sometimes surgery or hyperbaric oxygen therapy.

28. C ★★★

Acute invasive fungal rhinosinusitis should be high up on the list of differential diagnoses (which might also include lymphoma or carcinoma). Zygomycetes and species of *Aspergillus* are largely responsible for invasive fungal rhinosinusitis, which usually affects diabetics and other immunocompromised patients. Prompt diagnosis

and treatment are needed, as the disease is aggressive and
life-threatening. Histological examination of surgically debrided
tissue reveals necrosis and angio-invasive fungal hyphae. Treatment
in this case includes surgical debridement, intravenous amphotericin
and improved diabetic control.

29. B ★

Inhalation of racemic adrenaline is used to obtain symptomatic relief
from acute laryngotracheobronchitis (croup). Corticosteroids are also
used to reduce inflammation and oedema. Most cases are due to
parainfluenza type 1 virus, but other viral aetiologies include
respiratory syncytial virus (RSV), adenovirus and rhinovirus. Specific
antiviral therapy is generally not used.

30. E ★ ★ ★

Orbital cellulitis is a serious infection of orbital soft tissues posterior
to the orbital septum. It may arise from extension of infection from
the face, paranasal sinuses or lacrimal sac, trauma or surgery to the
orbit or from haematogenous spread. Common organisms include
Staphylococcus aureus and *Streptococcus* species. Intravenous,
in-hospital therapy is usually required and in a penicillin-allergic
patient, clindamycin may be an appropriate first choice (depending
on local guidelines and antimicrobial resistance).

General feedback on 26–30: OHMS 2nd edn → pp706–9;
OHCM → pp376, 379, 440, 480

Table 15.1 Question blueprint

	Mechanisms of disease	Investigation of disease and data interpretation	Diagnosis	Patient management
CVS	Amyloid	Hypertension		CVS drugs (EMQ)
RS	Pleural effusion	Obstructive lung disease	Lung function test Solitary lung nodule (EMQ)	Asthma
GIT	Colorectal Ca	Coeliac disease	Ischaemic bowel Coeliac disease	*H. pylori*
LIVER & PANCREAS		PBC Miscellanous (EMQ)	Miscellanous (EMQ)	
GU inc KIDNEY	PCKD		Glomerulonephritis	Minimal change disease Interstitial nephritis Urinary tract infection BPH

(*Continued*)

Clinical application of medical sciences

417

Table 15.1 (cont.)

	Mechanisms of disease	Investigation of disease and data interpretation	Diagnosis	Patient management
GYNAE & BREAST	CIN		Fat necrosis	Breast cancer
CNS inc PNS	Neurodegenerative disease Peripheral neuropathy	AIDS/PML	Meningitis Miscellaneous (EMQ)	
LYMPHORETIC	CML	Myeloma		
EYES EARS THROAT			Glaucoma	ENT infections (EMQ)
ENDO	Hypercalcaemia	Diabetes insipidus	Hyperparathyroidism	Miscellanous (EMQ)
SKIN BONE JOINTS	Monoarthritis		Osteomalacia	Osteoporosis

INDEX

Note: Page numbers in *italics* denote answers

435